SOCIAL SCIENCES IN HEALTH CARE AND MEDICINE

Social Sciences in Health Care and Medicine

Janet B. Garner
and Thelma C. Christiansen
Editors

Nova Science Publishers, Inc.
New York

For permission to use material from this book please contact us:
Telephone 631-231-7269; Fax 631-231-8175
Web Site: http://www.novapublishers.com

LIBRARY OF CONGRESS CATALOGING-IN-PUBLICATION DATA

Social sciences in health care and medicine / Janet B. Garner and Thelma C. Christiansen, editors.
p. ; cm.
Includes bibliographical references and index.
ISBN 978-1-60456-286-6 (hardcover)
1. Social medicine. I. Garner, Janet B. II. Christiansen, Thelma C.
[DNLM: 1. Social Medicine--methods. 2. Community Health Services. 3. Delivery of Health Care--organization & administration. 4. Social Problems. 5. Social Work. WA 31 S67804 2008]
RA418.S6485 2008
362.1--dc22

2007051480

Published by Nova Science Publishers, Inc. ≃ New York

CONTENTS

PREFACE

Health care and medicine are dependent upon a close interaction with social sciences and professions in order to effectively treat patients. Athough medicines have become more and more targeted in recent times, it is the recovery of the patient which is the true test of the system whether it be in a hospital setting or within a daily societal setting. Such interactions may be psychological or interactions with social organizations essential to phase the patient back into society. This book presents new issues, experiences and research in the field from around the globe.

Short Communication A - This study was designed to identify predictors of behavioral disorders in children with learning disabilities and children without learning disabilities in the UAE public school system. It examined the relative contributions of child characteristic (i.e., presence of learning disability, gender, age), parents sociodemographics.

and aspects of classroom environment (e.g, social support received from teachers ,peers and friends ,meaningful and genuine relationships with classmates ,teachers help in academic matters and use of educational resources , and cooperative learning, in addition to students satisfaction with the physical environment) to behavioral disorders such as internalizing and externalizing problems, and mixed syndromes, mainly anxious/depressed, withdrawn/ depressed, somatic complaints, social problems, thought problems, attention problems, rule breaking behavior, and aggressive behavior. The participants were 200 students from both sexes who ranged in age from 12 to 18 years. Structured interviews were carried out with students at schools. Practical implications to special education at the identification prevention and intervention level were discussed.

Chapter 1 - The significant association between an individual's social network and his or her health and mortality at old ages is well-documented in western societies. However, similar research from developing countries, especially among long-lived persons, is rare due to lack of data. The value of social support embedded in the social network for healthy longevity is generally more significant in developing countries given the lack of advanced and institutionalized social security systems. This chapter provides us with a good opportunity to address how social network types and intimacy are related to healthy longevity among Chinese elders.

Using the Chinese Longitudinal Healthy Longevity Survey (CLHLS), a unique specially designed nationwide survey with a sample of 15,232 community-residing Chinese elders, this chapter examines the associations between social network types and intimacy and subsequent healthy longevity from 2002 to 2005 within a multi-level context. The outcome variables include instrumental activities of daily living, activities of daily living, cognitive functioning, self-rated health, chronic diseases, frailty index, and mortality. The authors classified social networks into eight types based on living arrangement, number of frequently visiting children, and social connection (playing cards/mah-jong and involvement in religious and social activities): (1) isolated, (2) children-visiting-only, (3) family coresidence only, (4) family coresidence plus children-visiting only, (5) social connection only, (6) social connection plus children visiting, (7) social connection plus family coresidence, and (8) social connection plus family coresidence & children visiting. Source of intimacy was measured by the most frequent daily talking-person and grouped into (1) nobody/social service provider/matron, (2) spouse, (3) child, and (4) friend/neighbor. Other individual variables and community socioeconomic variables served as controls. The authors used multilevel logistic regression to examine the effects of social network types and source of intimacy on subsequent 3-year mortality and health status.

Our analyses show that compared to the isolated elders, elders in socially integrated networks had up to a 35% reduction in odds of mortality over a 3-year period, although such protection was diminished after controlling for baseline health. Elders in family-oriented networks, on the other hand, had up to a 51% increase in odds of mortality over the 3-year period independent of baseline health. Compared to those who did not have an intimate network alter, those whose source of intimacy was a friend/neighbor or spouse had 15-50% decreased odds of death in the presence of various confounders including baseline health. Socially integrated networks reduce the likelihood of poor health by up to 60% in terms of cognitive impairment, ADL/IADL disability, poor self-rated health, chronic diseases, and frailty. Similar results were found for having a friend/neighbor as the source of intimacy. These results suggest that the protective effects of network types and source of intimacy on healthy longevity still exist at advanced ages.

We further examined the patterns of social network types and source of intimacy by age, gender, childhood and adulthood SES, and community SES. The authors demonstrate there are substantial differences in network type and source of intimacy across ages, gender and SES. These findings are useful for the promotion of successful aging among the Chinese elderly in the context of largely reduced family size and greatly changing household structure due to population aging.

Chapter 2 - Long-term care is receiving increasing attention as population aging increases the demand for long-term care services and boosts the cost of health expenditures. Although China's old age support system has been studied, previous research has insufficiently examined the long-term care system and its related issues.

This chapter systematically evaluates long-term care needs, costs, unmet needs, provisions, finances, and their associated factors among the Chinese elderly population. The authors mainly use the data from the 2005 wave of the Chinese Longitudinal Healthy Longevity Survey (CLHLS) including 15,593 elders aged 65 and older with over-sampling of the oldest-old to investigate these issues. Additional data were analyzed including a nationwide survey on the elderly and the 2000 census.

We find that about 5-6% (or about 5.7 million) of the Chinese elderly needed long-term care in 2005 if the long-term care need was defined as a status in which a person has been disabled in any of six of activities of daily living for more than ninety days. That figure will reach 27 million in 2050 given the same age-sex-specific prevalence rates. Yearly long-term care expenditures reached 21 billion *Yuan* in 2005, accounting for 2.7% of total health expenditures. The proportion of unmet and undermet needs was nearly 60%. In other words, there were 3.5 million Chinese elders who needed long-term care services but could not access them. This number could climb to 16 million in 2050 given the same age-sex-specific rate.

Our results revealed that more than 80% of long-term care services were provided by family and more than 50% of costs were paid for by family. Our results further revealed that care needs, costs, unmet and undermet needs, provisions, and sources of payments varied across regions and between urban and rural areas, and that individual socioeconomic status and family/social resources were associated with long-term care needs, provisions, and finances, although such associations did not follow the same patterns across subpopulations. These findings are useful in identifying target populations, assessing the long-term care needed, and initiating appropriate services given that rapid population aging and dramatic social and demographic changes will bring great pressure on and challenges to the long-term care system in China.

Chapter 3 - Based on a recent evaluation, this chapter presents an account of the latest model of UK National Health Service (NHS)-led long-term care of older people. It reviews key aspects of the model which include a new role for primary care in anticipatory or preventive medicine for older people; mechanisms for co-ordinating health and social care; relationships between primary care practitioners and secondary care professionals; and the impact on older people's hospital admissions and length of stay. The chapter embeds this review in a historical account of theoretical, policy and service approaches to long-term care which enables the elements of continuity and change contained within the model to be picked up. This in turn permits the conclusion that the particular significance of this latest model in both theoretical and policy terms lies in the framing of illness in old age within the 'risk' paradigm that has come increasingly to characterize late modern society.

Chapter 4 - Programme budgeting and marginal analysis (PBMA) is as an explicit, robust, and practical tool to assist decision-makers in setting priorities in health care. The PBMA framework has been used in at least 70 health service organisations across the UK, Australia, and Canada over the last 25 years. In this chapter, the authors synthesise experiences from these countries in both developing the PBMA framework and implementing the results of PBMA exercises. In particular, they have found the methods used in PBMA are now less mechanistic than they have been in the past, recognising the need to balance pragmatic and ethical considerations with economic rationality. The authors identify and discuss international consistencies and controversies in the treatment of these considerations, as well as, international challenges in the application of the PBMA framework in local health service organisations. Finally, they describe a framework for pragmatic study design in PBMA studies, based on lessons learnt from the practical application of PBMA, including institutional and managerial challenges in health systems.

Chapter 5 - Self-rated health (SRH) has become an increasingly common measure used in population surveys because it has been proven to be a robust predictor of functional disability, mortality, morbidity, and health care use. The present study investigated the correlation of poor SRH in 2,205 randomly selected workers aged 16-83 years among 244 small- and medium-scale manufacturing enterprises (SMMEs) by means of a self-administered questionnaire. SRH was assessed with a question: How would you describe your health during the past 1-year period? Response options were 'very good', 'good', 'poor', and 'very poor.' Poor SRH was defined by rating the above question as 'poor' or 'very poor' (while good SRH was defined by ‘good’ or ‘very good’). Overall, 33.4% of men and 32.1% of women rated their health as poor. Multivariable logistic regression analysis was carried out to estimate the risk of having poor (against good) SRH. The analysis revealed that female gender, poor household financial situation, higher educational attainment, current smoking, insomnia symptoms, depressive symptoms, poor health condition, and long work hours are associated with poor SRH. Several industry sectors such as papermaking, printing and chemical had a higher prevalence of poor SRH as compared to the textile industry. Gender-specific analysis did not show much difference in associated factors between men and women in this sample, but men in the highest group of BMI and women working under a shift/night schedule were gender-unique factors related to poor SRH. Although the results should be interpreted cautiously because of self-reporting and cross-sectional study design, the authors conclude that poor SRH is prevalent among workers in SMMEs, and is associated with a number of modifiable factors at individual and organizational level.

Chapter 6 - Continuity of care is understood to be an enabling factor, leading to better health outcomes, and is positively correlated with having access to health services, increased patient satisfaction, and decreased emergency department use. More comprehensive care is viewed to be an outcome of having continuity of care. Further, continuity of care is also a core principle of health care planning. Central to establishing continuity of care is the development of a relationship between doctor and patient. The transfer of information between these parties facilitates the development of continuity in general and specifically informational continuity of care. Informational continuity of care refers to how well a patient’s health information is able to ‘travel’ with him/her throughout the health service system including over time with the same practitioner and between practitioners in different settings including through primary, secondary, and tertiary care.

In this chapter the authors draw on the findings of a study conducted in Ontario, Canada to support our contention that patients and family caregivers play a significant role in establishing informational continuity of care within family practice. The authors draw on findings from two primary datasets: (1) in-depth interviews (n=24) with both chronically ill patients and family caregivers who frequently speak on behalf of a chronically ill relative during medical appointments, and (2) a systematic review of the role that patients, doctors, and information technology play in establishing informational continuity of care. The authors combine the findings of these datasets in a methodologically innovative way in order to consider the use of computer technologies in information transfer and management in the interaction between doctor and patient/caregiver in the family practice setting. The findings reveal that chronically ill patients and family caregivers do indeed care about *how* information is recorded by doctors and that this shapes the doctor-patient interaction. The findings also show that they have strong opinions of the role(s) that computer technologies should play during the interaction specifically. The authors conclude this chapter by considering the implications of the findings for family doctors and the practice of family medicine.

Chapter 7 - Objective(s): (1) To examine concern for face and different forms of Intimate Partner Violence (IPV) on formal or informal help-seeking intention; and (2) To examine the moderating effect of concern for face on formal or informal help-seeking intention among different groups of pregnant women who suffer from IPV.

Design: A retrospective cross-sectional comparative quantitative study at a university-affiliated regional hospital among 1,200 Hong Kong Chinese pregnant women.

Measurements: The Protective and Acquisitive Face Orientation (PAFO) scale (Short Form) and the modified Cohen's Willingness to Seek Help scale were used to measure concern for face and help-seeking intention. The different forms of IPV were investigated by using the Revised Conflict Tactics Scale (CTS-2).

Results: The results of hierarchical regression models found that women with "Psychological Aggression" significantly negatively associate with formal help intention after adjusting for socio-demographic variables. Women with one subscale of Protective Face Concern: "Keep a low profile to avoid attention (KLP)" was found to negatively associate with formal and informal help-seeking intention after adjustment ($p < 0.05$). The moderating effects of "Physical Assault" and KLP on informal help-seeking intention were found.

Conclusion: IPV and concern for face have an inhibitive effect on the intention to seek help. Implications and limitations are also discussed.

Chapter 8 - Improvements in the quality of biomedical care have resulted in a change in disease trends. In the twenty-first century, in developed countries, it is estimated that 80% of healthcare funds are now being directed towards the care and support of those with chronic diseases. The last decade has seen a rapid change in the role of the community pharmacist. There is a pressing need for increasing healthcare professionals' theoretical and practical knowledge of patient self-management, as well as their skills in helping their patients who have a chronic disease to manage effectively their illness on a daily basis. Pharmacists have high levels of therapeutic knowledge and skills, and are very often the first, and most common, point of contact for people with chronic illness. Community pharmacies offer accessible and convenient venues for patients with chronic disease to gain support for improving their self-management skills. Thus, pharmacists are in an ideal position to contribute to the improved quality of care of patients with a chronic disease. This chapter will discuss the theoretical issues surrounding self-regulation of illness behavior, the concept of illness self-management, and how these constructs can be applied to deliver effective self-management programs. The methods the authors adopted for a number of our research projects trialing community pharmacy disease programs, along with the results, will be used to illustrate these ideas. Importantly, the generic application of these programs to a range of disease states, and healthcare settings, will also be discussed.

Chapter 9 - Much of the research on risk factors for substance use, mental health, and physical health in adults has largely focused on individual risk factors. Although of great importance, individual risk factors are only one component of understanding individuals' risk. Understanding other factors, such as relational influence processes (i.e., influence from family, peers, and the community) are also important for public health efforts. Among adult couples, an intimate partner can be a powerful influence of change, motivating an individual to make positive changes or seek treatment for problems; however, intimate partners can also be a source of negative influence causing the escalation or relapse of problematic or negative behaviors or blocking treatment and intervention efforts. The goal of this commentary is to provide background on why relational processes are important and to describe how these processes can be used to improve health. On the basis of empirical findings regarding relational processes, the authors make a number of recommendations for individuals and health care practitioners to begin to consider the larger domain of risk and protective factors.

Chapter 10 - In Africa, it was very common that older family members make important health decisions when young members are sick. Traditionally, the extended family and clan had been the backbone of the African family system as they had provided help and support to its members whenever needed, especially in times of crises. However, because of the unprecedented demands and needs of people living with HIV/AIDS, these institutions may not be able to meet these challenges.

Additionally, because of modernization and individualism prevalent in urban areas, the roles of the extended family in times of need may be weakened. In fact, AIDS is an exorbitant disease, and currently, most Africans cannot afford effective antiviral therapies. Some families have spent their life savings on loved ones with AIDS but have not seen any improvement in the health of the sick. Also, stigma associated with HIV/AIDS has made it difficult for family members to cope with the disease and openly talk about their loved ones who are either HIV positive or have AIDS. Consequently, extended family members or clans may be reluctant to help because of fear of being stigmatized or the inability to care for a sick family or provide assistance because of poverty.

In general, caregiving has a negative impact on the health and well-being of caregivers. Caregiving to people living with AIDS is a stressful activity that can lead to anxiety and depression. Furthermore, caregiving to children with HIV/AIDS is believed to be extraordinarily challenging because when a child is affected usually one parent or both are affected as well. Thus, caring for a child with AIDS can threaten the family unit by creating additional medical, psychosomatic, and financial strains on the family. Living with AIDS affects the family unit as a whole. It changes behaviors of infected children and challenges their physical and mental abilities.

Caregivers of children living with AIDS face many demands on their families' limited resources, both from the children as well as from other infected family members. This only adds to the burden of stress that the caregivers may already be experiencing. However, studies have indicated that effective coping strategies may reduce the level of stress and anxiety among caregivers. Furthermore, a few studies report that caregiving has some positive influences on caregivers.

The study proposes to examine informal caregiving to children with HIV or AIDS in Togo in order to generate empirical indicators that will be used to develop caregiving measures. Informal caregiving has become an important outlet for people living with AIDS since AIDS is a chronic disease that eventually incapacitates its victims. Moreover, the health care system is poorly developed in Africa, with scarce resources for people with AIDS. Thus, the plight of family members and friends who are caretakers of a loved one with AIDS is compounded.

Researchers have developed instruments to measure the level of stress and anxiety among people giving care to loved ones or close relatives afflicted with chronic and debilitating illnesses; for example the Hopkins Symptom Checklist; the CES-D measure and measures of stress by Pearlin, et al. Unfortunately, these measures of caregiving experiences have all been developed in the western societies which are economically and culturally different from African societies. Because these measures tend to be culture specific, they cannot adequately assess the experiences of informal caregivers in Africa where the effects of HIV/AIDS has been the most severe. Transporting measures from non-African settings may not translate the concepts and experiences of the caregivers in ways that are intelligible and meaningful to African caregivers. Thus, developing instruments to measure caregivers to children with HIV/AIDS is necessary to make intervention programs efficacious. This study attempts to develop an instrument that will measure caregiving experiences of people caring for children with HIV or AIDS in Togo.

Chapter 11 - Regardless of whether health care is funded by government or private insurance, general practitioners (GPs) often act as gatekeepers in restricting access to specialized medical resources in many countries. The current literature on referrals suggests that factors other than a patient's health care needs affect a doctor's decision to refer that individual to a medical specialist. This essay investigates a range of mechanisms that help explain the general practitioner's referral decisions in the Norwegian public health care system. In particular, the focus is on the consequences of a major health policy reform in Norwegian general practice, the introduction of a patient list system in 2001.

Data was obtained from the Statistics Norway's Level of Living Household Panel Study, which includes a representative sample of 3,500 individuals interviewed annually. After introduction of the patient list system, GP referrals appeared to be less influenced by the patient's health condition. In particular, after the reform and after accounting for health condition, patients with low educational qualifications were less likely to be referred to specialist treatment, and patients living in major city regions or using a female GP were more likely to receive a referral. The data also suggest that the incentive structure associated with a patient list system increases competition between practitioners. Consequently, a patient's request is more difficult to reject, and this diminishes the GP's commitment to the gatekeeper role.

This essay analyzed these changes further by exploring the physician's performance of the gatekeeping role within different institutional work settings and with different workloads.

In: Social Sciences in Health Care and Medicine
Editors: J. B. Garner, T. C. Christiansen, pp. 1-10
ISBN: 978-1-60456-286-6

Short Communication A

CLASSROOM ENVIRONMENT AS A PREDICTOR OF BEHAVIOR DISORDERS AMONG CHILDREN WITH LEARNING DISABILITIES IN THE UAE

Vivian Khamis
United Arab Emirates University
College of Education
P.O. Box 17551
Al-Ain, Abu Dhabi, United Arab Emirates
E-mail vkhamis@uaeu.ac.ae

ABSTRACT

This study was designed to identify predictors of behavioral disorders in children with learning disabilities and children without learning disabilities in the UAE public school system. It examined the relative contributions of child characteristic (i.e., presence of learning disability, gender, age), parents sociodemographics.

and aspects of classroom environment (e.g, social support received from teachers ,peers and friends ,meaningful and genuine relationships with classmates ,teachers help in academic matters and use of educational resources , and cooperative learning, in addition to students satisfaction with the physical environment) to behavioral disorders such as internalizing and externalizing problems, and mixed syndromes, mainly anxious/depressed, withdrawn/ depressed, somatic complaints, social problems, thought problems, attention problems, rule breaking behavior, and aggressive behavior. The participants were 200 students from both sexes who ranged in age from 12 to 18 years. Structured interviews were carried out with students at schools. Practical implications to special education at the identification prevention and intervention level were discussed.

Keywords: Behavior Disorders, Learning Disabilities, United Arab Emirates Children, Classroom Environment.

INTRODUCTION

Learning disabilities and other developmental difficulties of children represent social events with ramifications for their social system. The effect of a learning disability on children is profound. Children with learning disabilities (LD) have significant social and emotional problems; they do run a greater risk than their nondisabled peers of having these types of problems (Lerner, 1997).They have a tendency to be rejected by their peers and to have a poor self concept. One plausible reason for the social problems of some students with LD is that they have deficits in social cognition which make them misread social cues and may misinterpret the feelings and emotions of others. It may be also that some of the behavioral characteristics of children with LD annoy others and /or make it more difficult for others to interact with them (Hallahan & Kauffman, 1997; Lerner, 1997).

Although children with LD exhibit a lot of problems, they do have a great deal of inter- and itra-individual variation in their psychological and behavioral characteristics. Some of these differences have been viewed as originating primarily within the child. However, such person centered views of human behavior cannot account for all possible varieties of behavior in all possible situations. A number of researches have noted that classroom environment contributes significantly to the number and seriousness of behavioral and emotional problems (Jones & Jones, 1990, 2001; Lerner, 1997). In fact, the school setting and classroom environment have particular importance for children with learning disabilities because it is in this context that they are defined as learning disabled. Attributes of the classroom setting may interact with a student's attributes to contribute to the emotional and behavioral disorders. Classroom environment settings, therefore, are important factors in "making it or breaking it" for the learning disabled child (Freiberg, 1999; Thomas, 2002, Zabel, & Zabel, 1996). Evaluation of physical, organizational, and human classroom settings attributes gives clues regarding the ways these settings can be modified to provide healthy and productive change for children with learning disabilities (Doyle1986; Jones & Jones, 1990, 2001).

Although the problem of children with learning disabilities is not a new one, psychological research on this disorder among *UAE*_children is non-existent. Most of the studies in the area of special education in UAE have dealt with surveys that investigate the efficacy of the special education placement of disabled children (El-Sweidi & Abu Shehab, 1995) , teaching effectiveness of special education teachers (Dukmak & Alghazo, 2004) and coping with stress among parents of children with mental retardation (Khamis, 2005).Also, no effort has been devoted to the identification, prevention, and intervention of childhood emotional and behavioral disorders primarily because of the absence of the screening procedures as well as the unavailability of the empirically based assessment instruments in the UAE public school system. Consequently, there is no information available that can provide insight into the broad spectrum of competencies, adaptive functioning and problems of children with LD in the United Arab Emirates or on the causes and correlates (e.g., classroom environment) that may have influenced them. The further study of the effect of various aspects of classroom environment on behavior disorders in children with learning disabilities in the UAE public school system will help professionals to diagnose problems, monitor and promote change and program improvement, appraise and improve leadership.

Method

Participants

The participants were 200 students from the public school system, of whom 101 were males and 99 were females representing the various United Arab Emirates (i.e., Abu Dhabi, Dubai, Sharjah, and Ras Al-Khaima). They ranged in age from 12 to 18 years (*M* = 14.44, *SD* = 2.16) and their grade level varied from grade 6 to 12. In this sample students GPA ranged from 41 to 99(*M* = 69.27, *SD* = 21.53). According to teachers records and students' reports 56.5% (n= 113) of these children had learning disabilities, mainly in mathematics (25.5%), and language (18 %), or in both mathematics and language (17.5%).

For the entire sample, the mean level of education for mothers and fathers was some preparatory, with the range extending from illiteracy to post-graduate study. Approximately 61.5 % of these students were from intact families, 8 % reported that their parents were divorced, 7 % were widowed and 23.5 % their fathers had more than one wife. Most of the mothers were housewives (73 %) and the remaining were working either as teachers or employees. On the other hand, the majority of the fathers (85.5 %) were working, mainly in the army or police or as employees in the business sector. The number of family members living in the household ranged from 2 to 31 (*M* =11.35, *SD* =5.51). The student's average number of siblings was 9.15 (range, 1 to 27). Families' combined gross income ranged from 1000 to 42000 UAE Dirham.

Sample Selection

The design for sample selection was based on four primary stratified variables: gender, age of the child, presence of learning disability, and various Emirates (i.e. Abu Dhabi, Dubai etc). Data from the Ministry of Education and Youth (MOEY) was used to allocate schools that provide regular and special education for children with learning disabilities in the various United Arab Emirates. Children then were selected randomly from each school with the help of school personnel and these students were asked for an interview.

Procedure

Informed consent was obtained from the Ministry of Education, school directors and the participants. They were given a full explanation of the study, assured of the anonymity of their responses, and were ensured confidentiality of all information collected. Five female special education graduates who were trained by the author carried out the interviews with the student at school.

Instrumentation

Child and Family Data Sheet

A brief questionnaire was developed to secure demographic and background information about the child and the family from mothers and fathers. The child variables considered for this study were age, gender, type and presence of learning disability. The families' sociodemographics were level of education completed by parents, marital status, employment, family size, and total household income.

Behavioral and Emotional Disorders

Behavioral and emotional disorders were assessed using the Youth Self Report Form (YSR; Achenbach, 1999, 2002) of the Achenbach System of Empirically Based Assessment (ASEBA). The YSR consists of 101 problem behaviors reflecting internalizing and externalizing problems such as anxious/depressed, withdrawn/ depressed, somatic complaints, social problems, thought problems, attention problems, rule breaking behavior, and aggressive behavior. Behavioral and emotional problems are rated by children aged 12 to 16 using a 3-point scale ranging from not true to very true or often true. Cronbach's alpha is .91.

Classroom Environment Scale (CEC)

The classroom environment scale (CEC) was designed for the purpose of this study to measure the students' perception of classroom environment such as social support received from teachers ,peers and friends (emotional support, advice, encouragement, companionship, and boosting morale), meaningful and genuine relationships with classmates ,teachers help in academic matters and use of educational resources , and cooperative learning, in addition to students satisfaction with the physical environment(seating arrangements, comfortable chairs, air ,light). The items of the scale were declarative statements to which the students answered "not true" (0), "somewhat true" (1), or "certainly true" (2). A factor analysis of twenty-one items, using a principal-component analysis with a varimax rotation of eigenvalues greater than or equal to 1.0, generated five factors that explained 57.39 % of the variance. Only factor loadings of .50 were selected to represent factors. Cronbach's alpha for the total scale is .80.

Statistical Analyses

Multivariate analysis of variance (MANOVA) was employed to examine the differences in behavioral and emotional disorders in UAE school age children such as internalizing and externalizing problems, mixed syndromes and total problems scale, as a function of child-related variables, parent's sociodemographics, learning disabilities and classroom environment. Resulting significant differences were tested using the Scheffe test. Pearson correlation coefficients were conducted, correlating the previously mentioned variables with classroom environment and parent's socio-demographic variables such as parent's education, number of siblings and family income. Hierarchical multiple regression was used to predict behavioral and emotional disorders of children from four blocks of predictor variables. The four-predictor blocks were: a) child characteristics b) parents' sociodemographics, c) presence of LD, and d) classroom environment.

RESULTS

Child Characteristics and Behavioral and Emotional Disorders

Behavioral and emotional disorders were determined by using the three domains of YSR and the total problems scale. Multivariate analysis of variance (MANOVA) was employed to examine differences between males and females, age, and learning disabilities on internalizing and externalizing problems, mixed syndromes and total problems scale (YSR). The results revealed no significant interactions among the groups on the YSR nor on any of the YSR domains $F(3, 187) = 1.21$, $p < .29$. However ,Multivariate analysis of variance (MANOVA) showed significant main effect for gender on internalizing behavior problems , $F(3, 187) = 3.67$, $p < .05$, with females experiencing more internalizing problems (i.e., depression, anxiety and withdrawal) than males . No significant differences were found on any of the YSR domains nor on the total problems scale (YSR) as a function of child's age (see Table 1).

Also significant main effect were found for learning disabilities on internalizing behavior problems, $F(3, 187) = 7.28$, $p < .0001$; externalizing behavior problems, $F(3, 187) = 16.71$, $p < .0001$; mixed syndromes , $F(3, 187) = 24.13$, $p < .0001$, and total problems, $F(3, 187) = 19.14$, $p < .0001$ with children who had LD exhibiting more internalizing problems (i.e., depression, anxiety and withdrawal) , externalizing problems (i.e., aggression, rule breaking) , mixed syndromes (i.e., attention ,thought and social problems) than children without LD (see Table 1).

Parents Sociodemographics and Behavioral and Emotional Disorders

Correlation coefficients also showed significant positive association between number of siblings and externalizing problems ($r = .20$, $p < .05$), and total problems ($r = .16$, $p < .05$) .Children who have large number of siblings exhibit more externalizing problems such as aggression and rule breaking. Also significant positive relationship was found between fathers' education and children's internalizing problems ($r = .15$, $p < .05$). Fathers with higher levels of education have children with more internalizing problems.

Table 1. Means and Standard Deviations of YSR dimensions and total problem scale by Child Characteristics

Variable/ Child Characteristics	Internalizing		Externalizing		Mixed Syndromes		Total Problems	
	M	*SD*	*M*	*SD*	*M*	*SD*	*M*	*SD*
Child's Gender								
Male {n=101)	15.46	9.46	15.79	12.13	18.15	10.84	49.40	29.59
Female {n=99)	17.94	7.78	12.81	9.84	15.39	8.84	46.63	23.92
Child's Age								
12-13 {n=75)	17.00	9.03	16.34	11.62	17.71	10.64	51.30	29.03
14-15 {n=58)	16.92	7.73	14.09	10.63	17.10	9.22	48.12	24.25
16 & above {n=67)	16.01	9.36	12.41	10.42	15.58	9.91	44.47	26.96
Academic Status								
Students with LD {n=113)	18.32	8.75	17.26	11.59	20.07	9.96	55.68	27.04
Students without LD {n=87)	14.35	8.28	10.44	8.84	12.51	8.32	37.42	23.32

*Indicates p< 0.05;** Indicates <0.01;***Indicates<0.001;****Indicates<0.0001

Classroom Environment and Behavioral and Emotional Disorders

Correlation coefficients also showed significant negative association between classroom environment and internalizing problems ($r = -.23$, $p < .01$), externalizing problems ($r = -.49$, $p < .01$) , mixed syndromes ($r = -.43$, $p < .01$) and total problems ($r = -.43$, $p < .01$). Children who perceived their classroom environment negatively in terms of lack of support from teachers, negative patterns of interaction and relationships with peers and teachers tended to report higher levels of emotional and behavioral disorders including higher scores on the three YSR dimensions internalizing, externalizing and mixed syndromes as well as the total problems scores.

The Prediction of Child Behavioral and Emotional Disorders

Hierarchical multiple regression was used to predict behavioral and emotional disorders of children from four blocks of predictor variables. The four-predictor blocks were: a) child characteristics b) parents' sociodemographics, c) presence of LD, and d) classroom environment.

The predictor blocks were entered in the order listed. This order was based upon chronology of occurrence. The early entry of a variable block into the regression equation provided a statistics control for the impact of those variables upon behavioral and emotional problems.

Table 2, indicates that the model containing all four predictor blocks accounts for 33.8 % of behavioral and emotional problems variance. Each predictor block separately accounted for the following percentage of child behavioral and emotional disorders variance: 2.1% by child characteristics, 5.1% by parent's sociodemographics, 13.9 % by presence of LD, and 12.7% by classroom environment.

Table 2. Prediction of behavioral and emotional disorders by child characteristics, parents' sociodemographics, presence of LD, and classroom environment

Predictor Variable	*B*	*R*	R^2	*F*	*df*	*p*<
Block 1: Child Characteristics		.144	.021	1.83	2.174	.16
Child's Gender	2.07					
Child's Age	-1.06					
Block 2 : Parents Demographics		.267	.072	2.18	6.170	.04
Father's Education	-.06					
Mother's Education	.38					
Number of Siblings	.73*					
Family Income	.000					
Block 3 : Presence of LD	15.45****	.459	.211	6.44	7.169	.0001
Block 4: Classroom Environment	-1.55****	.582	.338	10.73	8.168	.0001

Gender is coded: Male=1; Female=0. Age is coded: Age in Years. Level of Education is coded: Level of Education in years. Presence of LD is coded: Students with LD=1; non-LD =0. Classroom Environment is coded: 5-point scale ranging from 21 to 105.

*Indicates $p< 0.05$;** Indicates <0.01;***Indicates<0.001;****Indicates<0.0001

The absolute increase in R^2 is small for child characteristics, .021; parents' sociodemographics, .051; presence of LD, .139; and medium for classroom environment .16 obtained by dividing the percentage of additional variance by the percentage of unexplained variance prior to entry. Cohen's (1988) guidelines for small, medium (those typical in behavioral research) and large effect sizes are .02, .15, and .35, respectively.

In Table 2, the column denoted beta contains the standardized or beta coefficients of the eight individual variables contained in the model. The absolute magnitude of the emotional and behavioral disorders. Beta coefficients are particularly good indexes of the relative importance of variables as they express the unique variance attributable to a predictor while controlling for all other predictors within the final regression model.

Of the child characteristics none of the variables was significantly associated with child emotional and behavioral disorders. Among parent's sociodemographic variables, only one stood out as a significant predictor of more child emotional and behavioral disorders. Children who had a large number of siblings appeared to exhibit more emotional and behavioral disorders. As for learning disabilities, children who had LD were more likely to suffer from emotional and behavioral disorders.

In addition, classroom environment appeared to be a salient predictor of emotional and behavioral disorders in children. Children who perceived their classroom environment negatively tended to report higher levels of emotional and behavioral disorders. Therefore, negative patterns of interaction between children and peers as well as teachers, and lack of teacher's academic support were associated with emotional and behavioral disorders in UAE school-aged children.

CONCLUSION

The pattern of results from this study provides evidence that the number of UAE school age children who could be considered learning disabled is alarmingly high. A significant proportion of this sample (56.5 %) were identified as having learning disabilities based on students self report data and informal methods of academic assessment by their teachers especially in language and mathematics.

Consistent with previous findings (Anderson,, Kutash, & Duchnowski, 2001; Bower, 1995; Elbaum, 2002; Pavri & Monda-Amaya, 2000), the results of this study indicated that learning disabilities are characteristics of students with emotional and behavioral disorders. Although having academic difficulties is not known to cause emotional and behavioral disorders in children, it frequently accompanies maladaptive behavior and possibly contributes to maladjustment. On the other hand, it could be argued that maladaptive behavior makes academic success unlikely and contributes to school failure. Previous researchers have indicated that disordered behavior and underachievement appear to influence each other reciprocally (Kauffman, 2001).

Consistent with previous research (Kasen, Johnson, &Cohen, 1990; Walker, 1995; Walker, Colvin, & Ramsey, 1995) the analyses of the results emphasized the crucial role of classroom environment in predicting emotional and behavioral disorders in school age children. Children who perceived their classroom environment negatively were more likely to report higher levels of emotional and behavioral disorders. While behavioral and emotional disorders are effected by the presence of learning disabilities in UAE school age children, , it is also true that the presence of learning difficulties may have very different effects on students if they occur in different classroom environment. Consequently, classroom environment may contribute to the development of emotional or behavioral disorders in children.

In this study, children who reported that they lack : a) social support from teachers ,peers and friends (emotional support, advice, encouragement, companionship, and boosting morale);b) meaningful and genuine relationships with classmates c)teachers help in academic matters and use of educational resources ; d) cooperative learning; and e) dissatisfaction with the physical environment (seating arrangements, comfortable chairs, air, light) were more likely to report suffering from emotional and behavioral disorders.

The different patterns of predictor-outcome relations have practical as well as theoretical implications. In the light of the present findings, many supports and strategies may be used to promote good classroom behavior and reduce emotional and behavioral disorders in children. They include relationship building strategies, antecedents-based interventions, and behavior-reduction techniques. Building meaningful and genuine relationships with and among students is an essential aspect of creating a learning environment that supports their learning and promotes their positive classroom behavior. Teachers can do this by collaborating and communicating with others, fostering an acceptance of individual differences, friendships and mutual respect and employing cooperative learning.

ACKNOWLEDGMENT

This research was supported by a grant provided by the United Arab Emirates University, under the terms of Award No.03-03-3-11/05. The completion of this work was greatly facilitated by the institutional support of the scientific research affairs at UAEU.

REFERENCES

Achenback, T.M. (1991). *Manual for the Youth Self Report and 1991 profile.* Burlington, VT: University of Vermont, Department of Psychiatry.

Achenback, T.M. & Rescorla, L.A. (2001). *Manual for the ASEAB School-Age Forms and Profiles.* Burlington, VT: University of Vermont, Research Center for Children, Youth, and Families.

Anderson, J.A., Kutash, K. & Duchnowski, A.J. (2001). A comparison of the academic progress of students with EBD and students with LD. *Journal of Emotional and Behavioral Disorders, 9*, 106-115.

Bower, B. (1995). Criminal intellects: Researchers look at why lawbreakers often brandish low IQs. *Science News,* 147, 232-233.

Cohen, J. (1988). *Statistical power analysis for the behavioral sciences* (2nd Ed.). Hillsdale, NJ: Erlbaum.

Doyle, W. (1986). Classroom management techniques. In O. C. Moles (Ed.), *Handbook of Research on Teaching* (pp.392-431). New York: McMillan.

Dukmak, S. & Alghazo, I. (April, 2004).The teaching effectiveness of special education teachers in the United Arab Emirates. Paper presented at the 5th Annual UAE University Research Conference.

Elbaum, B. (2002) .The self concept of students with learning disabilities: A meta analysis of comparisons across different placements. *Learning disabilities Research and Practice, 17*, 216-226.

El-Sweidi, M. & Abu Shehab, A. (1995). *Survey of disabilities in the United Arab Emirates families.UAE*: Ministry of Labor and Social Welfare.

Freiberg, J.H. (1999). *School climate: measuring, improving, and sustaining healthy learning environments* . London ; Philadelphia : Falmer Press.

Hallahan, D. & Kauffman, J. (1997). *Exceptional Learners: Introduction to Special Education* (7th Ed.). Boston, MA: Allyn and Bacon.

Jones, V.F. & Jones, L.S. (1990).*Comprehensive classroom management.* Boston: Allyn and Bacon.

Jones, V.F. & Jones, L.S. (2001).*Comprehensive classroom management. Creating community of support and solving problems.* (6th Ed.) Boston: Allyn and Bacon.

Kasen, S., Johnson, J. & Cohen, P. (1990). The impact of school emotional climate on student pathology. *Journal of Abnormal Psychology, 18*, 165-177.

Kauffman, J. (2001). *Characteristics of emotional and behavioral disorders of children and youth.* (7th Ed.) .New Jersey: Merrill Prentice Hall.

Khamis, V. (2005).*Coping with Stress among Parents of Children with Mental Retardation in the United Arab Emirates.* Paper presented at the 6th Annual UAE University Research Conference.

Lerner, J.W. (1997). *Learning disabilities: theories, diagnosis, and teaching strategies* . Boston: Houghton Mifflin.

Pavri, S. & Monda-Amaya, L. (2000). Social support in inclusive schools: Student and teacher perspectives. *Exceptional children, 67*,391-411.

Thomas, B. (2002). *Classroom environment in child education.* Jaipur, India: Aavishkar Publishers.

Walker, H.M. (1995). *The acting out child: Coping with classroom disruption* (2nd Ed.). Longmont, CO: Sopris West.

Walker, H.M., Colvin, G., & Ramsey, E. (1995). *Antisocial behavior in schools: strategies and best practices.* Pacific Grove, CA: Brooks/Cole.

Zabel, R.H. & Zabel, M.K. (1996). *Classroom management in context: orchestrating positive learning environments.* Boston, MA : Houghton Mifflin, c1996.

In: Social Sciences in Health Care and Medicine
Editors: J. B. Garner, T. C. Christiansen, pp. 11-49
ISBN: 978-1-60456-286-6

Chapter 1

SOCIAL NETWORK TYPES, INTIMACY AND HEALTHY LONGEVITY AMONG THE CHINESE ELDERLY

Danan Gu[1], Qiushi Feng[2] and Jessica Sautter[3]
Duke University, USA

ABSTRACT

The significant association between an individual's social network and his or her health and mortality at old ages is well-documented in western societies. However, similar research from developing countries, especially among long-lived persons, is rare due to lack of data. The value of social support embedded in the social network for healthy longevity is generally more significant in developing countries given the lack of advanced and institutionalized social security systems. This chapter provides us with a good opportunity to address how social network types and intimacy are related to healthy longevity among Chinese elders.

Using the Chinese Longitudinal Healthy Longevity Survey (CLHLS), a unique specially designed nationwide survey with a sample of 15,232 community-residing Chinese elders, this chapter examines the associations between social network types and intimacy and subsequent healthy longevity from 2002 to 2005 within a multi-level context. The outcome variables include instrumental activities of daily living, activities of daily living, cognitive functioning, self-rated health, chronic diseases, frailty index, and mortality. We classified social networks into eight types based on living arrangement, number of frequently visiting children, and social connection (playing cards/mah-jong and involvement in religious and social activities): (1) isolated, (2) children-visiting-only, (3) family coresidence only, (4) family coresidence plus children-visiting only, (5) social connection only, (6) social connection plus children visiting, (7) social connection plus family coresidence, and (8) social connection plus family coresidence & children visiting. Source of intimacy was measured by the most frequent daily talking-person and grouped into (1) nobody/social service provider/matron, (2) spouse, (3) child, and (4) friend/neighbor. Other individual variables and community socioeconomic

[1] (Corresponding author), 200 Trent Dr. Rm 1506 Busse BLDG
Medical Center, Duke University, Durham, NC 27710, USA, Tel: 1-919-660-7532
Fax: 1-919-668-0453, Email: gudanan@duke.edu, gudanan@yahoo.com.

[2] Department of Sociology, qiushi@soc.duke.edu.

[3] Department of Sociology, Jsautter@soc.duke.edu.

variables served as controls. We used multilevel logistic regression to examine the effects of social network types and source of intimacy on subsequent 3-year mortality and health status.

Our analyses show that compared to the isolated elders, elders in socially integrated networks had up to a 35% reduction in odds of mortality over a 3-year period, although such protection was diminished after controlling for baseline health. Elders in family-oriented networks, on the other hand, had up to a 51% increase in odds of mortality over the 3-year period independent of baseline health. Compared to those who did not have an intimate network alter, those whose source of intimacy was a friend/neighbor or spouse had 15-50% decreased odds of death in the presence of various confounders including baseline health. Socially integrated networks reduce the likelihood of poor health by up to 60% in terms of cognitive impairment, ADL/IADL disability, poor self-rated health, chronic diseases, and frailty. Similar results were found for having a friend/neighbor as the source of intimacy. These results suggest that the protective effects of network types and source of intimacy on healthy longevity still exist at advanced ages.

We further examined the patterns of social network types and source of intimacy by age, gender, childhood and adulthood SES, and community SES. We demonstrate there are substantial differences in network type and source of intimacy across ages, gender and SES. These findings are useful for the promotion of successful aging among the Chinese elderly in the context of largely reduced family size and greatly changing household structure due to population aging.

Keywords: China, Chinese elderly, oldest-old, healthy longevity, social relationships, social network, network type, social support, longitudinal survey, intimacy, culture, determinant.

INTRODUCTION

In this chapter we will discuss the effects of social networks and sources of intimacy on health outcomes among the Chinese elderly. We will first review the existing literature on the structure of social networks, the effects of social networks on health, and sociodemographic differentials in social networks and their effects on health. We will then review limitations of previous research to set the stage for our analyses, and provide necessary context for the study of social networks in China, a developing country in East Asia with a unique culture of social networks. We then present the Chinese Longitudinal Healthy Longevity Survey (CLHLS) and the measures of social network types, sources of intimacy, individual and community-level sociodemographic characteristics, health behaviors, and psychological attitudes. We then describe results addressing the following research questions: (1) What effects do social network types and sources of intimacy have on health outcomes? (2) What effects do social network types and sources of intimacy have on health behaviors and psychological attitudes that may influence health outcomes? (3) What sociodemographic factors predict social network types and sources of intimacy? Finally we discuss these results, which mostly indicate that the relationships found in research in developed countries also apply to China, a developing country.

Characteristics of Social Networks

A social network is defined as a web, collection, or set of linkages of interpersonal relationships and the characteristics of those ties in varying contexts (Berkman et al. 2000; Fischer 1982; Litwin 2001). Social networks connect an elder to society, enhancing his or her social integration and continuity (Inglehart & Baker 2000). The social network perspective emphasizes not the attributes of each individual, but rather their embeddedness in the social environment, specifically the structural characteristics of interpersonal connections. More broadly speaking, social networks tap the structural pattern of interpersonal relations and the content of social linkages among elders and persons linked to the network (i.e., individuals and organizations) (Luke and Harris 2007).

Our understanding of how social networks influence health and mortality has been substantially advanced and extended in recent decades by cross-sectional and longitudinal empirical research across different populations. Social network analyses of health and mortality often examine two central properties, the structure and function of social networks (Kang et al. 2007). The structural features include network size, density or frequency of contact, homogeneity (similarities among network members), duration of ties (the length of time contacts have known each other), reciprocity, and geographic proximity (Berkman et al. 2000; Burt 2001; Castilla et al. 2000; Litwin 1995; Wenger 1991). Functional aspects of social networks, also called social support, represent the health-promoting resources channeled through the structure of the social network, either actual or subjective. The social support functions realized through the social network encompass emotional, instrumental, appraisal and informational components (Kang et al. 2007).

Social networks and embedded social support attain even more importance for people at advanced ages because of increased rates of disease and disability (Bosworth & Schaie 1997). At old ages, environmental support (including from family, friends, and others), social ties, and assistance from others become critical factors in the maintenance of individuals' independence (Bosworth & Schaie 1997).

Social Networks and Health Outcomes

Over the past few decades, many studies have explored the potential associations among social networks, social support, and health outcomes, especially among elders (for some recent reviews, see Berkman et al. 2000; Giles et al. 2005; Seeman & Crimmins 2001). There is widespread agreement that better social linkages could result in a decreased mortality hazard, whereas social isolation increases the mortality risk (Berkman & Glass 2000; House, Landis, & Umberson 1988; LaVeist et al. 1997; Uchino, Cacioppo, & Kiecolt-Glaser 1996). With few exceptions (e.g., Jorm et al. 1991), most studies have been conducted in the United States (Seeman et al. 1993), European countries (Penninx, van Tilburg, & Kriegsman 1997), Australia (Giles et al. 2005), and Asia (Sugisawa, Liang, & Liu 1994). These studies have consistently indicated that structural and functional social network characteristics have significant effects on survival among old adults; higher levels of social connection, participation, and support greatly improve the longevity of aged people. The corroboration of the protective effects of social networks on survival is impressive given that the socio-cultural context of the target population, follow-up time, sample size, and participants' ages vary considerably across different studies (see Giles et al. 2005).

Most studies have found a negative association between structural and functional network characteristics and disability among elders. For example, Mendes de Leon and colleagues (2001) report that, (1) network size and social interaction reduce disability risk, (2) friend ties are associated with decreased disability, and (3) emotional support lowers the rate of activities of daily living (ADL) dependency. Mendes de Leon and colleagues (2001) also find that network size and emotional support are negatively associated with prevalence of ADL impairment. However, they also report that instrumental support increases the risk of disability. Such an increased risk might be either because the instrumental support increases the "dependency," or because disabled people need more instrumental support. Some other studies find no significant relationship between network size and social support and the onset of ADL disability (e.g., Seeman, Bruce, & McAvay 1996).

Research shows that the social networks of the elderly are strongly related to their perceived health status, but the association may vary in different cultures and populations. This is because macro-level social forces, especially inequality, cultural orientations, and processes of social change, shape individuals' social networks. Cultural variations in social networks produce differential effects on health through varied psychological mechanisms and psychobiological process (Berkman et al. 2000; Litwin 2006). For example, Litwin (2006) finds that frequent contact with children and friends/neighbors improves self-rated health (SRH) among Western-oriented Jewish-Israeli elders, but proximity to children is negatively related to SRH among this group of elders. On the other hand, proximity to children has no significant effect on SRH among the Arab-Israeli minority that has mainly family-based networks. In a study comparing two French-speaking Canadian communities, Zunzunegui and colleagues (2004) find that there is a consistent positive impact of social network on SRH. However, the importance of support from children varied by community. In addition, Zunzunegui and colleagues (2004) find evidence for the importance of the friend network in both of the two Canadian communities, but not in a similar study in Spain (Zunzunegui et al. 2001).

Social networks may influence many other health outcomes among elderly people. For instance, social networks reduce the likelihood of cognitive decline (Bassuk et al 1999; Seeman et al 2001). Social networks are also well known to positively affect mental health: fewer social ties are often linked to depressive symptoms (Kawachi & Berkman 2001), whereas greater social ties reduce risk of depression among the elderly and boost their self-confidence (Bondevik & Skogstad 1998; Newsom & Schulz 1996). Lack of social contacts or low levels of social contacts are linked to higher risks of disease incidences such as coronary heart diseases (Vogt et al 1992) and a higher likelihood of low health related quality of life (López García et al. 2005).

The protective effects of social network on health and mortality are also evident among patients with specific diseases. For example, breast cancer patients who were socially isolated had a 66% higher risk of all-cause mortality and 100% higher risk of breast cancer mortality than those who were non-isolated (Kroenke et al. 2006). Individuals with a large social network have a better possibility of recovery or survival after stroke (Glass & Maddox 1992) and better possibility of recovery from various illnesses (Ruberman et al 1984; Williams et al 1992). Social network is further associated with healthcare service use and care expenditure, although this association is complicated (Bosworth & Schaie 1997; Kang et al. 2007).

Literature on the association between intimacy and health outcomes focusing on elderly people is relatively rare. Intimacy refers to the willingness to disclose information about private topics to another person (Clark & Reis 1988), or to emotional and physical closeness (Mattiasson & Hemberg 1998). Studies focusing on non-elderly populations show that a lack of interpersonal intimacy can inhibit mental health, development and maturity (Mattiasson & Hemberg 1998). Disclosure of stressful events improves physical functioning, self-reported health (Pennebaker 1993; Pennebaker & Susman 1988), and psychosocial well-being (Harvey, Curry, & Bray 1991), and is associated with fewer symptoms of illness (Reis et al 1985). Such effects are also evident among rheumatoid arthritis patients (Kelley, Lumley, & Leisen 1997). Empirical studies further report that different sources of intimacy (e.g., spouse, family, or friends) may have different meanings, provide different kinds of assistance, and meet different needs (Weiss 1982; Hobfoll, 1985). For example, studies focusing on adult women reveal that those considering spouse or friends as sources of intimacy are more satisfied with social support, as compared to those naming family members as sources of intimacy (Hobfoll, Nadler, & Leiberman 1986).

The mechanisms driving the associations between social networks and health outcomes work mainly through adaptation of behavior and biopsychosocial pathways (Berkman et al 2000; Luke & Harris 2007; Lang 2001; McAuley 1993; Seeman & Crimmins 2001). According to Berkman and colleagues (2000), networks operate at the behavioral level through four primary pathways: (1) social support; (2) social influence; (3) social engagement and participation; and (4) access to material goods and resources. These micro-psychosocial and behavioral processes ultimately influence more proximate pathways to health status and mortality, including: (1) buffering of stress; (2) increase in self-esteem, self-efficacy, sense of morale, and security; (3) promotion of healthy lifestyle and awareness of utilization of healthcare services; (4) regulation of contact with infectious diseases; and (5) improvement of immune system function (Ajrouch, Blandon, & Antonucci 2005; Berkman et al. 2000; Litwin 2001; Unger et al. 1999; Seeman & Crimmins 2001).

Sociodemographic Differentials in Social Networks and Health

Both structural and functional characteristics of social networks and their impacts on health and mortality vary significantly by age, gender, socioeconomic status (SES), and other individual or community-level factors.

There is robust evidence that number of social ties often decreases gradually at old ages due to detachment from socioeconomic activities, widowhood, disabilities and illness, death of other network members, and deliberate discontinuation of weak ties (Ajrouch, Blandon, & Antonucci 2005; Lang 2000; Lang & Carstensen 1994). Empirical studies using similar assessment methods have consistently found that older people have, on average, about half as many social contacts as adults who are in their 20s or 30s have (for a review, see Lang and Carstensen 1998). Not only does network size decrease with advanced age, but the structure of the network, through which resources are mobilized, also changes. Elderly people's social support mainly comes through family ties, while younger adults tend to rely more on their friends (Levitt, Weber, & Guacci 1993; Olsen et al 1991). Age-related changes are not only driven by structural changes across the life span, but also stem from adaptive strategies of aged people themselves. That is, purposeful actions by aging individuals may alter the structure of social relationships. Since emotional needs become more valued in later life, aging people may intentionally drop periphery contacts in the social network and focus on more intimate relationships as sources of emotional support (Baltes & Carstensen 1996; Carstensen 1991, 1992). Regardless of the pathway, aging people often lose social contacts with age, and social relationships may play a much more important role in maintaining health status (Sherbourne et al 1992; Yasuda et al 1997).

Gender differentials in social networks have been widely recognized, particularly in relation to life stage (Antonucci 2001; Ajrouch, Blandon, & Antonucci 2005; Due et al. 1999). Research focusing on young adults has shown that while adult men and women generally report a similar number of persons in their network, men's networks consist of fewer kin and neighbors, but more non-kin, coworkers, and friends in both Oriental and Western societies (Cheng and Chan 2006; Due et al 1999; Lee, Ruan, & Lai 2005; Moore 1990; Yeung, Fung, & Lang 2007). Research shows similar patterns among old adults and further reveals that old women are more likely than old men to develop supportive networks (Ajrouch, Blandon, & Antonucci 2005; Unger et al. 1999). Accordingly, women tend to mobilize and receive more emotional and instrumental social support through these social networks than men do (Hays and Oxley 1986; Okamoto and Tanaka 2004; Yeung, Fung, & Lang 2007). In addition to gender differentials in the structure of social networks, the positive effects of social networks on health are generally significant among men, but commonly non-significant among women, especially in the case of marriage (House, Robbins, & Meltzner 1981; Pilisuk et al 1993; Shye et al 1995; Okamoto & Tanaka 2004). As a consequence, lack or loss of social ties leads to higher risks of poor health and mortality among men as compared to women (Seeman 1996; Unger et al 1999).

Although there has been relatively little research on socio-economic differences in the social networks of older people, there is a consensus among researchers that SES influences the structure of social networks and mediates the impacts of social networks on health and mortality. On average, people with a lower SES have a smaller network with a larger portion of kin ties as compared to those with a higher SES (Ajrouch, Blandon, & Antonucci 2005; van Groenou and van Tilburg 2003). High-status occupations seem to confer greater opportunities for individuals to form ties with high-status coworkers than low-status positions do (Ajrouch, Blandon, & Antonucci 2005). People with higher education levels tend to have more diverse, less family-based networks because greater cognitive resources and skills are needed to develop and sustain social relationships (van Groenou & van Tilburg 2003; Wenger 1995). Low income indicates a lower ability to buy good food, live in quality housing, and join clubs and organizations, reducing social participation and personal network size (van Groenou & van Tilburg 2003). Thus, people without adequate economic and educational resources may suffer more in the absence of social support (Robert & House 1996; Unger et al. 1999). However, Kubzansky and colleagues (1998) found that lower levels of education were associated with larger social networks among adults aged 70 to 79. And Rosengren and colleagues (1988) argue that the highest SES individuals are the most affected by poorer social network. A few researchers have recently reported significant effects of childhood SES on network characteristics at old ages, although such effects are less important compared to adulthood SES (van Groenou & van Tilburg 2003).

Research on urban/rural residential differences in social networks is relatively rare given that urban/rural differences are relatively insignificant in developed countries. These few studies show that urban dwellers have more geographically dispersed networks consisting of more non-family and/or single-stranded relationships than did the respondents living in rural areas (Fischer 1982; Wenger 1995).

The association between community characteristics and individual social networks is becoming more prominent (see Thomése & van Tilburg 2000). Researchers view local communities as a set of social structural opportunities to maintain personal relationships (Thomése & van Tilburg 2000). A study from The Netherlands shows that urbanization affects the physical distance of networks. Elders from more urbanized communities tend to have fewer social ties within the community they live in, but more core ties within one-hour's travel (Thomése & van Tilburg 2000). One recent study from the U.S. also demonstrates that elders from communities with higher SES tend to have few social ties within the community but more ties outside the community (Wen, Cagney, & Christakis 2005). Indeed, macro social-structural factors such as employment opportunities, economic modernization, urbanization, and the societal unionization of work, can affect the nature and quality of personal networks and support (Berkman et al. 2000; House, Landis, & Umberson 1988; Lee, Ruan, & Lai 2005).

Measurement of Social Networks

Researchers have used a variety of approaches and methods to measure the characteristics of personal networks. Yet, both the measurement instruments and procedures tend to be too complicated, thus making them subject to interview bias. It remains uncertain how well the estimates obtained from these instruments and procedures approximate actual personal networks (Fu 2005). Thus, in measuring the huge body of information in a social network, some social gerontologists have recently developed the concept of a network typology to identify common characteristics from numerous social ties and from various measurements in a parsimonious manner based on latent or cluster analysis techniques (Litwin 2001; Wenger 1991). For example, Litwin (2001) summarizes seven variables (marital status, number of children living nearby, frequency of contact with children, friends, and neighbors, frequency of synagogue and social club attendance) into a single network type variable with five categories: diverse, friends, neighbors, family, and restricted. The concept of network types summarizes social network information and implies differential availability of social support according to one's particular network constellation (Litwin & Landau 2000). This approach also borrows insights from the convoy model, which suggests that people take on different sets of roles in their life spans, which correspondingly accompany different sets of social ties (Kahn & Antonucci 1980). The network types identified in the various typologies in different populations across continents exhibit several similarities, especially regarding composition (see Litwin 2001), indicating significant potential for use by gerontological practitioners and researchers. The resource of intimacy is studied less frequently among elders, as noted earlier. One study focusing on non-elderly women classifies source of intimacy as spouse, family member, and friends/neighbors (Hobfoll, Nadler, & Leiberman 1986).

Limitations of Previous Research

To date, several limitations of existing literature are noticeable. First, although the effects of social networks on health outcomes have been examined throughout multiple countries, much of the research focuses on the Western advanced countries. There is less empirical research in the context of developing countries, where social support embedded in the social network may be important due to lack of advanced and institutionalized social security systems. Indeed, the underlying association between type of social network and healthy longevity among elders and the oldest-old in developing countries remains largely unexplored. Some research has demonstrated that the value of social network types to health may vary in different populations (Fischer & Shavit 1995; Grossetti 2007). As noted by Litwin (2007), recent studies in developed nations have discovered different patterns of valuable network factors in different countries. Friends play a significant role in promoting survival rates for the Swiss, while spouses are more important for Danish people. Emotional support leads to lower mortality rates in Amsterdam, while social participation significantly reduces death among Jewish-Israelis. As we will detail below, studies have demonstrated the difference in the composition of personal support networks between the Chinese and the westerners (Lee, Ruan, & Lai 2005). We speculate that some of the basic hypotheses about social networks and health outcomes in the Western nations may not be applicable in China.

Second, early life SES is likely to play some direct or indirect role in determining the structure and function of social networks at late ages given that personal network in later life reflects opportunities and choices made earlier in life about developing and maintaining certain personal relationships. Changes in SES during the life-course, from childhood to late adulthood, represent changing opportunities and may thus affect personal network (van Groenou & van Tilburg 2003), but this issue is seldom examined in the social network literature.

Third, there is a dearth of research on the influence of community factors on social network formation (Berkman et al. 2000). To our knowledge, this kind of research is almost completely absent in developing countries.

The fourth limitation is that, although a number of recent studies have stressed the importance of diversity of types of social network (Agneessens, Waege, & Lievens 2006), intimacy (see Hale, Hannum, & Espelage 2005), and size of support network in affecting health and mortality, the majority of studies are based on latent class models that are largely determined by the variables and specific methods employed. No study has ever looked at the differential effects of source of intimacy (i.e., intimacy with spouse, children, friends/neighbors, etc.). Indeed, few studies have distinguished differentials in health and mortality between kin and non-kin sources of intimacy.

The fifth limitation of existing research is that most studies analyze only one dimension of health and overlook the multidimensionality of health outcomes associated with social networks and health. The benefit of social support embedded in social networks for one health condition may not translate into a benefit for another health outcome. It is imperative to examine various dimensions of health to tap the full spectrum of associations between social networks and health and mortality.

Social Networks in China

The Chinese live in a network of *guanxi,* which is regulated by the Confucian ethical system of benevolence-righteousness-propriety (Hwang 1997-8). According to Fei (1948), the uniqueness of the Chinese social network lies in the binding of the actor to others. Specifically, each person is situated at the center of a concentric network circle and the extent of intimacy with someone else is determined by the relative position of that person within the concentric circles of one's psychological field (Hwang 2000). The importance of taking appropriate action at one's position embedded in one's social network is highly emphasized, and the roles and relationships between the actor and others within the network are interdependent. This is drastically different from the Western social network in which people are more independent (Hwang 1997-8; Hwang 2000; Markus & Kitayama 1991). This unique feature of social networks profoundly influences social-economic activities in Chinese livies, even as the society of China is becoming increasingly modernized and westernized (Lin 1995, 2001; Bian 1997).

Family ties are deeply rooted in China and are the center of social networks for many Chinese. Traditionally, these strong family ties have led to social norms whereby spouses and daughters take care of elders and maintain frequent contact with them (Hwang 1997-8). About 77% of the Chinese adult sample in the 1995-98 World Values Survey reported family as "very important" in their life domains.[4] Empirical studies on Chinese kinship ties confirm the prominent role of family or close kin in social support networks in contemporary China (Freeman & Ruan 1997; Lee, Ruan, & Lai 2005; Lai 2001; Yan 1996).

However, some studies find that Chinese people prefer turning to non-kin such as friends and coworkers when confronting emotional issues. One study compares China with many other Western nations and shows that Chinese familial roles are less diffuse than in the West, especially in the provision of instrumental support, and that the function of the Chinese family in providing emotional support is relatively weak (Freeman & Ruan 1997). Such a feature is probably due to a central feature of Chinese family tradition; the paternalistic and hierarchical kinship structure in China may discourage the sharing of emotional problems among close relatives (Freeman & Ruan 1997).

Several studies have explored the characteristics of social networks among the general adult population in China (e.g., Lai 2001; Lee, Ruan, & Lai 2005; Yan 1996), and a few studies have investigated the association between social support and mortality at adult ages (Yip et al. 2007) and old ages (Liu, Liang, & Gu 1995). However, most of these studies are locally based and lack a systematic examination of characteristics of social networks and their association with various health outcomes among Chinese elders.

There are many reasons why an investigation of social networks and health outcomes in China is important. Social networks play a significant role in social and economic activities in the Chinese cultural context; China has the largest aging population in the world; and most of the care of elders in China is provided via social ties in the absence of a welfare state system. As the number of elders in China rapidly increases in coming decades, understanding of the effect of social networks on healthy longevity will become increasingly important.

---

[4] The corresponding number for Vietnamese, Korea, and Japan are 82%, 90%, and 91%, respectively.

Research Questions

In this chapter we will address the following research questions to examine the effects of social networks and source of intimacy on health outcomes among the Chinese elderly:

- What effects do social network types and sources of intimacy have on 3-year mortality and other health outcomes?
- What effects do social network types and sources of intimacy have on health behaviors and psychological attitudes that may influence health outcomes?
- What sociodemographic factors predict social network type and source of intimacy?

In summary, by using the Chinese Longitudinal Healthy Longevity Survey (CLHLS), a unique specially designed nationwide survey of the elderly, this chapter aims to examine the associations among network types, sources of intimacy, and health in terms of activities of daily living (ADL) impairment, instrumental activities of daily living (IADL) impairment, cognitive function, chronic disease, SRH, frailty index, and mortality. We will include measures of childhood, adulthood, and community SES in the analysis, given that these factors are related to health and mortality at old ages (see Subramanian et al. 2006; Zeng, Gu, & Land 2007). We also examine the factors associated with social network types and source of intimacy within a multilevel, life course context. To our knowledge, this is the only study in China on this topic with a nationwide sample of older adults, and the first study to include childhood SES, adulthood SES, and community SES to analyze characteristics of social networks and their associations with mortality and various health outcomes among the elderly.

DATA AND METHODS

Data

This study uses data from the 2002 and 2005 waves of the Chinese Longitudinal Healthy Longevity Survey (CLHLS).[5] The CLHLS, which began in 1998, is the first nation-wide longitudinal survey ever conducted in a developing country to have a very large sample of the oldest-old. Interviews were conducted in randomly selected half of the counties/cities in 22 provinces in China with an attempt to interview all centenarians in the sampled counties/cities with informed consent. For each centenarian with a pre-designated random code, one nearby octogenarian and one nonagenarian of pre-designated age and sex were randomly interviewed. The term ‘nearby’ refers to the same village or street, or the same town, county or city, when applicable. This sampling strategy is designed to ensure comparable numbers of randomly selected male and female octogenarians and nonagenarians at each age from 80 to 99. The second wave was conducted in 2000. The CLHLS has started to include young elders aged 65-79 in the sample since the third wave in 2002. Excluding those institutionalized

---

[5] We did not use the four waves of data available so far. This is because the first two waves only sampled elders aged 80 and older and did not include data on source of intimacy.

elders, the 2002 wave interviewed 4,739 young seniors and 10,493 oldest-old seniors aged 80-109, with 6,484 men and 8,748 women. Of the total 15,232 community-residing interviewees in the 2002 wave, 7,842 (51.5%) were re-interviewed in the 2005 wave, 5,343 (35.1%) died before the 2005 wave, and 2,045 (13.4%) were lost to follow-up.

The data relevant to social network structure include living arrangement, number of living children and their frequency of visits, playing cards/mah-jong, involvement in religious and social activities, and source of intimacy. Other intensive data cover demographic characteristics, family and household characteristics, lifestyle, diet, psychological characteristics, economic resources, self-reported health, self-reported life satisfaction, lower and upper extremities performance, instrumental activities of daily living (IADL), activities of daily living (ADL), cognitive functioning, and chronic disease. All information was obtained through in-home interviews. The date of death for deceased respondents was collected from various sources including death certificates, next-of-kin, and neighborhood committees. All dates at death were validated and the dates reported on death certificates were ultimately used when available – otherwise the next-of-kin's report was used, followed by neighborhood registries. Systematic assessments of the CLHLS regarding the accuracy of age reporting, the reliability, validity, and consistency of numerous measures, and the randomness of attrition show that data quality in the CLHLS is quite good (Gu 2008a, 2008b; Gu & Dupre 2008; Zeng & Gu 2008).

Measurements

Health Outcomes

We attempt to capture a relatively full spectrum of the associations between social network and health outcomes by including 3-year mortality and six health measures in the analysis. Activities of daily living (ADL) refer to basic personal care tasks of every day life. In this study, ADL disability is defined as self-reported difficulty with any of the following ADL items: (a) bathing, (b) dressing, (c) eating, (d) indoor transferring, (e) toileting, and (f) continence. The high validity and reliability of self-reported ADL disability in the 2002 wave of the CLHLS has been reported (Gu 2008a). Following previous studies (Crimmins, Hayward, & Saito 1996), we dichotomize ADL functional capacity into "active" (no ADL limitation) and "disabled" (at least one ADL limitation).

Instrumental activities of daily living (IADL) disability is defined as self-reported difficulty with any of the following IADL items: (a) visiting neighbors, (b) shopping, (c) cooking, (d) washing clothes, (e) walking for 1 km, (f) lifting 5kg weight, (g) crouching and standing up three times, and (h) taking public transportation. The reliability and validity of IADL measures are reasonably good (Gu and Dupre 2008). We dichotomize IADL functional capacity into "active" (no IADL limitation) and "disabled" (at least one IADL limitation).

Cognitive impairment is measured by the Chinese version of the Mini-Mental Status Examination (MMSE), which is adapted from the work of Folstein and his colleagues (Folstein, Folstein, & McHugh 1975) and tests the following aspects of cognitive functioning: orientation, registration, copy and design, calculation, recall, naming, language (repetition, read and obey, write, and command). The Chinese version of the MMSE is intended to meet the cultural and socioeconomic conditions in China and to make the questions easily understandable and answerable among normally functioning oldest-old Chinese (Zeng &

Vaupel 2002). The Chinese version of the MMSE has proven to be reliable and valid (Gu 2008a; Zhang, Gu, and Hayward 2008). Given generally low levels of education among Chinese elders, we use a score of 18 or higher out of total 30 as the cutoff value to classify the respondent as cognitively unimpaired (Zhang et al. 2008).

Chronic illness is measured by a single dummy variable that indicates whether the respondent has any of twenty major chronic diseases such as hypertension, diabetes, heart disease, cerebrovascular disease, arthritis, cataracts, cancer, pneumonia, or Parkinson's disease. The prevalence of chronic disease in the CLHLS is highly reliable as compared to other Chinese nationwide surveys (Gu & Dupre 2008).

Self-rated health (SRH) is assessed using a single item. Subjects were asked "In general, would you say your health is: (1) very good, (2) good (3) so so (4) bad or (5) very bad?" We dichotomize the measure of self-rated health into very good/good health versus so so/bad/very bad health, and treat it as a binary outcome to correct for its highly skewed distribution. Self-rated health has high predictive validity for mortality, physical disability, chronic disease status, health behaviors, and health care utilization (Chen and Wu 2008; Ferraro, Farmer, & Wybraniec 1997; Idler and Benyamini 1997). It may also better capture a sense of overall well-being, commensurate with the WHO's definition of health in which health is more than simply the absence of disease but also includes mental, physical, and social dimensions of well-being (Hill, Ross, & Angel 2005).

We also include a frailty index, which captures the cumulative health deficits of an individual (Mitnitski et al. 2005), to measure overall health condition. The validity of frailty as a proxy for biological age and as a predictor of mortality and health change has been well-documented (Mitnitski, et al. 2005; Yashin et al. 2007). Despite some modest restrictions on how to construct a frailty index, the majority of existing studies calculate a frailty index based on variables available in the dataset used (Mitnitski et al. 2005). Consistent with the established literature, we construct a frailty index based on 39 variables from various dimensions of self-rated health, cognitive functioning, disability, auditory and visual ability, depression, heart rhythm, and numerous chronic diseases. Each item is dichotomized and coded as 1 when the deficit is present and 0 when the deficit is absent. We assign a score of two if the sampled person had a serious illness that caused him/her to be hospitalized or bedridden two or more times (Goggins et al. 2005). The frailty index was constructed by summing all deficits and dividing by the number of total possible deficits, thus it ranges from 0 to 1. Please refer to Gu and colleagues (2007) for the validity of frailty index in the CLHLS. We then classified those respondents who survived to the 2005 follow-up wave into healthy survivors and non-healthy survivors based on the quartile of their frailty index in 2005.[6] Those with frailty index in the lowest quartile were considered as healthy survivors. Otherwise, they were regarded as non-healthy survivors. In addition to health conditions, we also examine mortality risk across the three-year follow-up period from 2002 to 2005.

Independent Variables

As noted earlier, there is no gold standard in measuring social networks, and new approaches are constantly being developed to capture different dimensions of the concept (Berkman et al. 2000; Litwin 2001). Based on living arrangements, having frequently visiting

---

[6] We also used the quantile of the frailty index as the criterion of healthy and non-healthy survival. The patterns are the same.

children, and social connection in terms of playing cards/mah-jong, involvement in religious and organized social activities,[7] we generate a single variable of types of social networks. We did not apply the latent class analysis method, which is increasingly used in recent literature to generate a typology of social network, because such a classification is not fully clear-cut and is also unable to distinguish full membership and partial membership like the Grade of Membership method (see Manton, Woodbury, & Tolley 1994). Therefore, we decided to use a simplified way to define social network types.

We classified social network among Chinese community-residing elders into eight types in this chapter:

1) *Isolated*: live alone, not married, no living children, and no social connection;
2) *Children-visiting-only*: live alone or with spouse only, have children visiting, and no social connection;
3) *Family coresidence only*: live with children or grandchildren and/or their spouses, but no children visiting, and no social connection;
4) *Family coresidence plus children-visiting*: live with children or grandchildren and/or their spouses, have children visiting, and no social connection;
5) *Social connection only:* participate in at least one of three measured social activities, but not living with offspring, and no children visiting;
6) *Social connection plus children-visiting*: participate in social activities and have children visiting, but not living with offspring;
7) *Social connection plus family coresidence*: participate in social activities, live with offspring, but have no children visiting;
8) *Social connection plus family coresidence & children-visiting*: participate in social activities, live with offspring, and have children visiting;

Except for Type one, an elder in each type may or may not live with his/her spouse. Types two through four are characterized by family contacts, while types five through eight are characterized by both family and social connections. Therefore, these eight types could be grouped into three larger types: isolated, family-oriented, and socially integrated.

Source of intimacy was measured by a question in the CLHLS "who is the most frequent talking-person in your daily life?" Responses were collapsed from eight categories into four categories: (1) spouse, (2) children and other family member, (3) friends/neighbors, and (4) social service providers/matron/nobody.[8] The distributions of types of social networks and sources of intimacy among the Chinese elders are listed in Table 1.

To ensure robust results, we controlled for numerous factors that have been reported to be associated with healthy longevity (e.g., Anderson et al. 1997) and with social network (e.g., Litwin & Landau 2000), as reviewed above. Control variables at the individual level include demographic, childhood and adulthood socioeconomic status (SES), psychological disposition, and health practice. Demographic variables include age, sex, ethnicity (Han vs Non-Han), and urban/rural residence (Urban=1, Rural=0). Childhood SES is measured by

---

[7] Organized activities normally include activities organized by clubs, non-governmental organizations, senior associations, formal or informal social entities, etc.

[8] The frequency in the category of social service providers/matron is very small (n=208) which causes convergence problems when we examine the factors associated with sources of intimacy. After statistical test, we find that it has no significant difference from the category of nobody. Therefore, we combined these two categories.

whether the interviewee was born in an urban area and by his or her father's primary occupation when the respondent was a child (white-collar occupation vs other).[9] Adult SES is measured by education (1+ years of schooling vs 0), primary lifetime occupation (white-collar occupation vs other), and family economic condition as compared to others (good=1, so so/poor=0). The adequacy of these childhood and adulthood SES measures in the CLHLS has been well addressed in the literature (e.g., Zeng, Gu, & Land 2007; Zhu & Xie 2007). Psychological disposition includes optimistic attitudes (Yes vs No), loneliness (Yes vs No), and feeling of usefulness (Yes vs No).[10] Health practice measures include whether the respondent is a current smoker (Yes vs No), whether the respondent is a current drinker of any alcohol (Yes vs No), and whether the respondent regularly exercises (Yes vs No). We control for each health condition at the 2002 wave when we address the associations between types of social network and six health indicators in 2005. We control for frailty index in the 2002 wave when we explore associations between type of social network and mortality from 2002-2005.

At the community level (a county/district of a city),[11] we controlled for GDP per capita and percentage of urban population to account for an important environmental factor for social network and health (Anderson et al. 1997; Sandtröm et al. 2003). These two variables mainly reflect the level of socioeconomic development in a community and were obtained from the National Bureau of Statistics of China (2003). Detailed coding for all control variables is available upon request.

Methods

We used multilevel random intercept logistic regressions to examine the effects of type of social network and source of intimacy on subsequent 3-year mortality rate and health status. With the random intercept design, we assume that the effect of each individual factor is the same across communities: the level-one (individual) coefficient of each covariate is fixed across level-two units (community). This design is called random-intercept and fixed-slope model and is widely used in multilevel analyses (Raudenbush, Bryke, & Cheong 2004). We also tested for multicollinearity of covariates in the models. The largest value of variance inflation factors was lower than 3, indicating there was no serious multicollinearity problem (Chandola 2001).

In mortality analyses, those who were lost to follow-up in 2005 were dropped, leaving a total sample of 13,187 respondents (7,550 women and 9,126 oldest-old aged 80 and older) consisting of 7,844 survivors and 4,882 decedents. Sequential models were designed to investigate how these factors mediate the associations between social networks and mortality.

---

[9] The correlation between being born in an urban area and current residence in an urban area is 0.33. Although it is higher than any other correlation in the dataset, such a correlation is mild and unlikely to introduce large bias in estimation.

[10] Each variable has five categories: Always, often, so so, seldom, and never. We code always and often as 1 and 0 otherwise.

[11] In western developed countries, most studies have used census tract, electoral ward, or zip code to define a community (Kawachi & Berkman 2003), largely due to conveniently available census data in Western societies. While this approach may generate misspecification problems, and thus underestimate neighborhood effects, it is a conservative strategy that takes advantage of existing data sources to study place effects on health. In our study, census data does not allow us to examine such a small unit. Therefore, we use county as a proxy for community. More importantly, the SES and environmental data are available only at the county level or higher.

Model I controls for demographic factors. Model II adds community level factors into Model I, while Model III additionally controls for childhood SES. Model IV additionally controls for adult SES. Model V adds psychological disposition and health practice and Model VI further adjusts for the frailty index in 2002 in Model V. The same analytical strategies were used with a sub-sample of respondents aged 80 and older to examine differentials between the oldest-old sample and the entire sample.

In analyzing health indicators, we include only those who survived to the 2005 wave (8,157 respondents). Two sequential models are employed to test the effects of type of social network and source of intimacy on each of six subsequent health outcomes. Model I controls for all individual level factors and two community-level factors. Model II further includes baseline health status in 2002.[12] Interactions between social network type and age, gender, urban/rural residence, and both adult and childhood SES were tested and found to be non-significant. Therefore, no interactions were added to the model, and no separate models were run for these sub-samples.

We used multilevel random intercept multinomial logistic regressions to investigate the factors associated with type of network and source of intimacy, based on the whole sample in 2002. In order to simplify the analysis, we group the eight network types into three large types of networks: isolated, family-oriented, and socially integrated. We retain four categories for source of intimacy. Sequential models were designed to test the effect of individual demographics, childhood SES, adult SES, and community SES on social networks at old ages. Model I only includes demographics. Model II includes community SES into Model II. Model III adds childhood SES into Model II, and Model IV further controls for adult SES.

To distinguish different samples and facilitate the description, we define three sub-samples for analyses. The network-mortality sub-sample is used for analyzing associations between network type or intimacy and mortality. The network-health sub-sample is used for analyzing associations between network type or intimacy and health measures. The network type/intimacy sub-sample is used to examine factors affecting network type or intimacy (cf. Table 1).

To reduce the possible influence of missing items (although only about 2% of the data) on our data analysis and inferences, we imputed missing values for continuous variables with the variable mean, and missing values for categorical variables with the mode of the variable. Other imputation approaches were also tested and yielded similar results. Given that the sampling weight variable in the publicly released CLHLS dataset is calculated based on the age-sex-urban/rural residence-specific distribution of the population and does not capture other important compositional variables, such as marital status, economic status, etc., the weight was not applied in the current study. Research has shown that including variables related to sample selection produces unbiased coefficients without weights (Winship & Radbill 1994). All analyses were performed using HLM 6.01 (Raudenbush, Bryke, & Cheong 2004).

---

[12] We run six models for each health measure as for network-mortality sample. Since the results for some models are almost identical, we decided to present two models to simplify the analysis. The results for the rest four models are available upon request.

RESULTS

Description of the Sample

Table 1 presents the unweighted sample distributions for three samples that are used for analyses in this chapter. Clearly, the most frequent type of social network among the CLHLS samples is coresidence with family plus children visiting but no social contact in terms of playing mah-jong, religious involvement, or participation in organized social activities. The social network of the majority of Chinese elders is family-centered. About 2% of respondents in the samples have no contact with family or friends, which is similar to some findings in developed countries (Bowling, Grundy, & Farquhar 1995:331). Approximately 25-30% of the sample list friends/neighbors as a source of intimacy. Approximately 9% of respondents report that they have no family member or friend/neighbor that they talk to frequently as a source of intimacy. About 35% to 44% of intimacy comes from children and other family members. The patterns for social network structure and intimacy sources across the three samples are similar, with a slight difference in the network-health sample. In this sub-sample, friend/neighbors and spouses account for a relatively higher proportion as the source of intimacy, relatively more elders have social contacts, and a smaller portion of elders have no intimate family members or friends/neighbors. The network-health sub-sample is much younger than the other two, with relatively higher SES, better psychological disposition, and more men.

Table 1. Distribution of the sample population aged 65 and older, the CLHLS 2002 -2005

	Network-mortality analysis sample	Network-health analysis sample (in 2005)	Network type/ intimacy analysis sample
Individual level factors			
Total No. of respondents	13,187	7,845	15,232
Social network types			
Isolated	2.3	2.1	2.4
Children-visiting only	15.6	17.7	15.6
Family coresidence only	7.1	4.3	7.0
Family coresidence plus children-visiting only	39.7	32.0	38.8
Social connection only	1.6	1.8	1.8
Social connection plus children-visiting	12.4	16.9	12.6
Social connection plus family coresidence	2.3	2.3	2.3
Social connection plus family coresidence & children visiting	19.1	22.9	19.4
Source of intimacy (Daily most frequent talking-person)			
Nobody/social service provider/matron	8.5	5.1	8.6
Spouse	21.9	29.3	22.2
Children or family member	43.7	35.2	43.4
Friends/neighbors	25.9	29.8	25.7

	Network-mortality analysis sample	Network-health analysis sample (in 2005)	Network type/ intimacy analysis sample
All other variables			
Age [a]	86.3	81.6	86.2
Men	42.8	45.3	42.6
Urban	42.2	43.2	44.9
Han ethnicity	93.8	93.6	94.3
Born in urban	13.6	14.4	15.0
Father's occupation was white-collar job	3.7	3.9	3.9
1+ years of schooling	37.6	42.5	38.1
White-collar job	8.0	10.0	8.6
Good family economic condition	17.3	17.6	17.4
Current smoker	18.8	21.3	18.6
Current drinker (any alcohol)	21.4	23.2	---
Regular exercise	31.0	36.8	---
Optimistic	69.5	75.1	---
Loneliness	39.9	32.6	---
Uselessness	66.9	61.6	---
IADL disabled in 2005	70.2	66.2	---
ADL disabled in 2005	29.3	23.0	---
Cognitively impaired in 2005	41.1	35.5	---
Having 1+ diseases in 2005	60.6	62.7	---
Self-rated poor health in 2005	23.1	24.2	---
Frailty index in 2005 [a]	---	0.20	---
IADL disabled in 2002	---	56.7	---
ADL disabled in 2002	---	16.3	---
Cognitively impaired in 2002	---	25.6	---
Having 1+ diseases in 2002	---	59.1	---
Self-rated poor health in 2002	---	16.4	---
Frailty index in 2002 [a]	0.23	0.18	---
% deceased	40.5	---	---
Community level factors			
Total No. of communities	845	845	845
Per capita GDP (in 1000 *RMB*) [a]	6.4	6.4	6.4
% of urban population [a]	30.5	30.5	30.5

Note: (1) Figures in the table are all percentages in 2002 except as indicated. All percentages and means are unweighted (2) a, mean. (3) ---, not used in analysis models; therefore, omitted.

Effects on Mortality

Table 2 illustrates how different types of social networks are associated with three-year mortality risk among Chinese elders. Adjusting for demographic factors, Model I (upper panel of Table 2) reveals that, with the exception of the children-visiting only type, elders whose social relationships are characterized by family connection only were 40-60% more likely to die compared to isolated seniors. The family coresidence without children's visiting type has the highest mortality risk. These findings are unexpected but possible, as we explain in the discussion. On the other hand, socially integrated elders are 15-34% less likely to die than isolated elders. But social connection only without family connection does not significantly reduce mortality risk. These effects persist even if community level factors (Model II), childhood SES (Model III), and adult SES (Model IV) are additionally added into analysis. Further controlling for health practice and psychological disposition (Model V) slightly increases the effect of network types without social connection, and slightly reduces the protective effect of network types with social connection. Once baseline overall health condition in 2002 is controlled (Model VI), the protective effect of social connection on the likelihood of three-year mortality is not significant. These findings suggest that the protective effects of social connection on mortality operate mainly through health practice and health condition. The lower panel of Table 2 indicates that these patterns still hold among the oldest-old population.

Similarly, Table 3 presents the effects of source of intimacy on three-year mortality risk for the whole elder sample and the oldest-old sample. Compared to those who have nobody or has only social service providers/matrons to talk to, those whose source of intimacy is a spouse or friend/neighbor have nearly half the odds of death during a three-year period; those whose source of intimacy is a child or other family member have 20% lower odds of death. The presence of community SES (Model II) and individual SES (Model III and Model IV) do not alter the effect. After adjusting for health practice, the protective effects are slightly modified (Model V). Further controlling for overall health condition in 2002, the effects of having a spouse or friend/neighbor as a source of intimacy is moderately modified down to 17-25%, but still significant (Model VI). The effect of having a child or family member as the source of intimacy is not significant in the presence of the baseline overall health status, however. Results among the oldest-old are more or less the same (lower panel of Table 3). These findings suggest that having an intimate spouse or friends/neighbors might be more important than children in providing emotional support that mediates mortality risk.

Table 2. Effects of types of social network on subsequent 3-year mortality among the Chinese elders, the CLHLS 2002-2005

	Models					
	I	II	III	IV	V	VI
Age 65+						
Isolated (reference)	1.00	1.00	1.00	1.00	1.00	1.00
Children-visiting only	1.00	1.00	1.00	0.99	1.09	1.08
Family coresidence only	1.53**	1.54**	1.54**	1.51**	1.62**	1.52**
Family coresidence plus children-visiting only	1.37*	1.36*	1.36*	1.36*	1.50*	1.41*
Social connection only	0.84	0.84	0.84	0.84	0.93	0.97
Social connection plus children-visiting	0.66**	0.66**	0.66**	0.66**	0.78	0.86
Social connection plus family coresidence	0.78	0.77	0.77	0.76	0.90	0.96
Social connection plus family coresidence & children visiting	0.79+	0.79+	0.79+	0.79	0.97	1.06
-LL	7061.9	7061.8	7061.3	7016.5	6922.3	6726.7
rho	0.03***	0.03***	0.03***	0.03***	0.03***	0.03***

	Models					
	I	II	III	IV	V	VI
Age 80+						
Isolated (reference)	1.00	1.00	1.00	1.00	1.00	1.00
Children-visiting only	0.98	0.98	0.98	0.97	1.05	1.04
Family coresidence only	1.45*	1.45*	1.45*	1.43*	1.53**	1.44*
Family coresidence plus children-visiting only	1.26	1.26	1.26	1.24	1.37*	1.28+
Social connection only	0.80	0.80	0.79	0.78	0.88	0.93
Social connection plus children-visiting	0.64**	0.64**	0.64**	0.63**	0.75+	0.85
Social connection plus family coresidence	0.72+	0.72+	0.72+	0.70+	0.84	0.88
Social connection plus family coresidence & children visiting	0.70*	0.70*	0.70*	0.70*	0.87	0.94
-LL	5672.3	5672.1	5671.4	5628.6	5543.4	5374.7
rho	0.02***	0.02***	0.02***	0.02***	0.02***	0.03***

Note: (1) The numbers in the table are odds ratios. The odds ratios of all covariates are not presented in the table but are available upon request. (2) Model I controls for demographic factors. Model II adds community level factors, while Model III additionally controls for childhood SES. Model IV additionally controls for adulthood SES. Model V adds health practice variables and psychological disposition into Model IV, and Model VI further adjusts for the frailty index in 2002. (3) +, p<0.1; *, p<0.05; **, p<0.01; ***, p<0.001.

Table 3. Effects of sources of intimacy on subsequent 3-year mortality among the Chinese elders, the CLHLS 2002-2005

	Models					
	I	II	III	IV	V	VI
Age 65+						
Daily most frequent-talking person						
Nobody/social service provider/matron (reference)	1.00	1.00	1.00	1.00	1.00	1.00
Spouse	0.54***	0.54***	0.54***	0.55***	0.66***	0.77**
Children or family members	0.81**	0.81**	0.81**	0.82**	0.93	1.10
Friends/neighbors	0.54***	0.54***	0.54***	0.54***	0.64***	0.84*
-LL	7093.7	7093.1	7092.8	7045.2	6946.9	6739.3
rho	0.03***	0.03***	0.03***	0.03***	0.03***	0.03***
Age 80+						
Daily most frequent-talking person						
Nobody/social service provider/matron (reference)	1.00	1.00	1.00	1.00	1.00	1.00
Spouse	0.58***	0.58***	0.58***	0.59***	0.71**	0.82+
Children or family members	0.82*	0.82**	0.82**	0.82*	0.94	1.09
Friends/neighbors	0.54***	0.54***	0.54***	0.54***	0.65***	0.85+

Table 3. Continued.

	Models					
	I	II	III	IV	V	VI
-LL	5700.1	65699.9	5699.5	5654.7	5563.3	5384.8
rho	0.02***	0.02***	0.02***	0.02***	0.02***	0.02***

Note: (1) Intimacy is measured by the daily most frequently talking to person (2) The numbers in the table are odds ratios. The odds ratios of all covariates are not presented in the table but are available upon request. (3) Model I controls for demographic factors. Model II adds community level factors, while Model III additionally controls for childhood SES. Model IV additionally controls for adulthood SES. Model V adds health practice variables and psychological disposition into Model IV, and Model VI further adjusts for the frailty index in 2002. (4) +, p<0.1; *, p<0.05; **, p<0.01; ***, p<0.001.

Effects on Health Status

The results in Table 4 show that the positive effects of the socially integrated network types on IADL and ADL impairment are limited when compared to the isolated network. However, those who are socially integrated tend to have better cognitive function compared to those isolated seniors. For example, the odds ratios of being cognitively impaired among the social integrated elders is 7-40% (Model I) or 7-38% (Model II) lower as compared to those isolated elders. There is no significant difference between family-oriented network types and the isolated network on cognitive function. Although the odds of having chronic diseases are lower for all family-oriented and socially integrated network types as compared to the isolated network, most are not significant. With two exceptions (i.e., family coresidence only and social connection only), all types of social networks tend to reduce the odds of having poor self-rated health as compared with the isolated network; most are significant. The reduction is slightly larger among the socially integrated types (44-55% in Model I and 43-55% in Model II) than among family-oriented types (30-39% in Model I and 32-39% in Model II). In terms of frailty index, all seniors tended to be healthier than their isolated counterparts, although the difference is not significant for those whose network type is either family coresidence only or family coresidence with social contacts but no children visiting. On average, the socially integrated network types produce more benefits than family-oriented types for overall health status.

Table 5 demonstrates how having a spouse, child, or friend/neighbor as the source of intimacy affected six health indicators. Results in Model I reveal that, except in the case of having chronic diseases, having a friend/neighbor as the source of intimacy significantly reduce subsequent risk of IADL disability, ADL disability, cognitive impairment, and poor self-rated health by 35%, 48%, 49% and 33%, respectively. The protective effects of having a spouse as the source of intimacy are slightly smaller; the protective effects of having a child or family member as the source of intimacy are moderately smaller. For overall health condition, only those having a friend/neighbor as the source of intimacy have a significantly lower likelihood (31%) of having a frailty index score larger than 0.1. No significant difference is found between having a spouse or a child and having nobody to talk to, however. These protective effects are mildly mediated by earlier health conditions (Model II).

Table 4. Effects of types of social relationships on six subsequent health outcomes among the Chinese elders aged 65 and older, the CLHLS 2002-2005

	IADL disabled	ADL disabled	Cognitive impaired	1+ chronic diseases	Self-rated poor health	Frailty Index >=0.1
Model I						
Isolated (reference)	1.00	1.00	1.00	1.00	1.00	1.00
Children-visiting only	0.85	1.12	0.83	0.79	0.70+	0.64+
Family coresidence only	1.00	1.17	0.91	0.77	0.77	0.79
Family coresidence plus children-visiting only	1.04	1.68*	1.00	0.73	0.61**	0.67+
Social connection only	0.89	1.47	0.78	0.79	0.73	0.54+
Social connection plus children-visiting	0.58*	0.86	0.53**	0.86	0.55**	0.48**
Social connection plus family coresidence	0.93	1.41	0.93	0.73	0.55*	0.65
Social connection plus family coresidence & children visiting	0.72	1.11	0.60*	0.71+	0.46***	0.44**
-LL	3647.9	3320.5	3762.3	4844.7	4036.3	4066.1
rho	0.13***	0.14***	0.18***	0.18***	0.11***	0.10***
Model II						
Isolated (reference)	1.00	1.00	1.00	1.00	1.00	1.00
Children-visiting only	0.79	1.11	0.81	0.73	0.68*	0.65+
Family coresidence only	0.82	0.97	0.88	0.72	0.74	0.78
Family coresidence plus children-visiting only	0.89	1.34	0.96	0.68+	0.61**	0.67+
Social connection only	0.97	1.27	0.80	0.75	0.72	0.53*
Social connection plus children-visiting	0.59*	0.79	0.54**	0.82	0.55**	0.51**
Social connection plus family coresidence	0.86	1.22	0.93	0.68	0.55*	0.68
Social connection plus family coresidence & children visiting	0.71	0.99	0.62*	0.68+	0.47***	0.47**
-LL	3517.7	3162.1	3675.4	4744.7	3982.8	3983.3
rho	0.12***	0.13***	0.18***	0.18***	0.10***	0.10***

Note: (1) The numbers in the table are odds ratios. The odds ratios of all covariates are not presented in the table but are available upon request. (2) Model I controls for all factors at the individual level and two indicators at the community level. Model II further includes the corresponding health measure in 2002. (3) +, p<0.1; *, p<0.05; **, p<0.01; ***, p<0.001.

In summary, most types of social network, especially the socially integrated types, tend to exert protective effects on subsequent health status as compared to the isolated type. The socially integrated types also have protective effects on mortality risk, although controlling for baseline health seems to diminish such effects. Having a friend/neighbor or spouse or child/family member as the source of intimacy substantially improves subsequent survivorship and various health conditions as compared to those who have nobody to talk to.

The protective effects of having a friend/neighbor as the source of intimacy on mortality and most health indicators are significant in all cases as long as having a spouse as the source of intimacy is significant. However, the effect of having a spouse as the source of intimacy is not always significant when the effect of having a friend/neighbor as the source of intimacy is significant. The effects of having a child as the source of intimacy are significant in most cases when the effects of having a spouse are significant. Given the above findings, it might be true that the overall effect of having a friend/neighbor as the source of intimacy on healthy longevity was the largest, followed by spouse and then by children.

Table 5. Effects of source of intimacy (most frequently talking to person)on six subsequent health outcomes among the Chinese elders aged 65 and older, the CLHLS 2002-2005

	IADL disabled	ADL disabled	Cognitively impaired	1+ chronic diseases	Poor Self-rated health	Frailty Index >=0.1
Model I						
Daily most frequent-talking person						
Nobody/social service provider/matron (reference)	1.00	1.00	1.00	1.00	1.00	1.00
Spouse	0.75+	0.71*	0.54***	1.24+	0.73*	0.88
Children or family members	0.87	0.82	0.64***	1.12	0.68**	0.85
Friends/neighbors	0.65**	0.52***	0.51***	1.08	0.67**	0.69*
-LL	3661.5	3323.8	3775.8	4846.0	4047.7	4080.4
rho	0.12***	0.15***	0.18***	0.18***	0.11***	0.10***
Model II						
Daily most frequent-talking person						
Nobody/social service provider/matron (reference)	1.00	1.00	1.00	1.00	1.00	1.00
Spouse	0.89	0.76+	0.59***	1.29+	0.80+	0.93
Children or family members	0.97	0.85	0.71**	1.16	0.77*	0.89
Friends/neighbors	0.82	0.60***	0.58***	1.14	0.76*	0.74*
-LL	3526.6	3163.9	3687.1	4746.9	3994.0	3994.1
rho	0.12***	0.14***	0.18***	0.18***	0.10***	0.10***

Note: (1) Intimacy is measured by the daily most frequently talk to person. (2) The numbers in the table are odds ratios. The odds ratios of all covariates are not presented in the table but are available upon request. (3) Model I controls for all individual level factors and two community level factors. Model II further includes the corresponding health measure in 2002. (4) +, p<0.1; *, p<0.05; **, p<0.01; ***, p<0.001.

Association with Behavior and Psychological Attributes

Given that social networks may impact health through behavioral and psychological pathways (Berkman & Glass 2000), we further explore the associations of network types and sources of intimacy with health practice and several psychological characteristics. Results in Table 6 demonstrate that socially integrated elders are more likely to do regular exercises, more optimistic, and less likely to feel lonely and useless as compared to those who are isolated or whose networks are family-oriented. However, socially integrated elders are more likely to smoke and drink alcohol, possibly because of Chinese social-interaction culture. Those who have friends/neighbors as the source of intimacy are more likely to exercise regularly and be optimistic, while they are less likely to feel lonely and useless as compared to those who have nobody to talk to.

Table 6. Associations of network types and source of intimacy with health behaviors and psychological attitudes among elders aged 65 and older, the CLHLS 2002

	Health practice			Psychological characteristics		
	Smoking	Drinking	Exercising	Optimistic	Lonely	Useless
Network type						
Isolated (reference)	1.00	1.00	1.00	1.00	1.00	1.00
Children-visiting only	0.90	1.07	1.70**	1.24+	0.42***	0.69*
Family coresidence only	1.08	0.87	1.18	0.96	0.47***	0.68*
Family coresidence plus children-visiting only	0.93	0.96	1.33+	1.28+	0.39***	0.63**
Social connection only	1.78**	1.42	2.44***	1.33	0.60**	0.61*
Social connection plus children-visiting	1.29	1.35+	2.83***	1.91***	0.30***	0.41***
Social connection plus family coresidence	1.45+	1.52*	3.07***	1.90***	0.27***	0.48***
Social connection plus family coresidence & children visiting	1.14	1.32+	3.16***	2.32***	0.25***	0.41***
-LL	6143.0	6963.7	7753.6	8599.4	9314.8	8813.8
rho	0.07***	0.10***	0.24***	0.12***	0.10***	0.15***
Source of intimacy						
Nobody/social service provider/matron (reference)	1.00	1.00	1.00	1.00	1.00	1.00
Spouse	0.93	1.23*	2.21***	2.77***	0.20***	0.48***
Children or family members	0.88	1.16+	1.88***	2.43***	0.44***	0.52***
Friends/neighbors	1.14	1.33**	3.19***	2.74***	0.42***	0.53***
-LL	6154.9	6980.5	7804.9	8580.0	9204.5	8841.8
rho	0.06***	0.10***	0.24***	0.11***	0.10***	0.14***

Note: (1) Intimacy is measured by the daily most frequent talking-person. (2) The numbers in the table are odds ratios adjusted community-level factors and individual demographics and SES. The odds ratios of all covariates are not presented in the table but are available upon request. (3) +, $p<0.1$; *, $p<0.05$; **, $p<0.01$; ***, $p<0.001$.

Factors Associated with Network Type and Source of Intimacy

As indicated in the literature, there is some evidence that both individual and community characteristics are associated with the structure of social networks. We examined how each of these major characteristics is related to one's network type and source of intimacy. Table 7 reports odds ratios from multinomial logistic regression showing the effect of various factors on network type (family-oriented, socially integrated, and isolated). Several patterns are noteworthy. Age increases the likelihood of having a family-oriented network, and decreases the likelihood of having a socially integrated network. Urban seniors are more likely to have socially integrated network types and less likely to have family-oriented types as compared to rural seniors. As compared to old women, old men are less likely to be socially isolated, but are more likely to have family-oriented or socially integrated networks. The high possibility of having a socially integrated network among old men is due to their higher SES in adulthood (see Model IV). There is no difference between Han and non-Han ethnicities. Higher childhood SES is related to socially integrated networks, but such effects are largely offset by adulthood SES. Higher adulthood SES increases the likelihood of having a socially integrated network. Finally, higher community per capita GDP of a community increases the chance of social contacts for its senior residents, whereas urbanization reduces such a possibility.

Table 7. Factors associated with types of social network among the elders aged 65 and older, the CLHLS 2002

	Model I	Model II	Model III	Model IV
Family-oriented VS isolated				
Age	1.02**	1.02**	1.02**	1.02**
Men (women)	1.27*	1.27*	1.27*	1.32*
Urban (rural)	0.73**	0.68**	0.67**	0.73*
Han ethnicity (non-Han)	0.72	0.69	0.70	0.67
Born in urban (no)			1.11	1.16
Father's job was white-collar (no)			0.82	0.92
1+ years of schooling (no)				0.96
White-collar job (no)				0.78
Good family economic condition				0.40***
Per capita GDP (in 1000 *RMB*)		1.01	1.01	1.00
% of urban population		1.01+	1.01+	1.01+
Socially integrated VS isolated				
Age	0.94***	0.94***	0.94***	0.94***
Men (women)	1.17**	1.17**	1.17**	0.92
Urban (rural)	1.45***	1.44***	1.36***	1.24***
Han ethnicity (non-Han)	1.14	1.10	1.10	1.12
Born in urban (no)			1.30***	1.18*
Father's job was white-collar (no)			1.25*	0.96
1+ years of schooling (no)				1.37***
White-collar job (no)				1.84***
Good family economic condition				1.45***
Per capita GDP (in 1000 *RMB*)		1.06***	1.07***	1.07***
% of urban population		0.99*	0.99*	0.99*
-LL	27326.7	27381.7	27375.9	27070.1

Note: (1) The numbers in the table are odds ratios. Category of a variable in the parentheses is the reference. (2) Model I includes demographics. Model II adds community SES into Model I. Model

III additionally controls for childhood SES, and Model IV further controls for adulthood SES. (3) +, p<0.1; *, p<0.05; **, p<0.01; ***, p<0.001.

Table 8 similarly presents the effect of individual and community characteristics on source of intimacy. Likewise, several clear patterns are evident. First, age decreases the likelihood of having a spouse, friend/neighbor, or child as the source of intimacy. Urban seniors are less likely to have a child/family member or friend/neighbor as the source of intimacy as compared rural elders. As compared to old women, old men are more likely to have a spouse or friend/neighbor as the source of intimacy and less likely to have a child/family member as the source of intimacy. No difference is found between Han and non-Han ethnicities. Similar to current residential status, being born in an urban area reduces the likelihood of having a friend/neighbor, or child/family member as the source of intimacy. Elders who had a white-collar job are less likely to have a friend/neighbor or child as the source of intimacy. Better family economic condition increases the likelihood of having a spouse or child as the source of intimacy. Education has no significant effects on source of intimacy. Finally, community per capita GDP has no effect on the source of intimacy, but urbanization slightly reduces the likelihood of having a child or friend/neighbor as the source of intimacy.

Table 8. Factors associated with source of intimacy of social network among the elders aged 65 and older, the CLHLS 2002

	Model I	Model II	Model III	Model IV
Spouse VS nobody/social service providers/matron				
Age	0.87***	0.87***	0.87***	0.87***
Men (women)	3.74***	3.75***	3.75***	3.47***
Urban (rural)	0.99	1.01	1.01	0.94
Han ethnicity (non-Han)	1.52+	1.54+	1.53+	1.54+
Born in urban (no)			0.96	0.94
Father's job was white-collar (no)			0.99	0.92
1+ years of schooling (no)				1.07
White-collar job (no)				1.12
Good family economic condition				1.41**
Per capita GDP (in 1000 *RMB*)		1.02	1.02	1.02
% of urban population		1.00	1.00	1.00
Children/family member VS nobody/social service providers/matron				
Age	0.99***	0.99***	0.99***	0.98***
Men (women)	0.69***	0.69***	0.69***	0.71***
Urban (rural)	0.80**	0.80*	0.88+	0.87+
Han ethnicity (non-Han)	0.97	0.99	0.99	1.00
Born in urban (no)			0.81*	0.82
Father's job was white-collar (no)			0.91	1.02
1+ years of schooling (no)				1.00
White-collar job (no)				0.61**
Good family economic condition				1.42***

Table 8. Continued.

	Model I	Model II	Model III	Model IV
Per capita GDP (in 1000 *RMB*)		1.02	1.02	1.02
% of urban population		0.99**	0.99**	0.99**
Friends/neighbors VS nobody/social service providers/matron				
Age	0.92***	0.93***	0.93***	0.93***
Men (women)	1.30***	1.31***	1.31***	1.31**
Urban (rural)	0.80**	0.85*	0.90	0.89
Han ethnicity (non-Han)	0.97	1.00	0.99	1.00
Born in urban (no)			0.80*	0.81*
Father's job was white-collar (no)			0.95	1.03
1+ years of schooling (no)				1.05
White-collar job (no)				0.75*
Good family economic condition				1.06
Per capita GDP (in 1000 *RMB*)		1.02	1.02	1.02
% of urban population		0.99***	0.99***	0.99***
-LL	34064.3	34112.7	34129.3	33884.5

Note: (1) Intimacy is measured by the daily most frequently talking to person. (2) The numbers in the table are odds ratios. Category of a variable in the parentheses is the reference. (3) Model I includes demographics. Model II adds community SES into Model I. Model III additionally controls for childhood SES, and Model IV further controls for adult SES. (4) +, p<0.1; *, p<0.05; **, p<0.01; ***, p<0.001.

DISCUSSION

Drawing from the world's largest aging population, we analyzed data from a nationwide longitudinal survey in China, a developing country with a unique culture and institutional arrangement, to investigate the short-term effects of social network types and source of intimacy on subsequent health status and survival at old ages. We also analyzed individual and community factors that affect the social network itself. To our knowledge, this study is the first to use nationally representative data to examine such effects under a multilevel context in China. Building on previous work concerning social networks and health outcomes, our empirical results show that type of social network and source of intimacy determine subsequent health conditions and survivorship independent of individual sociodemographic characteristics. As illustrated by our study, the relationships reported in developed countries hold well in China. Based on the uniqueness of Chinese population, institutions, socioeconomics and culture, such a result greatly expands the validity of previous knowledge on the relationship between social network and health.

Our study indicates that socially integrated network types are more likely to provide substantial protection against poor health and mortality among the Chinese elderly population, even at oldest-old ages. This suggests that social integration is a very important factor in determining healthy longevity. On the other hand, we find that isolation increased risk of morbidity and mortality. These findings support previous work from developed countries (Giles et al. 2005; Litwin 2001), and extend some local findings in China (Liu, Liang, & Gu 1995). Social integration has been shown to promote healthy behavior (Uchino

2004), psychological well-being (McAuley 1993), and metabolism and immune function (Seeman & Crimmins 2001), which enables elders to maintain good health. Isolation may disconnect elders from social support (LaVeist et al. 1997), which expedites the rate of aging and deregulates the immune mechanism, thus producing deleterious effects on health (Berkman et al. 2000; Cohen et al. 1997).

One unexpected but interesting finding is that those who have family-oriented network types are disadvantaged in subsequent three-year survival. There are many possible reasons for this finding. First, every relation embedded in a social network involves costs and benefits (Bosworth & Schaie 1997), and relational strain from conflicts and excessive demands is very common (Due et al. 1999). One study shows that approximately 10-25% of Danish elders have conflicts with family and 20-35% have conflicts with partners (Due et al. 1999). Similar patterns are also found regarding intergenerational conflicts among Chinese coresiding families, especially between daughter-in-law and mother-in-law, which is mainly due to a reduction of parents' power and prestige in decision making within the family and empowerment of young women (Pearson et al. 2002; Zheng & Lin 1994). Second, the elders have to face or bear inescapable family conflicts since it is difficult to voluntarily leave family-centered social networks, while it is relatively easy to get rid of non-family-centered relations and elderly people may have abandoned contact with conflicts over the years (Due et al. 1999).Third, as evidenced in the literature (Freeman & Ruan 1997), most Chinese seek emotional support from friends or neighbors rather than family due to a paternalistic and hierarchical nature. This implies that the exclusively family-oriented network might be the poorest vehicle for transmitting social support. Fourth, elders who live alone might be robust due to earlier mortality selection, and a greater proportion of them may have genes favorable to longevity. This may make them more advantageous in comparison to elders with an exclusively family-oriented network. It is possible that those who have an exclusively family-oriented network may have a higher proportion of introvert-personality, which may negatively affect healthy longevity. We encourage additional research to validate these explanations.

Our results further reveal that those who have friends/neighbors (namely non-family ties) as the source of intimacy are most advantaged in health and survival among the Chinese elderly, indicating that friends convey more benefits than family members to health and survivorship at old ages in China. This is in accordance with some previous findings from Western elderly populations, where friends or neighbors are found to be more helpful in emotional support, companionship, and daily activities, and shed more influence on one's health behaviors such as smoking, alcohol consumption, and exercise (e.g., Giles et al. 2005; Litwin 2001). Some studies further suggest that lack of supportive family resources can be mitigated by converting close friends into semi-family ties among old people (MacRae 1992; Lang, Staudinger, & Carstensen 1998). The protective effect of friends and neighbors might also be due to the fact that, unlike family/kin, contact with friends/neighbors usually entails no obligations. One recent comparative study reports that the unique social organizational and control system in mainland China makes it relatively easy for people lacking kin resources to strengthen supportive ties through workplace ties and neighboring relations, while this is less likely in Westernized Hong Kong (Lee, Ruan, & Lai 2005).

Our findings may support the socioemotional selectivity hypothesis, which argues that with increasing age, one's social choices are likely to become more selective as a means of emotional regulation (Carstensen, Fung, & Charles 2003). Our findings also provide additional evidence in support of the potential compensation mechanism in the absence of normative family resources (Lang 2001). All of this, of course, does not underrate the importance of family support in old age. A great deal of research has found that the family is the principal provider of healthcare when needed (López García et al. 2005; Kawachi & Berkman 2001; Seeman, Bruce, & McAvey 1996).

The protective effects of socially integrated network types and having friends/neighbors as intimate ties on health and survival are apparent. Yet, it is not the structural characteristics of the network, but rather the functional characteristics (e.g., social support) embedded in the network and many other intermediate factors that drive such benefits to health and survival. Although we are unable to provide a complete and defined answer, we have shown positive associations between socially integrated network types and having close friends/neighbors and good heath behaviors and psychological attitudes.

One issue requires special attention here. The relatively high prevalence of smoking among the socially integrated network types is likely due to the unique culture in China. As noted in literature (e.g., Tu, et al. 2000), smoking is regarded as a form of etiquette in social contact, and even represents success in career and business, and affluence and sophistication. Although this is indeed a negative aspect of social connections, we believe that the overall protective effects of social contact on promotion of other healthy behaviors are much larger than its negative effects, and thus its net effect should be positive. Quantitative analysis in further research will be helpful in evaluating the net effect size of social contact on health behaviors.

We further test how individual demographics, individual SES, and community SES are associated with network types and source of intimacy. Consistent with the literature (Ajrouch, Blandon, & Antonucci 2005; Lang 2000), older people are less likely to have/maintain non-family ties in their social network. This is mainly because decreasing functional capacity with age prohibits some elders from broad social contacts. Given the high mortality of spouses in old age, older elders on average are less likely to have a spouse as an intimate person in their social network.

The finding of gender differentials in network types is in line with studies focusing on both young and old adults (Cheng & Chan 2006; Lee, Ruan, & Lai 2005; Moore 1990). We find that old women are more likely to formulate family-based network types and have children/family members as their intimates, while men often have networks consisting of colleagues and friends. This pattern is largely determined by the gender role. Women are likely to be care providers (Kawachi & Berkman 2001), even among women with a high SES (Moen, Robinson, & Fields 2000). The feminine role is supposed to be more emotion-dependent, whereas the masculine role stresses individuality (Addis & Mahalik 2003; van Emmerik 2006). The finding that spouse is more likely to be a source of intimacy among men than women is associated with the higher level of widowhood among women.

Our results show that, on average, individuals belonging to the lowest social class have a lower degree of social integration, which is consistent with other studies (van Groenou & van Tilburg 2003; Rosengren et al. 1998). Early childhood SES continues to play some role in determining characteristics of social network structure at old ages. This is because one's network at old ages reflects opportunities and choices made earlier in his/her life about development of and maintenance of certain personal ties, which are constrained by SES (van Groenou & van Tilburg 2003). However, one's adult SES had a greater impact on type of network than childhood SES, which provides additional evidence from a developing country to support the finding based on the Netherlands (van Groenou & van Tilburg 2003).

Elders from more economically developed communities are more likely to have socially integrated networks, confirming the previous study in Western society (Thomése & van Tilburg 2000). This finding partly supports the commonly recognized notion that, during the course of economic modernization, family ties are loosened while non-family ties tend to gain importance (Lee, Ruan, & Lai 2005).

Urban elders in our sample are more likely to develop/maintain socially integrated network types, confirming earlier findings from other populations (Fischer 1982; Wenger 1995). However, community-level urbanization tends to reduce such likelihood. These seemingly contradictory results are not unexplainable. On one hand, urban elders are more likely than rural seniors to participate in organized group activities due to their greater organizational access to facilities or resources. On the other hand, people in highly urbanized communities (i.e., more densely populous areas) tend to avoid their neighbors because they do not like strangers nearby (Thomése & van Tilburg 2000). More urbanized communities also attend to have greater population mobility, which may reduce people's social networks within their residing community. Our finding is partly supported by two recent studies. One study on Dutch elders finds a smaller neighboring network among elders in more urbanized communities (Thomése & van Tilburg 2000), while the other finds a smaller network size among elder Americans in socio-economically developed communities (Wen, Cagney, & Christakis 2005). However, more research is required to further articulate the finding at a relatively smaller community level (e.g., town/township).

It is noteworthy to discuss the measurements of social network applied in the present study. Unlike most previous studies using numerous variables with traditional latent class analyses to generate a typology of social networks, we simplify the procedure by depending on several very clear-cut variables that are relevant to networks. We use this method because the traditional latent class models suffer from increasingly noted limitations (Manton et al. 1994). Many variables related to size and quality of ties suffer from recall biases and dynamic changes (Due et al. 1999; Fu 2005). Research has reported that respondents are more likely to report strong ties and tend to neglect weak ties in their social networks. Thus, the reliability of complete network measurement is influenced by data collection techniques, personality, measurement instruments, and network size (see Kogovšek & Ferligoj 2005), which could lead to substantial biases in the estimates (see Kossinets 2006). On the other hand, a global or single-item measurement is far less subject to these interviewer effects and minimizes recall biases (Fu 2005). Some researchers argue that living arrangements and major social contacts are the essential components that constitute social interactions and formulate and maintain personal networks (Fu 2005). Further, unlike the size and frequency of contact in a social network, the source of intimacy is relatively stable at old ages (Due et al. 1999). The above evidence has led us to believe that our classification of social network types directly identified by several clear-cut variables and the intimacy measure captures the major information reflected in the network structure well. Of course, we are fully aware that social network should be seen as a complex phenomenon (Agneessens, Waege, & Lievens 2006) and that differences in measurement of social network and analytical strategies would contribute to disparities in research findings (Litwin 2001). Therefore, further research is clearly warranted to generate different measures of social network structure among the Chinese elderly population to better clarify causal linkages between social networks and health outcomes, and thus to explore the underlying mechanism among that population.

Several limitations in this study deserve additional attention. First, dynamic change in one's social network is very likely, especially at old ages (Monge & Contractor 2003). However, we could not address the effects of network dynamics on health outcomes due to unavailability of data in the CLHLS.

Second, the level of exposure (duration) to the specific type of social network, which is a component of network, has not been studied because of the data availability.

Third, we did not distinguish marital status within each network type given our concerns about small cell size. For the same reason, we did not distinguish the family ties and kinship ties. Thus, we are unable to explore the healthfulness and deleteriousness of each family tie, which would be a research direction in the future.

Fourth, the social support embedded in each type of social network was not quantitatively defined nor examined due to lack of information. It is indeed the function of the network, not the structure, that confers benefit to health and survival (Berkman et al. 2000), and different types of social support have different effects on health and longevity (van Groenou & van Tilburg 2003). Lack of multiple measures of social support may underestimate the effect of each network type on health outcomes, although overestimation cannot be excluded.

Fifth, some personality factors such as coping resources and strategies may mediate the relationship between social networks and social support, and may affect the way of seeking social support (Reich & Zautra 1991). Fortunately, such a bias is likely to be minor among old adults (Lang 2001; Litwin and Landau 2000) and thus we believe omission of personality variables in the models does not cast a substantial bias in the estimates.

Sixth, the definition of community, geographically defined at the county level, is a relatively large unit as compared to neighborhood, blocks, census-track, or small areas that are frequently used in western research. Given the large variation within a county, smaller units of analysis would produce more robust results if the sample in each unit is sufficiently large.

Finally, we are unable to include social capital factors (e.g., individual's organizational membership) to adjust for their effect on healthy longevity. These are important components of social networks that have been associated with health outcomes in recent research (Islam et al 2006). We agree that the inclusion of additional measures would improve our understanding of the mechanisms involved in the relationship between social networks and healthy longevity. Clearly, our preliminary findings deserve further evaluation in future work.

In spite of limitations, the results of the present study have advanced our understanding of the richness and complexity of the effect of social networks on healthy longevity. Those who are living alone, childless, have low lifetime SES, and no social contacts would seem to be principal targets for support provision. Given that China is experiencing rapid population aging and urbanization, reduced household size and caregiving resources, and large-scale social transformation, these findings have significant policy implications for the promotion of successful aging.

ACKNOWLEDGEMENT

The dataset used in this chapter is from the fourth waves of the Chinese Longitudinal Healthy Longevity Survey (CLHLS) in 2005, which was funded by the National Institute on Aging (R01 AG023627-01, PI: Zeng Yi), and the China Natural Science Foundation, China Social Science Foundation, UNFPA, and Hong Kong Research Grant Council. This chapter was reviewed by Prof. Ming Wen at the Department of Sociology, University of Utah and Prof. Zhenmei Zhang at the Department of Sociology, Michigan State University.

REFERENCES

Addis, M.E. & Mahalik, J.R. (2003). Men, masculinity, and the contexts of help seeking. *American Psychologist*, 58(1), 5-14.

Agneessens, F., Waege, H. & Lievens, J. (2006). Diversity in social support by role relations: A typology. *Social Networks,* 28, 427-441.

Ajrouch, K.J., Blandon, A.Y. & Antonucci, T.C. (2005). Social networks among men and women: the effects of age and socioeconomic status. *Journal of Gerontology: Social Sciences*, 60B, 311-317.

Anderson, R.T., Sorlie, P., Backlund, E., Johnson, N., & Kaplan, G. A. (1997). Mortality effects of community socioeconomic status. *Epidemiology*, 8, 42-47.

Antonucci, T.C. (2001). Social relations: an examination of social networks, social support and sense of control. In J. E. Birren (Eds.) *Handbook of the Psychology of Aging* (pp. 427-453), San Diego, CA: Academic Press.

Baltes, M.M. & Carstensen, L.L. (1996). The process of successful aging. *Ageing and Society,* 16, 397-422.

Bassuk, S., Glass, T. & Berkman, L. (1999). Social disengagement, and incidence of cognitive decline in the community dwelling elderly. *Annals of Internal Medicine*, 131, 165-173.

Berkman, L.F. & Glass, T. (2000). Social integration, social networks, social support, and health. In L. F. Berkman & I. Kawachi (Eds.) *Social Epidemiology* (pp.137–173), Oxford: Oxford University Press.

Berkman, L.F., Glass, T., Brissette, I., & Seeman, T. E. (2000). From social integration to health: Durkheim in the new millennium. *Social Science and Medicine*, 51, 843–857.

Bian, Y. (1997) Bring strong tie back in: indirect connection, bridges, and job search in China. *American Sociological Review*, 62(3), 366-85.

Bondevik, M. & Skogstad, A. (1998). The oldest old, ADL, social network, and loneliness. *Western Journal of Nursing Research*, 20(3), 325–343.

Bosworth, H.B. & Schaie, K.W. (1997). The relationship of social environment, social networks, and health outcomes in the Seattle Longitudinal Study: two analytical approaches. *Journal of Gerontology*, 52B, 197-205.

Bowling, A., Grundy, E. & Farquhar, M. (1995). Changes in network composition among the very old living in inner London. *Journal of Cross-Cultural Gerontology*, 10, 331-347.

Burt, R.S. (2001). Structural holes versus network closure as social capital. In N. Lin, K. Cook, & R.S. Burt. (Eds.) *Social Capital* (pp. 31–56), New York: Aldine de Gruyter.

Carstensen, L.L. (1991). Socioemotional selectivity theory: social activity in life-span context. *Annual Review of Gerontology and Geriatrics*, 11, 195-217.

Carstensen, L.L. (1992). Social and emotional patterns in adulthood: support for socioemotional selectivity theory. *Psychology and Aging*, 7(3), 331-338.

Carstensen, L.L., Fung, H.H. & Charles, S. T. (2003). Socioemotional selectivity theory and the regulation of emotion in the second half of life. *Motivation and Emotion*, 27, 103–123.

Castilla, E.J., Hwang, H., Granovetter, E., & Granovetter, M. (2000). Social network in Silicon Valley. In C. M. Lee, W.F. Miller, H. Rowen, & M. Hancock. (Eds.) *The Silicon Valley Edge: A Habitat for Innovation and Entrepreneurship* (pp.218-247). CA: Stanford University Press.

Chandola, T. (2001). The fear of crime and area differences in health. *Health and Place*, 7, 105-116.

Chen, J. & Wu, Z. (2008). Gender differences in the effects of self-rated health status on mortality among the oldest-old in China. In Y. Zeng, D. L. Poston, D.A. Vlosky, & D. Gu. (Eds.). *Healthy Longevity in China: Demographic, Socioeconomic, and Psychological Dimensions*(pp.397-418). Dordrecht, The Netherlands: Springer Publisher.

Cheng, S.T. & Chan, A.C.M. (2006). Relationship with others and life satis faction in later life: do gender and widowhood make a difference? *Journal of Gerotology: Psychological Science*, 61B (1), 46-53.

Clark, M.S. & Reis, H.T. (1988). Interpersonal processes in close relationships. A*nnual Review of Psychology*, 39, 609-672.

Cohen, S., Doyle, W.J., Skoner, D.P., Rabin, B. S., & Gwaltney Jr, J. M. (1997). Social ties and susceptibility to the common cold. *Journal of American Medical Association*, 277, 1940-1944.

Crimmins, E.M., Hayward, M.D. & Saito, Y. (1996). Differentials in active life expectancy in the older population of the United States. *Journal of Gerontology: Social Sciences*, 51B(3), S111-S120.

Due, P., Holstein, B., Lund, R., Modvig, J., & Avlund, K. (1999). Social relations: network, support and relational strain. *Social Science and Medicine*, 48, 661-673.

Fei, X.T. (1948). *Rural China*. Shanghai: Observer. (in Chinese)

Ferraro, K.F., Farmer, M.M. & Wybraniec, J. (1997). Health trajectories: long-term dynamics among black and white adults. *Journal of Health and Social Behavior*, 38, 38-54.

Fischer, C.S. (1982). *To Dwell among Friends: Personal Networks in Town and City*. Chicago: University of Chicago Press.

Fischer, C.S. & Shavit, Y. (1995). National differences in network density: Israel and the United States. *Social Networks*, 17(2), 129–145.

Folstein, M.F., Folstein, S.E. & McHugh, P. R. (1975). Mini-mental state: a practical method for grading the cognitive state of patients for the clinician. *Journal of Psychiatric Research*, 12, 189-198.

Freeman, L.C. & Ruan, D. (1997). An international comparative study of interpersonal behavior and role relationships. *L'Ann'ee Sociologique*, 47, 89-115.

Fu, Y. (2005). Measuring personal networks with daily contacts: a single-item survey question and the contact diary. *Social Networks*, 27, 169-186.

Giles, L.C., Glonek, G.F.V., Luszcz, M.A., & Andrews, G. R. (2005). Effect of social networks on 10 year survival in very old Australians: the Australian longitudinal study of aging. *Journal of Epidemiology and Community Health*, 59, 574–579.

Glass, T.A. & Maddox, G.L. (1992). The quality and quantity of social support: stroke recovery as psycho-social transition. *Social Science and Medicine*, 34, 1249-1261.

Goggins, W.B., Woo, J., Sham, A., & Ho, S. C. (2005). Frailty index as a measure of biological age in a Chinese population. *Journal of Gerontology: Biological Sciences and Medical Sciences*, 60A, M1046-1051.

Grossetti, M. (2007). Are French networks different? *Social Networks*, 29, 391-404.

Gu, D. (2008a). General data assessment of the Chinese Longitudinal Healthy Longevity Survey in 2002. In Y. Zeng, D. L. Poston, D.A. Vlosky, & D. Gu. (Eds.). *Healthy Longevity in China: Demographic, Socioeconomic, and Psychological Dimensions* (pp.39-59). Dordrecht, The Netherlands: Springer Publisher.

Gu, D. (2008b). *Data Assessment for the 2005 Wave in the CLHLS*. The CLHLS technical report No.2007-01. Center for the Study of Aging and Human Development, Duke University, Durham, NC, USA. http://www.geri.duke.edu/china_study

Gu, D. & Dupre, M.E. (2008). Assessment of reliability of mortality and morbidity in the 1998-2002 CLHLS waves. In Y. Zeng, D. L. Poston, D.A. Vlosky, & D. Gu. (Eds.). *Healthy Longevity in China: Demographic, Socioeconomic, and Psychological Dimensions* (pp.99-115). Dordrecht, The Netherlands: Springer Publisher.

Gu, D., Zeng, Y, Liu, Y., & Zeng, X. (2007). Frailty index and their associations with mortality among the Chinese elderly. *Population Research*, 5, 35-41. (in Chinese).

Hale, C.J., Hannum, J.W. & Espelage, D.L. (2005). Social support and physical health: the importance of belonging. *Journal of American College Health*, 53(6), 276-284.

Harvey, D.M., Curry, C.J. & Bray, J.H. (1991). Individuation and intimacy in intergenerational relationships and health: Patters across two generations. *Journal of Family Psychology*, 5(2), 204-236.

Hays, R.B. & Oxley, D. (1986). Social network development and functioning during a life transition. *Journal of Personality and Social Psychology,* 50, 305-313.

Hill, T.D., Ross, C.E. & Angel, R.J. (2005). Neighborhood disorder, psychophysiological distress, and health. *Journal of Health and Social Behavior*, 46, 170-186.

Hobfoll, S.E. (1985). Limitations of social support in the stress process. In I. G. Sarason & B. R. Sarason (Eds.), *Socialsupport: Theory, Research and Application* (pp. 391-414). The Hague, the Netherlands: Martinus Nijhoff.

Hobfoll, S.E., Nadler, A., & Leiberman. J. (1986). Satisfaction with social support during crisis: Intimacy and self-esteem as critical determinants. *Journal of Personality and Social Psychology*, 51(2), 296-304.

House, J.S., Landis, K.R. & Umberson, D. (1988). Social relationships and health. *Science*, 241, 540-545.

House, J.S., Robbins, C. & Meltzner, H.L. (1981). The association of social relationships and activities with mortality: prospective evidence from the Tecumseh Community Health Study. *American Journal of Epidemiology*, 116, 123-140.

Hwang, K.K. (1997-8). Guanxi and Mientze: conflict resolution in Chinese society. *Intercultural Communication Studies*, VII (1), 17-29.

Hwang, K.K. (2000). Chinese relationalism: theoretical construction and methodological considerations. *Journal for the Theory of Social Behavior*, 30, 155-178.

Idler, E.L. & Benyamini, Y. (1997). Self-rated health and mortality: a review of twenty-seven community studies. *Journal of Health and Social Behavior*, 38, 21-37.

Inglehart, R. & Baker, W.E. (2000). Modernization, cultural change, and the persistence of traditional values. *American Sociological Review*, 65, 19–51.

Islam, M.K., Merlo, J. Kawachi, I. Lindström, M., & Gerdtham, U.G. (2006). Social capital and health: does egalitarianism matter? A literature review. *International Journal for Equity in Health*, Vol 5. Article No.3. (online journal)

Jorm, A.F., Henderson, A.S., Kav, D.W.K., & Jacomb, P. A. (1991). Mortality in relation to dementia, depression and social integration in an elderly community sample. *International Journal of Geriatric Psychiatry*, 6, 5–11.

Kahn, R.L. & Antonucci, T.C. (1980). Convoys over the life course: attachment, roles and social support. In: P. B. Baltes, & O.G. Brim. (Eds) *Life-span Development and Behavior* (pp. 254-283). San Diego, CA: Academic Press.

Kang, S.H., Wallace, N.T., Hyun, J.K., et al. (2007). Social networks and their relationship to mental health service use and expenditures among Medicaid beneficiaries. *Psychiatric Services*, 58(5), 689-695.

Kawachi, I. & Berkman, L.F. (2001). Social ties and mental health. *Journal of Urban Health: Bulletin of the New York Academy of Medicine*, 78(3), 458–467.

Kawachi, I. & Berkman, L.F. (2003). *Neighborhoods and Health*. New York: Oxford University Press.

Kelley, J.E., Lumley, M.A., & Leisen, J.C.C. (1997). Health effects of emotional disclosure in rheumatoid arthritis patients. *Health Psychology*, 16, 331-340.

Kogovšek, T., & Ferligoj, A. (2005). Effects on reliability and validity of egocentered network measurements. *Social Networks*, 27, 205–229.

Kossinets, G. (2006). Effects of missing data in social networks. *Social Networks*, 28, 247–268.

Kroenke, C.H., Kubzansky, L.D., Schernhammer, E.S., Holmes, M.D., & Kawachi, I. (2006). Social networks, social support, and survival after breast cancer diagnosis. *Journal of Clinical Oncology*, 24(7), 1105-1111.

Kubzansky, L.D., Berkman, L.F., Glass, T.A., & Seeman, T.E. (1998). Is education attainment associated with shared determinants of health in the elderly? Findings from the MacArthur Studies of Successful Aging. *Psychosomatic Medicine*, 60, 578–585

Lai, G. (2001). Social support networks in urban Shanghai. *Social Networks*, 371, 1–13.

Lang, F.R. (2000). Endings and continuity of social relationship: maximizing intrinsic benefits within personal networks when feeling near to death? *Journal of Social and Personal Relationship*, 17, 157-184.

Lang, F.R. (2001). Regulation of social relationships in later adulthood. *Journal of Gerontology*, 56B (6), 321-326.

Lang, F.R., & Carstensen, L.L. (1994). Close emotional relationship in late life: further support for proactive aging in the social domain. *Psychology and Aging*, 9, 315-324.

Lang, F.R., & Carstensen, L.L. (1998). Social relationships and adaptation in late life. In A. S. Bellack & M. Hersen (Eds.) *Comprehensive Clinical Psychology* (Vol.7, pp. 55-72). Oxford, England: Pergamon.

Lang, F.R., Staudinger, U.M., & Carstensen, L.L. (1998). Perspectives on socioemotional selectivity in late life: how personality and social context do (and do not) make a difference. *Journals of Gerontology: Psychological Science*, 53B, P21–P30.

LaVeist, T.A., Sellers, R.M., Brown, K A.E., & Nickerson, K.J. (1997). Extreme social isolation, use of community-based senior support service, and mortality among African American elderly women. *American Journal of Community Psychology*, 25(5), 721-732.

Lee, R.P.L., Ruan, D. & Lai, G. (2005). Social structure and support networks in Beijing and Hong Kong. *Social Networks*, 27, 249-274.

Levitt, M.J., Weber, R.A. & Guacci, N. (1993). Convoy of social support: an intergenerational analysis. *Psychology and Aging*, 8, 323-326.

Lin, N. (1995). Local market socialism: local corporatism in action in rural China. *Theory and Society*, 24, 301-354.

Lin, N. (2001). Guanxi: a conceptual analysis. In A. So, N. Lin, & D. L. Poston. (Eds.) *The Chinese Triangle of Mainland, Taiwan, and Hong Kong: Comparative Institutional Analysis* (pp. 153-166). Westport, CT: Greenwood.

Litwin, H. (1995). The social networks of elderly immigrants: an analytic typology. *Journal of Aging Studies*, 9(2), 155-174.

Litwin, H. (2001). Social network type and morale in old age. *Gerontologist*, 41, 516–524.

Litwin, H. (2006). Social networks and self-rated health: a cross-cultural examination among old Israelis. *Journal of Aging and Health*, 18(3), 335-358.

Litwin, H. (2007). What really matters in the social network-mortality association? a multivariate examination among older Jewish-Israelis. *European Journal of Ageing*, 4, 71-82.

Litwin, H. & Landau, R. (2000). Social network type and social support among the old-old. *Journal of Aging Studies*, 14(2), 213-228.

Liu, X., Liang, J. & Gu, S. (1995). Flow of social support and health status among older persons in China. *Social Science and Medicine*, 41(8), 1175-1184.

López García, E., Banegas, J.R., Graciani Pérez-Regadera, A., Herruzo Cabrera, R., & Rodríguez-Artalejo, F. (2005). Social network and health-related quality of life in older adults: a population-based study in Spain. *Quality of Life Research*, 14, 511–520.

Luke, D.A. & Harris, J.K. (2007). Network analysis in public health: history, methods and applications. *Annual Review of Public Health*, 28, 69-93.

MacRae, H. (1992). Fictive kin as a component of the social networks of older people. *Research on Aging*, 14(2), 226-247.

Manton, K.G., Woodbury, M.A. & Tolley, H.D. (1994). *Statistical Applications Using Fuzzy Sets*. New York: John Wiley & Sons Inc.

Markus, H. & Kitayama, S. (1991). Culture and the self: Implications for cognition, emotion, and motivation. *Psychological Review*, 98, 224-253.

Mattiasson, A.C. & Hemberg, M. (1998). Intimacy – meeting needs and respecting privacy in the care of elderly people: what is a good moral attitude on the part of the nurse/carer? *Nursing Ethics*, 5, 527-534.

McAuley, E. (1993). Self-efficacy, physical activity, and ageing. In: Kelly, J (Eds.) *Activity and Aging: Staying Involved in Later Life* (pp. 187-206). Newbury Park, CA: Sage.

Mendes de Leon, C.F., Gold, D.T., Glass, T.A., Kaplan, L., & George, L.K. (2001). Disability as a function of social networks and support in elderly African American and whites: the Duke EPSES 1986-1992. *Journal of Gerontology*, 58(3), 179-190.

Mitnitski, A., Song, X., Skoog, I., Broe, G.A., Cox, J.L., Grunfeld, E., & Rockwood, K. (2005). Relative fitness and frailty of elderly men and women in developed countries and their relationship with mortality. *Journal of the American Geriatrics Society*, 35, 2184-2189.

Moen, P., Robinson, J. & Fields, V. (2000). Women's work and caregiving roles: a life course approach. In E. P. Stoller, & R. C. Gibson. (Eds.) *Worlds of Difference* (pp. 165–175). Thousand Oaks: Pine Forge Press.

Monge, P., & Contractor, N. (2003). *Theories of Communication Networks*. New York: Oxford University Press.

Moore, G. (1990). Structure determinants of men's and women's personal networks. *American Sociological Review*, 55, 726-735.

National Bureau of Statistics of China, (2003). *The electric data for the 2000 census* (CD). Beijing: National Bureau of Statistics of China.

Newsom, J.T. & Schulz, R. (1996). Social support as a mediator in the relation between functional status and quality of life in older adults. *Psychology and Aging*, 11(1), 34–44.

Okamoto, K. & Tanaka, Y. (2004) Gender differences in the relationship between social support and subjective health among elderly person in Japan. *Preventive Medicine*, 38, 318-322.

Olsen, O., Iversen, L. & Sabroe, S. (1991). Age and the operationalization of social support. *Social Science and Medicine*, 32(7), 767-771.

Pearson, V., Phillips, M. R., He, F., & Ji, H. (2002). Attempted suicide among young rural women in the People's Republic of China: possibilities for prevention. *Suicide Life-Threatening Behavior*, 32, 359.

Pennebaker, J.W. (1993). Putting stress into words: Health, linguistic, and therapeutic implications. *Behavior Research and Therapy*, 31, 539-548.

Pennebaker, J.W. & Susman, J.R. (1988). Disclosure of traumas and psychosomatic processes. *Social Science and Medicine*, 26, 327-332.

Penninx, B., van Tilburg, T. & Kriegsman, D. (1997). Effects of social support and personal coping resources on mortality in older age: the longitudinal aging study Amsterdam. *American Journal of Epidemiology*, 146, 510–519.

Pilisuk, M., Montgomery, M.B., Parks, S.H., & Acredolo, C. (1993). Locus of control, life stress, and social networks: gender differences in the health status of elderly. *Sex Roles*, 28, 147-166.

Raudenbush, S., Bryke, A. & Cheong, Y.F. (2004). *HLM: Hierarchical Linear and Nonlinear Modeling*. Linvolneoof, IL: Scientific Software International, Inc.

Reich, J.W. & Zautra, A.J. (1991). Experimental and measurement approaches to internal control in at-risk older adults. *Journal of Social Issues*, 47(4), 143-158.

Reis, H.T., Senchak, M. & Solomon, B. (1985). Sex differences in the intimacy of social interaction: further exploration of potential explanations. *Journal of Personality and Social Psychology*, 48, 1204-1217.

Ruberman, W., Weinblatt, E., Goldberg, J.D., & Chaudhary, B.S. (1984). Psychosocial influences on mortality after myocardial infarction. *The New England Journal of Medicine*, 311(9), 552-559.

Robert, S. & House, J. S. (1996). SES differentials in health by age and alternative indicators of SES. *Journal of Aging and Health*, 8, 359-388.

Rosengren, A., Orth-Gomér, K. & Wilhelmsen, L. (1998). Socioeconomic differences in health indices, social networks and mortality among Swedish men: A study of men born in 1933. *Scandinavian Journal of Public Health*, 26(4), 272–280.

Sandtröm, T., Frew, A.J., Svartengren, M., & Viegi, G. (2003). The need for a focus on air pollution research in the elderly. *European Respiratory Journal*, 21, 92S-95S.

Seeman, T.E. (1996). Social ties and health: the benefits of social integration. *Annals of Epidemiology*, 6(5), 442–451.

Seeman, T.E., Berkman, L., Kohout, F., LaCroix, A., Glynn, R., & Blazer, D. (1993). Intercommunity variation in the association between social ties and mortality in the elderly: a comparative analysis of three communities. *Annals of Epidemiology*, 3, 325-335.

Seeman, T.E., Lusignolo, T.M., Albert, M., & Berkman, L. (2001). Social relationships, social support, and patterns of cognitive aging in healthy, high-functioning older adults: MacArthur Studies of Successful Aging. *Health Psychology*, 20(4), 243-255.

Seeman, T.E., Bruce, M.L. & McAvay, G.J. (1996). Social network characteristics and onset of ADL disability: MacArthur Studies of Successful Aging. *Journals of Gerontology Series B: Psychological Sciences and Social Sciences*, 51(4), 191–200.

Seeman, T.E. & Crimmins, E. (2001). Social environment effects on health and aging: integrating Epidemiologic and Demographic approaches and perspectives. *Annals of the New York Academy of Sciences*, 954 (1), 88–117.

Sherbourne, C.D., Meredith, L.S., Rogers, W., & Ware Jr, J. E. (1992). Social support and stressful life events: age difference in their effects on health-related quality of life among the chronically ill. *Quality of Life Research*, 1, 235-246.

Shye, D., Mullooly, J.P., Freeborn, D.K., & Pope, C.R. (1995). Gender difference in the relationship between social network support and mortality: a longitudinal study of an elderly cohort. *Social Science and Medicine*, 41(7), 935-947.

Subramanian, S.V., Kubzansky, L., Berkman, L., Fay, M., & Kawachi, I. 2006). Neighborhood effects on the self-rated health of elders: uncovering the relative importance of structural and service-related neighborhood environments. *Journals of Gerontology: Social Sciences*, 61B, 153-160.

Sugisawa, H., Liang, J. & Liu, X. (1994). Social networks, social support and mortality among older people in Japan. *Journal of Gerontology*, 49(1), 3–13.

Taylor, S.E. & Seeman, T.E. (1999). Psychosocial resources and the SES-health relationship. *Annals of the New York Academic Sciences*, 896(1), 210-225.

Thomése, F. & van Tilburg, T. (2000). Neighboring networks and environmental dependency: differential effects of neighborhood characteristics on the relative size and composition of neighboring networks of older adults in The Netherlands. *Ageing and Society*, 20, 55-78.

Tu, S..P., Walsh, M., Tseng, B., & Thompson, B. (2000). Tobacco use by Chinese-American men: an exploratory study of the factors associated with cigarette use and smoking cessation. *Asian American Pacific Island Journal of Health*, 8(1), 46-57.

Uchino, B.N., Cacioppo, J.T. & Kiecolt-Glaser, J.K. (1996). The relationship between social support and physiological processes: a review with emphasis on underlying mechanisms and implications for health. *Psychological Bulletin*, 119(3), 488–531.

Uchino, B.N. (2004). *Social Support and Physical Health Outcomes: Understanding the Health Consequences of Our Relationships*. New Haven, CT: Yale University Press.

Unger J.B., McAvay, G., Bruce, M. L., Berkman, L., & Seeman, T. (1999). Variations in the impact of social network characteristics on physical functioning in elderly persons:

MacArthur Studies of Successful Aging. *Journals of Gerontology Series B: Psychological Sciences and Social Sciences*, 54B, 245–251.

van Emmerik, I. H. (2006). Gender differences in the creation of different types of social capital: a multilevel study. *Social Networks*, 28, 24-37.

van Groenou, M. I. B., & van Tilburg, T.G. (2003). Network size and support in old age: differentials by socio-economic status in childhood and adulthood. *Ageing & Society*, 23, 625–645.

Vogt, T.M., Mullooly, J.P., Ernst, D., Pope, C.R., & Hollis, J. F. (1992). Social networks as predictors of ischemic heart disease, cancer, stroke and hypertension: incidence, survival and mortality. *Journal of Clinical Epidemiology*, 45(6), 659-666.

Weiss, R.S. (1982). Relationships of social support and psychological well-being. In H. C. Schulberg & M. Killilea (Eds.), *The Modern Practice of Community Mental Health* (pp. 148-162). San Francisco: Jossey-Bass.

Wen, M., Cagney, K.A., & Christakis, N.A. (2005). Effect of specific aspects of community social environment on the mortality of individuals diagnosed with serious illness. *Social Science & Medicine*, 61, 1119-1134.

Wenger, G.C. (1991). A network typology: from theory to practice. *Journal of Aging Studies*, 5, 147–162.

Wenger, G.C. (1995). A comparison of urban with rural support networks: Liverpool and North Wales. *Ageing and Society*, 15, 59–81.

Williams, R.B., Barefoot, J.C., Califf, R.M., et al. (1992). Prognostic importance of social and economic resources among medically treated patients with angiographically documented coronary artery disease. *Journal of American Medical Association*, 267(4), 520-524.

Winship, C. & Radbill, L. (1994). Sampling weights and regression analysis. *Sociological Methods and Research*, 23, 230-257.

Yan, Y. (1996). *The Flow of Gift: Reciprocity and Social Networks in a Chinese Village.* Stanford: Stanford University Press.

Yashin, A.I., Arbeev, K.G., Kulminski, A., Akushevich, I., Akushevich, L, & Ukraintseva, S. V. (2007). Cumulative index of elderly disorders and its dynamic contribution to mortality and longevity. *Rejuvenation Research*, 10(1), 75-86.

Yasuda, N., Zimmerman, S.I., Hawkes, W., Fredman, L., Hebel, J.R., & Magaziner, J. (1997). Relation of social network characteristics to 5-year mortality among young-old versus old-old women in an urban community. *American Journal of Epidemiology*, 145(6), 516-523.

Yeung, D.Y., Fung, H.H. & Lang, F.R. (2007). Gender difference in social network characteristics and psychological well-being among Hong Kong Chinese: the role of future time perspective and adherence to Renqing. *Aging & Mental Health*, 11(1), 45-56.

Yip, W., Subramanian, S.V., Mitchell, A.D., Lee, D.T.S., Wang, J., & Kawachi, I. (2007). Does social capital enhance health and well-being? Evidence from rural China. *Social Science and Medicine*, 64, 35-49.

Zeng, Y. & Gu, D. (2008). Reliability of age reporting among the Chinese oldest-old in the CLHLS data sets. In Y. Zeng, D. L. Poston, D.A. Vlosky, & D. Gu. (Eds.). *Healthy Longevity in China: Demographic, Socioeconomic, and Psychological Dimensions* (pp. 61-78). Dordrecht, The Netherlands: Springer Publisher.

Zeng, Y., Gu, D. & Land, K.C. (2007). The association of childhood socioeconomic conditions with healthy longevity at the oldest-old ages in China. *Demography*, 3, 497-518.

Zeng, Y. & Vaupel, J.W. (2002). Functional capacity and self-evaluation of health and life of the oldest-old in China. *Journal of Social Issues,* 58, 733-748.

Zhang, Z., Gu, D., and Hayward, M. (2008). Early life influences on cognitive impairment among oldest old Chinese. *Journal of Gerontology: Social Sciences*, (in press).

Zheng, Y.P. & Lin, K.M. (1994). A nation-wide study of stressful life events in mainland China. *Psychosomatic Medicine*, 56, 296-305.

Zhu, H. & Xie, Y. (2007). Socioeconomic differentials in mortality among the oldest old in China. *Research on Aging*, 29, 125-143.

Zunzunegui, M.V., Béland, F. & Otero, A. (2001). Support from children, living arrangement, self-rated health and depression of the elderly in Spain. *International Journal of Epidemiology*, 30, 1090-1099.

Zunzunegui, M.V., Koné A., Johri, M., Béland, F., Wolfson, C., & Bergman, H. (2004). Social networks and self-rated health in two French-speaking Canadian community dwelling populations over 65. *Social Science and Medicine*, 58, 2069-2081.

In: Social Sciences in Health Care and Medicine
Editors: J. B. Garner, T. C. Christiansen, pp. 51-84
ISBN: 978-1-60456-286-6

Chapter 2

LONG-TERM CARE NEEDS AND RELATED ISSUES IN CHINA

***Danan Gu*[1] *& Denese Ashbaugh Vlosky*[2]**
Duke University
Louisiana State University

ABSTRACT

Long-term care is receiving increasing attention as population aging increases the demand for long-term care services and boosts the cost of health expenditures. Although China's old age support system has been studied, previous research has insufficiently examined the long-term care system and its related issues.

This chapter systematically evaluates long-term care needs, costs, unmet needs, provisions, finances, and their associated factors among the Chinese elderly population. We mainly use the data from the 2005 wave of the Chinese Longitudinal Healthy Longevity Survey (CLHLS) including 15,593 elders aged 65 and older with over-sampling of the oldest-old to investigate these issues. Additional data were analyzed including a nationwide survey on the elderly and the 2000 census.

We find that about 5-6% (or about 5.7 million) of the Chinese elderly needed long-term care in 2005 if the long-term care need was defined as a status in which a person has been disabled in any of six of activities of daily living for more than ninety days. That figure will reach 27 million in 2050 given the same age-sex-specific prevalence rates. Yearly long-term care expenditures reached 21 billion *Yuan* in 2005, accounting for 2.7% of total health expenditures. The proportion of unmet and undermet needs was nearly 60%. In other words, there were 3.5 million Chinese elders who needed long-term care services but could not access them. This number could climb to 16 million in 2050 given the same age-sex-specific rate.

---

[1] (Corresponding author), 200 Trent Dr. Rm 1506 Busse BLDG, Medical Center, Duke University, Durham, NC 27710, USA, Tel: 1-919-660-7532. Fax: 1-919-668-0453, Email: gudanan@duke.edu, gudanan@yahoo.com.

[2] School of Social Work, Louisiana State University, denese@lsu.edu

Our results revealed that more than 80% of long-term care services were provided by family and more than 50% of costs were paid for by family. Our results further revealed that care needs, costs, unmet and undermet needs, provisions, and sources of payments varied across regions and between urban and rural areas, and that individual socioeconomic status and family/social resources were associated with long-term care needs, provisions, and finances, although such associations did not follow the same patterns across subpopulations. These findings are useful in identifying target populations, assessing the long-term care needed, and initiating appropriate services given that rapid population aging and dramatic social and demographic changes will bring great pressure on and challenges to the long-term care system in China.

Keywords: China, the elderly, old age support, long-term care, long-term care cost, unmet need, human security, demographic security, population security, filial piety, health, mortality.

1. Introduction

Long-term care is receiving increasing attention in Western nations both in the research community and by policymakers as population aging swells the demand for long-term care services and boosts the cost of health expenses. People of any age can experience some degree of functional limitations that would require long-term care in an institution, in a home or residence, or in a community setting. The definition of long-term care has been broadened over time to include all health and health-related services, provided formally or informally, in an institution or at home, to functionally impaired or chronically ill individuals in addition to traditional nursing home care (Schwab et al. 2003). Among various definitions of long-term care (Institute of Medicine 1986; Karlsson et al. 2004; Norton 2000; WHO 2000), WHO's definition is relatively complete and concrete. WHO defines long-term care as a system of activities undertaken by informal caregivers (family, friends, and/or neighbors) and/or professionals (health, social, and others) to ensure that a person who is not fully capable of self-care can maintain the highest possible quality of life, according to his or her individual preferences, with the greatest possible degree of independence, autonomy, participation, personal fulfillment, and human dignity (WHO 2000:6).

Regardless of the definition, there is a consensus on its three major components: Needs assessment, service provision, and financing (Karlson et al. 2004). *Needs* represents the amount of services for people who need assistance in daily-based activities. *Provision* means the individual or entity that provides the services: family, public sector, or private companies, or a combination thereof. Services that are unpaid and provided by the family, friend, or neighbors are normally called informal services, while services that are paid and provided by some commercialized organizations are often called formal services. *Financing* indicates the person or institution that pays for these services: private insurance, out-of pocket payments, taxes or social insurance. In summary, long-term care encompasses a broad range of help with daily activities that disabled individuals need for a prolonged period of time (Stone 2000:2).

There is no gold standard to assess long-term care needs. Measures of long-term care needs vary across studies. The most frequently used measurement in the existing literature is the rate/level/severity of disability in activities of daily living (ADL) and instrumental activities of daily living (e.g., Manton, Gu, & Lamb 2006). For instance, the National Long-term Care Survey (NLTCS) in the United States defines a long-term care need if a person has been disabled in any of the six ADL tasks (eating, dressing, bathing, getting in and out of the bed, inside transferring, and toileting) and any of the eight IADL tasks (walking around, laundry, housekeeping, phone use, meal preparation, shopping, going places outside of walking distance, and managing money) for ninety days or more (Manton, Gu, & Lamb 2006).

These three components of the long-term care system have been widely studied. Data in the United States show that about two-third of elders who need long-term care live in the community, although they are less likely to be severely disabled as compared to the remaining one-third who normally live in nursing homes (Stone 2000). About 15% of ADL impaired elderly people living in the community report that they need help that they do not receive in performing ADL tasks (unmet) or receive less help than necessary (undermet) (Jackson & Doty, 1997; Stone 2000). Both formal and informal long-term care providers are overwhelmingly females and two-third of unpaid informal care are family members-primarily wives and adult daughters (Stone 2000). The average number of hours of caregiving received was 21.6 hours per week in 1994 with 58% receiving less than 24 hours, 10% receiving more than 57 hours, and 15% having needs but never receiving services (Liu, Manton, & Aragon 2000). These numbers slightly declined in 1999 (Gu, Wang, & Zeng 2005). Nearly 60% of long-term care needs are paid by Medicare and Medicaid, and around one-third of long-term care costs are paid by family and the rest by private insurance (Stone 2000).

Numerous studies have also examined the factors that are associated with long-term care needs, unmet and undermet needs, use, provision, costs and financing. For example, data from the U.S. show that age is one of the most important predictors in determining the needs for and the use of long-term care (FIFARS 2004). Elderly women, regardless of their marital status, receive 60% of the hours provided by family that elderly men receive, but no gender difference is observed in receiving social services (Katz, Kabeto, & Langa 2000). African Americans, Hispanics, and Asian Americans receive more family cares but fewer social services than their White counterparts (Chadiha et al. 1995; Mui & Burnette 1994). Number of living children is a primary resource for individuals in maintaining access to informal care, especially for unmarried persons (Jenkins 2001; Soldo, Wolf, & Agree 1990). The availability of an informal family caregiver reduces the cost of formal long-term care (Yoo et al. 2004). Unmarried elders, especially women are more likely to use formal care (Logan & Spitze 1994). Higher income above the mean increases the probability of nursing home use although nursing home use is reduced when income is below the mean (Jenkins 2001; Kemper 1992).

Academic research on long-term care in Western societies has produced useful guidance for policymaking. At least in partial response thereto, Western nations have been undergoing fundamental reforms of their long-term care systems (Gibson, Gregory, & Pandya 2003; Karlsson et al. 2004). Home- and community-based care, residential care, and continuing care retirement communities (CCRCs) have flourished in the U.S. as alternatives to traditional nursing home care to meet financing constraints and to improve quality of care (e.g., individuals' preferences). As a consequence, the use of traditional nursing home care has started to experience a downward trend (Schwab et al. 2003).

However, studies systematically examining China's long-term care and its related issues are relatively rare. Most existing studies are descriptive analyses (e.g., Wu et al. 2005; Zhang

2006) and mainly focus on the current status of and the future trends in the disabled elderly population (e.g., Arnsberger et al. 2000; Liu & Mackellar 2001), their financial supports (e.g., Liu & Mackellar 2001; Wu et al. 2000), the healthcare system (Dong 2003), family care provisions (Li 1999), and institutional care availability (Zhan, Liu, & Bai 2006) and are not addressed in a comprehensive way. Factors that are associated with long-term care needs, provisions, and financing have not been systematically addressed using data from China. In addition, many Chinese studies are confined to local data (e.g., Wu et al. 2005; Hua & Di 2003) and therefore are devoid of detailed nationwide data on long-term care needs and future trends. By taking advantage of the 2005 Chinese Longitudinal Healthy Longevity Survey (CLHLS) with aggregated tabulations from the Sample Survey on the Aged Population in Urban/Rural China in 2000, the 2000 census, and other data sources, we attempt to systematically assess: (1) the needs, unmet and undermet needs, provisions, costs, and financing of long-term care; (2) factors that are associated with long-term care; and (3) future trends and possible challenges in China in the context of human/demographic security. To our knowledge, this is first study to systematically address long-term care needs and related issues in China in a relatively integrated way drawing linkages with demographic and human security issues.

2. Long-Term Care System in China

As a component of the old age support system, long-term care has not received adequate attention in China and accordingly the long-term care system is fragmented or underdeveloped. Collecting data on long-term care needs, provisions, and financing in nationwide surveys is relatively new. So far there is no specific institute or network to conduct assessments for long-term care needs even at the national level, although one local study shows that those elders admitted to institutional care settings are assessed regularly (Wu et al. 2005). Topics such as daily caregiving, medical care provisions and payments, and daily economic supports that are relevant to long-term care are normally addressed under the old age support system. It is difficult to understand China's long-term care system without referring to the old age support system. Therefore, we briefly introduce the old age support system first.

2.1. Old Age Support System

As a tradition of Chinese society, the ethic of filial piety requires children to take care of their aged parents in terms of caregiving, medical care payment, and financial support, which shapes China's old age support system (Ikels 1993). This tradition is connected to the Confucian ideology and is written into the Elders' Protection Law and the Constitution. Normally, sons provide financial support, while daughters-in-law perform daily caregiving (Zhan & Montgomery 2003). Indeed, care provided by children in China today is still primarily practiced and is relied upon as a means of securing old age care (Ikels 1993). According to the CLHLS in 2005, more than 90% of Chinese elders' primary caregivers were spouses or children when they were sick. Social services accounted for less than 10% of care, although this has been growing in recent years (Wu et al. 2005).

Medical care in old ages is covered by a healthcare system with a notable urban and rural geographic disparity. In cities, a healthcare system for employees was implemented in the 1950s, which covered 100% of medical care expenses for almost all urban employees and 50% of the costs for all dependents of beneficiaries (thus this may cover some of the long-term care insurance for the elderly). However, the urban system was reformed in the 1980s (Dong 2003). After healthcare reform, the urban system shifted to cost-sharing and then to combining pooled funds and individual accounts (basic medical insurance system) (Shi 2003). By 2003, the healthcare system only covered 57% of urban residents (Nation Bureau of Statistics of China 2004).

In rural areas before 1979, residents were covered by the cooperative medical scheme (CMS) system, which was financed by the local community. Under this system, the majority of rural residents saw doctors free of charge, and were partly reimbursed for drugs and hospitalizations (Liu, Xu, & Wang 1996). After reform in 1979, the rural cooperative medical system collapsed and shifted to a fee-for-service system, which required a greater number of rural people to pay their own healthcare costs (Shi 1993). Yet, individuals in rural areas often lacked the resources necessary to purchase the same amount of health care previously allowed by the communist system. In response, the number of village health officials decreased by 18 to 33% and the number of hospitals and health care centers in towns and villages decreased significantly from the 1970s thru the 1990s (Lok 1995). The number of hospital beds per thousand persons in the population in rural areas was less than half of that in urban areas in 2004 (Ministry of Health of China 2005). Consequently, individuals in rural areas experienced reduced access to medical care and the proportion of rural residents covered by the CMS dropped from over 85% in 1975 to less than 10% in 1997 (Tomlinson 1997; Wang et al. 2005). In 2002, the Chinese government started to re-establish the CMS system for rural residents and intends to cover all rural residents by 2008. However, the benefits of this new scheme are very limited and only cover severe diseases; thus coverage is not even closely relevant to long-term care needs (Wang, Gu & Dupre 2008). According to the 2002 and 2005 waves of the CLHLS, 35% of urban seniors' medical expenses were paid by the free public medical program, whereas 64% were paid by their children or themselves. The corresponding figures for rural elders were 4% and 94%.

For urban residents, the old age financial support system was primarily covered by a pension system that was initiated at the same time as healthcare was implemented in the 1950s as a part of social security (Sha 2007). Under this pension system, retirees could get a 75-100% of the last basic wage they earned when they were in the labor force (Li 1999). However, urban economic reform in the 1980s required many enterprises to take over the responsibility of paying retirees' pensions, which nearly bankrupted them due to heavy pension liability (Li 1999). Therefore, various reforms were initiated since the 1980s to shift partial liability to workers themselves. In 1997, the Chinese Government instituted a unified old age insurance system for urban workers comprised of a social pool of funds and personal accounts (Gu 2004). After years of great effort and practice, the current Chinese old age framework has taken its initial shape (Sha 2007). However, since the state does not have a sufficient pool of funding, current employees' contributions in personal accounts are used to pay the benefits of the current retirees under the previous pay-as-you-go system, which results in most individual accounts in the current pension system remaining unfunded. Before the

1990, rural residents had to rely solely on family for financial support. Although the Chinese government launched an old age insurance program in the 1990s in which each enrollee could get a subsidy from the government equaling his/her contribution, the coverage and benefits continue to be low.[3]

Currently, while around 50-60% of elders in cities have pension or retirement wages, there is still little or no state support for long-term care expenses of rural elders, who are the majority of the elderly population. The CLHLS data show that more than 90% of rural elders do not have a pension and more than 20% of the sampled elderly do not have sufficient financial resources to pay their daily expenses. Most rural couples still expect their old age security to derive from sons rather than daughters, or in the alternative from extra-familial resources (Croll 2000). However, one recent study shows that daughters are more beneficial than sons as caregivers to elderly parents' healthy longevity (Zeng & Gu 2007). Indeed, in spite of the implementation of the old age insurance program in the 1990s and the new rural cooperative medical scheme since 2002, the coverage and benefits of programs remain at a miminal level (Information Office of the State Council of the People's Republic of China 2004; Wang et al. 2006). This suggests that the rural elderly continue to be almost fully supported by their families. The parent-child relationship (especially with sons) still constitutes the essential bedrock of old age support, which has been attributed as one of the major causes for the rapid unbalanced sex ratio of children by some scholars (Das Gupta et al. 2003; Riley 2004; Thorborg 2005).

At the time the healthcare system was being established in the 1950s, China began to establish elderly homes to house "Three-No" elders (no relative, no income, and no physical ability to work) in each urban residential neighborhood through funding and in-kind contributions from local residential committees and governmental units (Chen 1996). Institutionalized "Three-No" residents are socially disadvantaged and exclusively dependent on meager subsidies from the government or local community. Most "Three-No" elders residing in rural areas were generally cared for by the local village, and either continued to live alone or with a local family. The local governments provide "Five-Guarantee" services (clothing, shelter, medication, food, and funeral) to "Three-No" elders free of charge. Traditionally, except for those "Three-No" elders, institutionalized elders in China were considered abandoned by their children who had not fulfilled their filial obligations (Gu, Dupre, & Liu 2007). Recent data show that the number of urban elders with limited informal caregiving resources who prefer to use institutional care is increasing (Ding and Ye 2001). Currently, approximately 15% of institutionalized residents (roughly 20% urban and 10% rural) are persons not considered as "Three-No" elders (Ministry of Civil Affairs 2005). The cost of admission, boarding, and services are provided free to "Three-No" elders; however, monthly costs for non-"Three-No" elders vary depending upon the services provided and the regional location of the facility. The primary reason for institutionalization in China is mainly due to limited caregiving resources, which is very distinct from that in Western societies where institutionalized elders are normally in extremely poor health. The proportion institutionalized in contemporary China was only around 1-2% for both elders aged 65-79 and the oldest-old aged 80+ according to the latest census (Gu, Dupre, & Liu 2007), compared with 5% and 20% in the United States (FIFARS 2004).

---

[3] Source: Information Office of the State Council of the People's Republic of China, *China's Social Security and Its Policy*, September 2004, Beijing.

In summary, although China today is pragmatic and has adopted flexible approaches with both public and private resources to improve capacity in old age support, the majority of seniors (56% among urban elders and 82% among rural elders) consider children their main source of old age support (CNRCA 2003: 98-99); and much of old age support in terms of primary caregiving, medical care payments, and daily expenses are from family.

2.2. Long-Term Care System

It is clear that the long-term care system in China so far has not yet separated from the historical old age support system, and that the majority of daily care is still provided exclusively by family members. However, the long-term care system is being established and is expanding. Emergence in the 1990s of informal and home- and community-based services such as the service-reserve project, the friends and neighborhood mutual help project, elderly service centers, day care centers, meals on wheels, the elderly hotlines, and volunteers in urban areas have helped those who are in need of long-term care services (Chen, Du, & Chen 2001; Shanghai Civil Affairs 2002). In the service-reserve project, the number of hours of care provided by young or non-disabled elders are reserved or banked and working individuals will receive the same amount of services in the future when they are in need. Social insurance and commercialized insurance programs also increased in the 1990s (Li 1999). Recent research has shown that some organized home- and community-based programs and institutional care facilities are beginning to be established in megacities in China in various forms, such as elderly homes, senior centers, and nursing homes to provide long-term care services (Chen 1996; Ministry of Civil Affairs 2005; Wu et al. 2005; Zhan, Liu, & Bai 2005). At present, formal home- and community-based care and institutional care account for less than 10% of all care provided. Coordination among government agencies involved in providing long-term care is poor (Zhang 2006). Approximately 10% of these formal institutions are privately operated and are typically located in urban areas. Public institutions normally provide better facilities than those privately owned (Zhan et al. 2005), with occupancy rates of around 76% and 63%, respectively (Ministry of Civil Affairs 2005).The professional skills of service personnel both in public and private institutions and the quality of care still need substantial improvements (Wu et al. 2005).

The cost of social services is beyond the affordability of most elders. For example, several studies show that the average monthly cost for institutionalization with limited services was approximately RMB 400–600 *Yuan* (around $50–70) in some major cities in the late 1990s (Liu 2001; Zhang & Lv 2001). That same cost in 2000 would amount to 90% of the yearly retirement wage of an urban elder.[4] This amount was equal to 20–25% of the average employee's wage in major cities in 2005 (National Bureau of Statistics of China 2006). Monthly costs would increase to roughly $200 or more for full (or extra) services (Zhang & Lv 2001).

The role of long-term care financing in determining the use of care services by the elderly and their level of health and well-being, as well as the growth and development of the care

[4] According to the Sample Survey on Aged Population in Urban/Rural China in 2000 by the China National Research Center on Aging (CNRCA), the average retirement wage for urban elders was around RMB 7,980 *Yuan* in 2000 (CNRCA 2003: 85).

sector itself is well understood (Chen 2001). However, China has not developed a system to long-term care financing. Both pension and old age insurance do not cover long-term care for the elderly. Although a few cities (e.g., Shanghai) have initiated a social welfare lottery to pay for home- and community-based long-term care services for "Three-No" elders in poverty, and for those who have made a substantial contribution to society, the coverage is only around 0.1% of total elderly population (Wu & Xu 2007).

In summary, the delineation between old age care and long-term care is difficult to determine. By integrating all fragmented information on long-term care in China, we can conclude that long-term care provisions are dominated by informal family care supplemented by home- and community-based care, institutional care, and private sources in urban areas. Rural areas almost solely rely on family caregivers.

3. Long-Term Care and Associated Factors: Empirical Evidence

3.1. Data Sources and Methods

The data to address the needs, unmet and undermet needs, provisions, costs, financing of long-term care, factors that are associated with long-term care and future trends are primarily drawn from the fourth wave of the Chinese Longitudinal Healthy Longevity Survey (CLHLS) in 2005. The CLHLS was started in 1998 and was conducted in a randomly selected half of the counties/cities in 22 Han-dominated provinces in China. The CLHLS aims to interview all centenarians with informed consent in the sampled counties/cities. For each centenarian with a pre-designated random code, one nearby octogenarian and one nearby nonagenarian with a pre-designated age and sex were interviewed on a random basis with informed consent. The term 'nearby' mainly indicates the same village or the same street if applicable, or the same town, county or city. This special design is intended to ensure comparable numbers of randomly selected male and female octogenarians and nonagenarians at each age from 80 to 99. So far, four waves have been successfully conducted in 1998, 2000, 2002, and 2005. The fifth wave will be conducted in 2008. Starting from the third wave in 2002, the CLHLS expands its coverage to include elders aged 65 to 79. The 2005 wave collected data on 5,047 young seniors aged 65-79 and 10,556 oldest-old aged 80-109 with 3,870 octogenarians, 3,927 nonagenarians and 2,759 centenarians. Out of the total 15,603 interviewees, there are 6,687 (42.9%) men, 8,916 (57.1%) women, 8,637 (55.4 %) rural residents, and 6,966 (44.6%) urban residents.

The 2005 wave collected extensive questionnaire data that had been collected in previous waves comprising demographic, family households, life style, diet, and psychological characteristics, as well as economic resources, family support, self-reported health, self-reported life satisfaction, lower and upper extremities performance, instrumental activities of daily living (IADL), activities of daily (ADL), cognitive functioning, and chronic diseases suffered and their adverse impacts on daily life. In addition, the fourth wave collected relatively detailed data on days of assistance received in each of six ADL tasks (bathing, dressing, indoor transferring, toileting, incontinence, and eating), direct caregiving costs, unmet needs, and the primary caregivers to provide such assistances for the first time. These new data facilitate our research goals for this chapter. Long-term care need was measured by assistance needed in performing any of six ADL tasks. If a respondent needed assistance in performing any of six tasks for more than three-months, it was considered that he/she needed long-term care services (which we coded as 1). Otherwise, he/she was not considered needing long-term care services (which we coded as 0).[5] The question, "Who mainly provides such caregiving?" (spouse, sons, daughters-in-law, daughters, sons-in-law, sons and daughters equally, grandchildren and their spouses, other relatives, neighbors, social services, housekeeper, and nobody) was asked to collect the caregiver information.

Long-term care costs were approximately measured by a single question in the CLHLS questionnaire: "How much is the direct cost for such assistance?" The direct cost only includes out-of-pocket expenditure for informal care and excludes medical expenditures, prescriptions, and the wage loss of the caregiver due to caregiving. To determine the source of those payments the CLHLS also asked "Who mainly pays for the cost?" (self, spouse, children and their spouses, grandchildren and their spouses, the public or collectives, and others).

The unmet and undermet needs were measured by the question, "Does the assistance provided by caregivers meet your needs?" We dichotomized the answer into fully met (code=0) and not fully met (code=1) needs. This measure is based on an individuals' own perceptions of their need for more help, which is a valid indicator of unmet need (Gibson & Verma 2006; Morrow-Howell, Proctor, & Rozario 2001).

All information in the CLHLS has been obtained through in-home interviews. This is the first nation-wide longitudinal survey with such a large sample size of the oldest-old ever conducted in a developing country. The systematic assessments on data quality regarding accuracy of age-reporting, reliability, validity, and the consistency of numerous measures and the randomness of attrition show that the data quality is high in the CLHLS (Gu 2008; Gu & Dupre 2008; Zeng & Gu 2008; Zhang, Gu, Zeng, & Liu 2006).

In addition, we use limited aggregated data relevant to long-term care needs from the Sample Survey on the Aged Population in Urban/Rural China in 2000 by the China National Research Center on Aging (CNRCA) to supplement the CLHLS. Furthermore, will also use population distributions from the 2000 census and the projected elderly population from the United Nations Population Division to estimate current and future numbers of elders in need of long-term care.

Multivariable logistic regressions are employed to investigate the factors associated with long-term care needs, source of payment, and unmet needs in long-term care services. Given the highly skewed distribution and the cost fluctuations, we use a two-stage regression approach to estimate a smoothed age-sex-urban-rural specific average cost in terms of the Chinese currency (*RBM*; 1 US$=7.6 *Yuan)* among those who need long-term care. In the first stage, we code the weekly cost among those who need long-term care into four categories *RMB*: 0, 1-49, 50-149, and 150+ *Yuan*. We then use multivariable multinomial logistic regression to estimate the age-sex-urban/rural specific probability for the use of care needs within each category. In the second stage, we multiply the estimated probability by the observed mean of each category to obtain the estimated age-sex-urban/rural specific average

[5] Given the unavailability of data on days needing assistance for IADLs, we are unable to take IADLs into consideration in constructing the long-term care needs indicator. Therefore, the long-term care need is somewhat underestimated.

weekly long-term care costs. We assume that all other covariates in the model were held at their means in determining the regression-based estimates of the costs. Multinomial logistic regressions are used to explore how factors are associated with different caregivers.

In all regression models, the variables of interest are those that have been found to be associated with long-term care needs, costs, and unmet and undermet needs in previous empirical studies (Finlayson 2002; Liu, Manton, & Aragon 2000; Gibson & Verma 2006). These variables are age, sex, urban/rural residence, ethnicity, socioeconomic status (education, occupation, and economic independence), and social/family support. The social/family support variable contains marital status, number of living children, living arrangement, and whether or not individual received adequate medical care. The health practice variable consists of regular exercise, smoking, and drinking at present. The detailed coding for the covariates is available upon request. All variables of interest are added simultaneously in the model. A variable of region is included in every model to reflect regional variation. This analytical strategy is also in line with the empirical framework that predicts health care utilization and access to long-term services and supports, which results in needing, predisposition (e.g., age, sex), and enabling factors (Andersen 1995).

The largest proportion of missing values is around 3% in this dataset. Thus, we used the mode for categorical variables and mean for continuous variables to impute the missing values. The data in this study are not weighted because the weight in the publicly released CLHLS dataset is simply calculated based on the age-sex-urban/rural residence-specific distribution of the population, which is unable to capture other compositions of the population; and research shows that including variables related to sample selection in analyses produces unbiased coefficients when the weight is not applied (Winship & Radbill 1994). Indeed, the general patterns and conclusions are similar to those based on weighted data. All analyses were performed using Stata version 10.0 (Stata Corp 2007).

3.2. Long-Term Care Needs and Associated Factors

Because we do not have information on days of IADL disability, we have to rely on the number of ADL disabled days. If we use a cut-point of 90 disabled days in any of the six of ADL tasks as a criterion, the 2005 CLHLS data reveal that the prevalence rate of Chinese elders aged 65 and over who need long-term care is 5.5%. Figure 1 presents the observed age-sex-urban/rural residence-specific prevalence rates of long-term care needs from the CLHLS in 2005; and Figure 2 presents the estimated proportion and number of the elderly population needing long-term care in China in 2005 by applying the rates in Figure 1 to the total elderly population of China in 2005. Figure 2 shows that 4.9% of elderly men and 6.1% of elderly women in contemporary China need long-term care services; whereas 7.1% of urban elders and 4.3% rural elders need long-term care services. On average, although the percentage is relatively low as compared with those in the United States, the numbers are relatively large (nearly 6.0 million), close to those in the U.S. (FIFARS 2004).

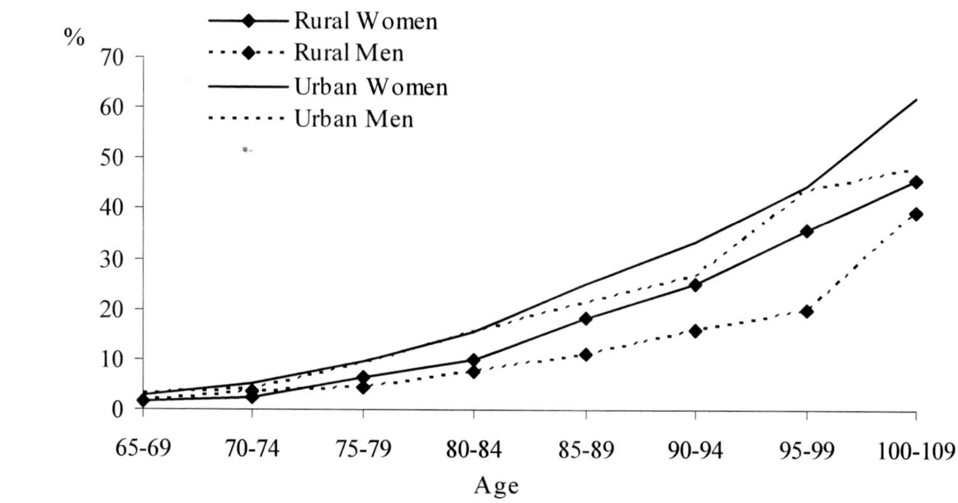

Figure 1. Age-sex-urban/rural-specific prevalence rates of long-term care needs, CLHLS 2005

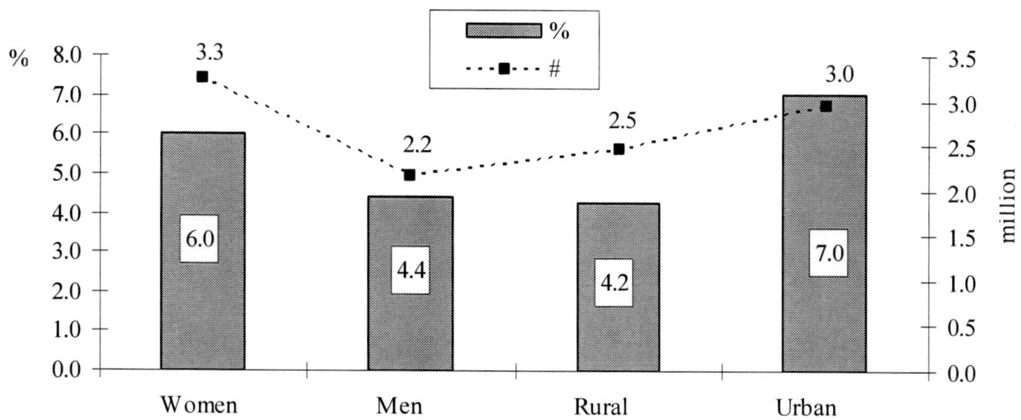

Figure 2. Estimated proportions and numbers of elders who need long-term care in China in 2005

Table 1 presents the factors that are associated with long-term care needs by sex and urban/rural residence. Several important patterns were found. An increase in each additional year of age increases the risk of having long-term care needs by 11%. Men are 35% less likely than women to need long-term care and this gender difference is similar for urban and rural seniors. As compared to rural seniors, urban seniors are 36% more likely to have long-term care needs and this urban/rural difference is similar for men and women. The finding that rural elders have a lower likelihood of long-term care need might be explained by mortality selection and differences in residential facilities and life styles between these two groups (Gu & Zeng 2004; Gu & Xu 2007).

The Han Chinese are more likely than non-Han Chinese to need long-term care. Possible interpretations for this finding include mortality selection and differences in life styles, living environments and/or age exaggeration between these two groups (Gu & Xu 2007:75-76). Education is not significantly associated with needing long-term care. This result is not in line with some findings in the U.S. showing that higher education is associated with low long-term care need (Crimmins, Hayward, & Saito 1996; Land, Guralnik, & Blazer 1994). This is possibly because mortality selection among uneducated elders in China is stronger than among American elders given that sanitation, medical technology, and socioeconomic development is less developed in China. Although economic independence has no impact on long-term care among urban or male elders, it reduces the likelihood of long-term care need by 26% among women and 46% among rural elders. Studies in the U.S. find that higher income reduces long-term care needs (Gornick, Eggers, & Riley 2001; Rautio et al. 2006). Poor elders may not have adequate financial resources to pay for treatment for their disabilities, thus their risk of needing long-term care is increased. Those who had white-collar jobs are 37% more likely to need long-term care as compared to those with non-white collar occupations, which is different from some Western studies find that elders with a higher occupational prestige are less likely to need long-term care (Grundy & Glaser 2000). The lower likelihood of having long-term care needs among Chinese elders with non-white collar occupations could be mainly due to mortality selection (higher mortality earlier in life). Marriage reduces the risk of having long-term care needs by 16%; this effect is more pronounced in women (33%) and in rural seniors (25%). Marriage promotes a healthy lifestyle and emotional support, which may yield physical benefits, which maintains daily functioning (e.g., House, Landis, & Umberson 1988). As compared to living alone, living with family or living in an institution increases the risk of long-term care needs by more than two-times. Having one or more living children increases the likelihood of needing long-term care by 4% for both men and women and for both urban and rural elders. Living with family or having more living children increases the likelihood that children perform daily activities for their elderly parents, which has resulted in the reduced functioning of the elder. Access to free public medical services reduces the likelihood of having long-term care needs (i.e., disability) by 20% and is more pronounced in men. This may be because access to these services improves physiological functioning which helps maintain good health. Regional differences are huge. Compared to North China, all region except Northeast China, have a substantially lower likelihood (OR=0.20-0.50) of having long-term care needs.

3.3. Long-Term Care Service Providers and Associated Factors

As indicated above, the majority (nearly 90%) of caregiving was provided by family members, especially by children. Figure 3 presents the distribution of primary long-term care helpers by current residence. The results in Table 2 are summarized as follows and involve comparisons using the category of 'children as long-term care provider' as the reference group. Men are 55% less likely than elderly women to use social services (versus children) for long-term care, possibly because they are normally cared for by their spouses. Elderly men are 3.6 times more likely than elderly women to have a spouse as a long-term care provider. Urban seniors are 4.1 times as likely as rural seniors to use social services. Elders with higher socioeconomic status (SES) are more likely to use social services as compared to those with lower SES. Lack of family caregiving resources increases the chances of using of social services; and high accessibility to free public medical service also increases the use of social services. These finding are in line with findings in the U.S. showing that age, gender, SES, and care resources are significant predictors of utilization of social services (see Finlayson 2002).

Table 1. Odds ratios of having long-term care need among the Chinese elderly, the 2005 CLHLS

	Total	Women	Men	Rural	Urban
Age	1.11***	1.11***	1.11***	1.10***	1.12***
Men (women)	0.65***	---	---	0.66***	0.63***
Urban (rural)	1.36***	1.33***	1.41***	---	---
Han ethnicity (non-Han)	1.67***	1.90***	1.32	2.13***	1.29
1+ years of schooling (0)	1.03	1.15	0.95	0.99	1.02
Economic independent(no)	0.93	0.74**	1.06	0.54***	1.11
White-collar job (no)	1.37***	1.28*	1.46***	1.54**	1.29***
Currently married (no)	0.84*	0.67***	0.93	0.75**	0.96
Number of living children	1.04***	1.04***	1.04*	1.03	1.05***
Living with family (alone)	2.65***	2.72***	2.50***	3.04***	2.25***
Living in an institution (alone)	2.94***	3.15***	2.71***	2.69***	2.82***
Covered by free public medical services (no)	0.79**	0.84*	0.67**	0.75**	0.86
Northeast China (north)	1.08	1.04	1.17	1.28	1.01
East China (north)	0.39***	0.36***	0.46***	0.42***	0.40***
Center and South China (north)	0.24***	0.23***	0.25***	0.30***	0.19***
West China (north)	0.26***	0.22***	0.35***	0.28***	0.25***
N	15,571	8,905	6,666	8,628	6,943
- Log pseudolikelihood	6295.9***	3980.2***	2297.1***	3207.6***	3064.0***

Note: (1) the category in the parentheses of each variable is the reference group. (2) +, p<0.1; *, p<0.05; **, p<0.01; ***, p<0.001.

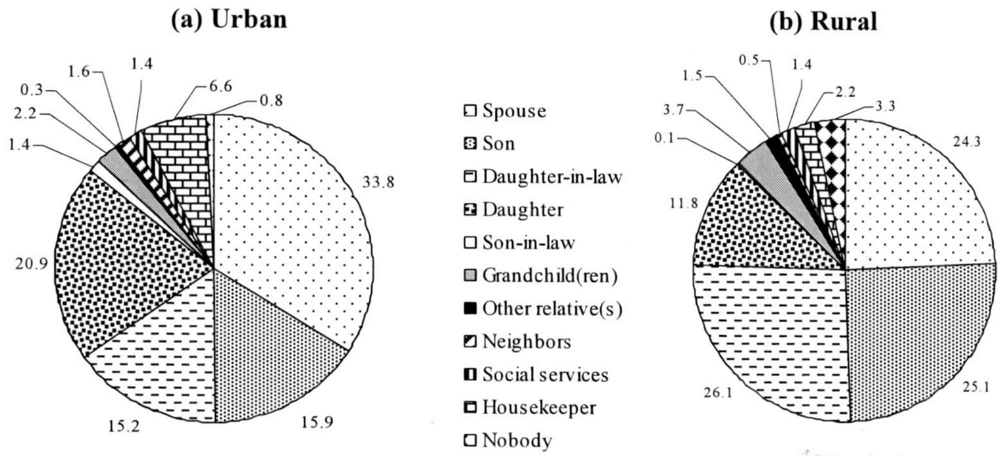

Figure 3. Observed percentage distribution of primary caregivers of the elders when they need long-term care in China by residence, the CLHLS 2005

Geographic differences in long-term care provisions are noteworthy. In the Northeast, elders are less likely to use children as long-term care providers, in comparison to the North. All other regions are similar to the North in that they are more likely to use social services for their long-term care needs. The elders in the Northeast, Central, Southern and Western regions are more likely to use their grandchildren as primary long-term caregivers.

Table 2. Relative risk ratios of having a caregiver among those who have long-term care needs, the 2005 CLHLS

	Spouse VS Children	Grandchildren VS Children	Social Service VS Children
Age	0.94***	1.05***	1.03**
Men (women)	4.03***	0.95	0.44*
Urban (rural)	1.10	1.08	4.14***
Han ethnicity (non-Han)	0.95	0.68+	4.68*
1+ years of schooling (0)	0.64+	0.99	2.67***
Economic independent(no)	1.18	1.34	2.21***
White-collar job (no)	0.95	0.81	1.37
Currently married (no)	---	1.30	1.37
Number of living children	0.96	0.66***	0.95
Living with family (alone)	1.29	0.70	0.15***
Living in an institution (alone)	10.3*	1.07	47.6***
Covered by free public medical services (no)	0.54*	1.00	2.14**
Northeast China (north)	0.49*	1.96*	0.40***
East China (north)	1.20	1.47	1.04
Center and South China (north)	0.91	2.07**	1.19
West China (north)	1.61	1.96*	0.96

Note: (1) The results are based on multinomial logistic regression. N=3,396 and - Log pseudolikelihood=2,304.4 ($p<0.001$). (2) Multinomial logistic regression in STATA produces relative risk ratio instead of odds ratio. (3) the category in the parentheses of each variable is the reference group. (4) +, $p<0.1$; *, $p<0.05$; **, $p<0.01$; ***, $p<0.001$.

3.4. Long-Term Care Costs and Associated Factors

According to the 2005 CLHLS data, the average observed yearly cost of long-term care among those who needed it was RBM 3,606 *Yuan* with 4,815 *Yuan* for urban elders and 2,707 *Yuan* for rural elders. In other words, the yearly long-term care cost could account for 20-30% of their annual incomes if we assume that the annual income of urban elders is 80% of that of current urban workers.[6] Note that such long-term care costs do not include the wage loss of the caregiver due to caregiving, which means that the real cost of long-term care and its

[6] The rate of 80% is estimated based on the survey data of the Sample Survey on the Aged Population in Urban/Rural China in 2000 by the China National Research Center on Aging (CNRCA) and average annual wage of employees in 2000 released by Ministry of Labor and Social Security, PRC (http://www.molss.gov.cn/gb/zwxx/ghytj.htm).

shared percentage of the elder's retirement wage would be even higher. By applying the model-based age-sex-urban /rural-specific schedule to the national population who had long-term care needs, we further estimated the average costs of long-term care per elder among the entire elderly population. The results show that each Chinese elder would spend nearly RBM 190 *Yuan* each year for long-term care services on average. The total long-term care expenditure accounted for about 3-4% of China's national total health expenditure in 2005.[7]

Table 3 further reports the estimated mean cost by age groups, SES factors, family/social supports, and region among those who need long-term care. Excluding young elders, variations in long-term care costs across ages were small; indicating age alone is not a significant predictor of long-term care expenditures among the oldest-old. Although the prevalence rate of long-term care in men is lower as compared to women, the cost of long-term care is higher once they are in need. Long-term care informal expenditures are much higher among urban elders than among rural elders. On average, those with higher SES spent more on long-term care. Married elders and those elders living with family tend to spend less on long-term care. Expectedly, institutionalized elders spent more on long-term care services, and those who are covered by free public medical services spend more on long-term care services as compared to those who are not. Elders in Eastern and Central/Southern China tend to spend more than elders from other regions. These patterns are related to patterns of use of long-term care services as noted above.

Table 3. Estimated yearly cost of long-term care (unit: *Yuan*), the 2005 CLHLS

	Cost		Cost
Age		Primary occupation	
Age 65-79	2,788.6	Non-white collar occupations	3,823.9
Age 80-89	3,967.0	White-collar occupation	2,513.4
Age 90-99	3,583.9	Currently marital status	
Age 100-109	3,464.5	Not married	3,792.5
Gender		Married	2,477.7
Women	3,227.0	Living arrangement	
Men	4,406.8	Living alone	3,482.4
Urban/rural residence		Living with family	3,552.0
Rural elders	3,064.1	Living in an institution	4,281.2
Urban elders	4,017.9	Covered by free public medical services	
Ethnicity		No	3,271.6
Non-Han Chinese	3,031.8	Yes	3,646.9
Han-Chinese	3,666.4	Region	
Years of schooling		North China	2,146.3
0	3,250.0	Northeast China	2,729.8
1+	4,331.5	East China	4,087.0
Economic independence		Center and South China	4,916.3
No	3,551.5	West China	2,107.9
Yes	3,630.6		
		Overall	3,606.0

Note: Numbers are estimated by using a two-step approach based on multinomial logistic regression. Except for overall cost, all estimates by adjusted for other covariates in the table.

[7] According to the CLHLS in 2005, total cost for daily care equals 1.3 times the cost for long-term care. In other words, the total cost of daily caregiving would around for 4-5% of the China's total health expenditure.

3.5. Source of Finance of Long-Term Care and Associated Factors

Figure 4 presents the distribution of the primary source of long-term care payments among those who paid out-of-pocket. At present, around 95% of long-term care expenditures are paid for out-of-pocket. The majority of payers are children, and less than 5% of costs are paid by the state and collectives. However, it is important to point out that since nearly 50% of the sample who received long-term care services did not pay any cost (family members provided the services), the proportion paid by the state and collective is actually much smaller.

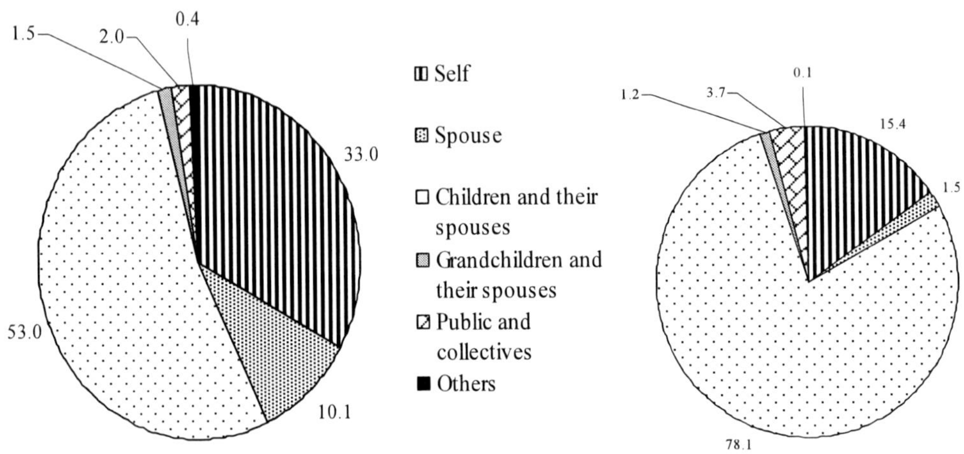

Figure 4. Distribution of primary source of long-term care payment among those who paid out-of-pocket by residence

Table 4 presents the odd ratios for factors that are associated with sources of payment. Except for age, marital status, and living arrangement, which are relevant to family caregiving resources, all other variables are not significantly associated with the source of payment. More family caregiving resource tends to increase the likelihood of long-term care costs paid by family.

Geographic differences are not significant, although the difference in odds is large, possibly because of the small sample size. We encourage further research with larger sample size.

Table 4. Odds ratios of source of long-term care payment, the 2005 CLHLS

	Paid by state/ collectives VS Family
Age	1.03+
Men (women)	1.06
Urban (rural)	0.77
Han ethnicity (non-Han)	0.58
1+ years of schooling (0)	1.34

	Paid by state/ collectives VS Family
Economic independent(no)	1.15
White-collar job (no)	0.74
Currently married (no)	1.88+
Number of living children	0.70+
Living with family (alone)	0.33**
Living in an institution (alone)	2.68*
Covered by free public medical services (no)	0.90
Northeast China (north)	1.38
East China (north)	0.88
Center and South China (north)	0.69
West China (north)	0.41
N	1,696
- Log pseudolikelihood	291.9***

Note: (1) Note: (1) the category in the parentheses of each variable is the reference group. (2) +, p<0.1; *, p<0.05; **, p<0.01; ***, p<0.001.

3.6. Unmet and Undermet Needs and Associated Factors

Unmet and undermet needs occur when long-term care services are unavailable or insufficient (Williams, Lyons, & Rowland 1997). The findings in the U.S. suggest that unmet needs can cause a range of negative consequences that include falling from insufficient human and physical supports, food insecurity, inability to use the toilet, low life satisfaction, or low quality of life (see Gibson & Verma 2006). According to the observed 2005 CLHLS data, nearly 60% of the Chinese elderly could not meet their long-term care needs.[8] No differences across ages and between sexes are found, but rural elders have a higher unmet need rate. Figure 5 reports the estimated number of elders who have unmet needs based on the age-sex-urban/rural residence prevalence rate in the 2005 CLHLS.

Table 5 presents the odds ratios of unmet needs (among those who need long-term care). Controlling for other covariates, both age and sex are not significant predictors of unmet long-term care needs. However, urban elders are 23% less likely to have an unmet need, and those of the Han ethnicity are 32% less likely to have an unmet need. SES variables have no significant relationships to unmet needs. Having more family/social resources reduces the risk of unmet needs, whereas institutionalization increases the risk of unmet needs. For example, each additional living child reduces the risk of having an unmet need by 5%; living with family reduces the risk by 32%; access to healthcare services reduces the risk by 59%. Institutionalization significantly increases the risk of having an unmet need by 91% (1.30/0.68) as compared to those living with family (not shown), although institutionalization is not significant compared to those living alone. These findings are consistent with the findings in the U.S. (see Gibson & Verma 2006; Kennedy 2001; Williams et al. 1997). Geographic variations are substantial except in rural areas. As compared to North China, all

[8] The prevalence of unmet needs among disabled old persons is around 30-40% in the U.S. (Gibson & Verma 2006; Williams et al. 1997).

regions are 60-70% more likely to have unmet needs, except the Northeast which was 23% less likely to have unmet needs. Interestingly, in the United States, regional differences are also associated with unmet and undermet needs (see Gibson & Verma 2006).

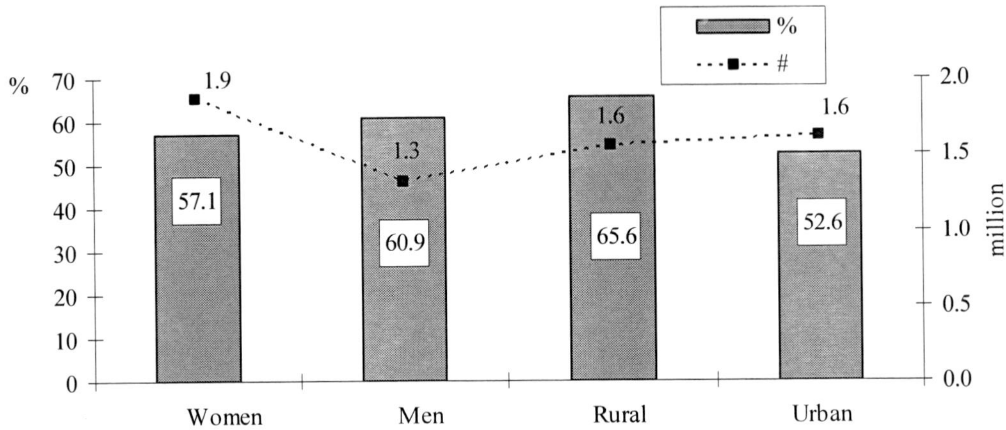

Figure 5. Estimated proportion and number of elders whose long-term care was unmet or undermet in China in 2005

In summary, in accordance with most literature in Western societies, these Chinese data show that predisposition and enabling resources are strongly associated with long-term care needs, service use, source of payment and unmet needs. Geographic differences are substantial. Although an increase in age increases long-term care needs, there is no significant association between age and the use of long-term care, primary source of payment and unmet and undermet needs. Compared to elderly Chinese women, elderly Chinese men have a lower long-term care need, a lower use of social services, and lower spending on long-term care. Elders with higher SES tend to have a higher long-term care need. They are also more likely to use long-term care services. Those living in poor economic conditions are less likely to use social services but they are more likely to experience unmet and undermet needs mainly due to limited resources. Those with limited family caregiving resources are more likely to use social services but are also more likely to have unmet/under needs. These findings are useful for policymakers to identify at-risk older persons who need long-term care.

Table 5. Odds ratios of unmet need, the 2005 CLHLS

	Total	Women	Men	Rural	Urban
Age	1.00	1.00	1.00	1.01	0.99
Men (women)	1.10	---	---	1.29	0.99
Urban (rural)	0.77***	0.79*	0.70*	---	---
Han ethnicity (non-Han)	0.68*	0.56**	1.00	0.66	0.71
1+ years of schooling (0)	1.08	1.05	1.10	0.90	1.19
Economic independent(no)	0.91	1.09	0.83	0.62	1.01
White-collar job (no)	0.96	0.83	1.10	0.88	1.00
Currently married (no)	1.15	0.98	1.22	1.60*	0.92
Number of living children	0.95**	0.94*	0.96	0.95+	0.94*

	Total	Women	Men	Rural	Urban
Living with family (alone)	0.68*	0.54**	1.09	0.62*	0.75
Living in an institution (alone)	1.30	1.24	1.45	0.73	1.68
Covered by free public medical services (no)	0.41***	0.42***	0.40**	0.48***	0.33***
Northeast China (north)	0.78+	0.78	0.75	0.62+	0.83
East China (north)	1.71***	1.73***	1.68*	1.04	2.16***
Center and South China (north)	1.63***	1.57**	1.88*	1.18	1.79**
West China (north)	1.62***	1.79**	1.32	1.11	1.84**
N	3,396	2,377	1,019	1,558	1,834
- Log pseudolikelihood	2186.5***	1527.0***	652.5***	974.0***	1200.1***

Note: (1) the category in the parentheses of each variable is the reference group. (2) +, p<0.1; *, p<0.05; **, p<0.01; ***, p<0.001.

4. Challenges of China's Long-Term Care System

Great challenges are inevitable for China's long-term care system (Wu et al. 2005; Wu & Xu 2007). In addition to the rapid growth of long-term care needs due to population aging, other factors are likely to make unmet and undermet needs worse. For example, there will be fewer family informal caregivers due to reduced fertility, declining family size, and higher mobility. Health care benefits and limited health care financing mechanisms make it impossible to acquire long-term care through other means. Provision networks are not well organized and the current long-term care workforce is inadequately trained.

4.1. Population Aging

Fertility decline and increased longevity in the fourth quarter of the last century have expedited the aging process in China (Gu 2004). The latest population projection released by the United Nations shows that the impending tempo of population aging in China is nearly as rapid as any country in history (UN Population Division 2007). It will be far faster than what was recorded in the more developed regions/countries over the past three decades and is exceeded only by Japan (Zeng & George 2000). While the number of Chinese aged 60 to 79 will grow nearly threefold between 2000 and 2050, the number of elders aged 80 and over will grow more than eightfold. This is the so-called aging of the aged. By 2050, there will be 103 million people aged 80 and over in China, more than there are in the entire world today. According to the UN's latest projection, the proportion of the elderly aged 65 and over will increase from 6.9% in 2000 to 16.2% and 23.7% in 2030 and 2050, respectively, while the proportion of the oldest-old aged 80 and over will climb from 0.9% in 2000 to 2.9% and 7.3% in 2030 and 2050, respectively (UN Population Division 2007).

While none of the aging countries has experienced unusual economic or political instability due to population aging thus far, social security reforms in most developed nations are underway in response to aging demographics. For instance, some European countries have worked to maintain lower ratios of workers to retirees by accepting more immigrants, extending the retirement age, and attracting more women into the workforce (Zoubanov 2000). Japan, while reluctant to accept a large number of immigrants, is adopting several of these options, as well as returning some of the responsibility for elder care to families (Zoubanov 2000). However, unlike most other countries, China's rapid population aging has its own unique characteristics: a high proportion of the oldest-old, a huge base, a high dependency ratio, large regional discrepancies, and an aging population not supported by economic vitality (Gu 2004). Therefore, China will face more constraints and challenges compared to other developed societies.

4.2. Growing Future Long-Term Care Needs

Although it is difficult to calculate future long-term care needs, the substantial recent increases in life expectancy in old age may lead to increasing demands for supportive services and programs for older persons and their family caregivers. The extent of the demand, however, will depend on the outcomes of current and future health promotion program and public health practices and their impact on disability-free life expectancy. Like studies in Western societies, studies from China also show a declining trend in disability among elders since the 1990s. For example, Gu & Zeng (2006) show that the age-specific prevalence rate of ADL disabilities declined by 1% each year from 1992 to 2002 for both elderly men and women. Some scholars argue that patterns of disability change are associated with the disability transition of a society (Myers, Lamb, and Agree 2003). Others argue that the trajectory of disability is determined by the progression of chronic diseases, medical improvements, and individual health practices (Robine & Michel 2004). This suggests that it is relatively difficult to estimate the future correct trajectory of disability, suggesting there is no guarantee that the disability decline trend will continue.

Given such uncertainties, we constructed four scenarios to capture the possible trajectory of long-term care needs in the future years. The first scenario assumes constant needs from 2005 to 2050. The second scenario assumes decreasing needs by 1% each year from 2005 to 2050. The third scenario assumes decreasing needs by 1% each year from 2005 to 2020, remaining constant thereafter. The fourth scenario assumes decreasing needs by 1% from 2005 to 2015 and constant needs from 2015 to 2025, and increasing again by 1% from 2025 to 2050. The age-sex-specific prevalence rate of long-term care need was fitted before it was used in the projection models to smooth minor fluctuations across observed age-specific rates. The 95% confidence interval of each scenario is also applied in projections to capture the stochastic shocks of the observed data. These scenarios and their 95% conference intervals are then incorporated into the population projection scenario that is obtained from the United Nations Population Division. Since the four population projection scenarios (low, medium, high, and constant fertility) available at the UN Population Division website are the same, we have only twelve possible projections for long-term care needs. We assume that these twelve projections capture 95% of all those possible trajectories of future long-term care needs for the Chinese elderly.

Figure 6 presents the projected number of elders who need long-term care under different scenarios with their confidence intervals from 2000 to 2050. Under Scenario One (constant scenario), elders who need long-term care services will climb from 5 million in 2005 to 15 million in 2030, and to 25 million in 2050. The average annual rate of increase is 3.6%, higher than the rate of increase (2.7%) of the entire elderly population in that period. The prevalence rate of long-term care need will climb from 5.5% (3.2%-8.5%) in 2005 to 7.5% (95% CI: 4.6%-11.7%) in 2050. These increases are merely due to changes in the age structure of the elderly population (i.e., elders become older). The situation could be worse under Scenario Four (i.e., a disability increase after 2025) in which the number of future elders needing long-term care services is projected to reach as high as 30 million in 2050, with 18 million and 45 million as its 95% low boundary and upper boundary, respectively. The prevalence rate of needing long-term care services in 2050 will be 8.6% (95% CI: 5.4%-13.5%). In other words, the number of elders needing long-term care will inevitably witness a substantial increase due to population aging unless the disability rate decreases. From these long-term care need projections, we find that the number of elders with unmet and undermet needs will reach 15 million in 2050 under the disability constant scenario and 18 million under the disability increase scenario with a disability increase after 2025. These trends suggest that China will face great challenges in providing further long-term care services and meeting elders' needs.

It is noteworthy that our projected number of disabled elders is only based on the age-sex-specific prevalence rate of disability without considering changes in other covariates such as socioeconomic status, living arrangement, psychosocial factors, access to medical care, and health practices that are associated with disability (Stuck et al. 1999). Indeed, even if it is possible to estimate the number of disabled elders accurately, it would still be insufficient to determine the level of *unmet* long-term care need, because the definition of unmet need contains both health and social components (Arnsberger et al. 2000). Therefore, our projections for long-term care needs are more like approximated estimates for the future trend rather than projections.

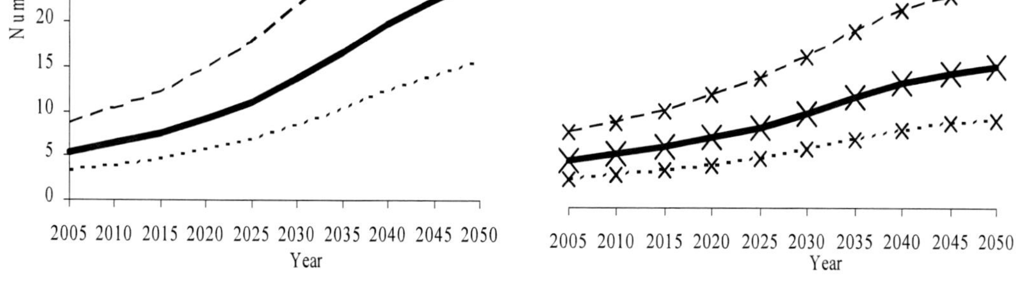

Figure 6. Continued on next page.

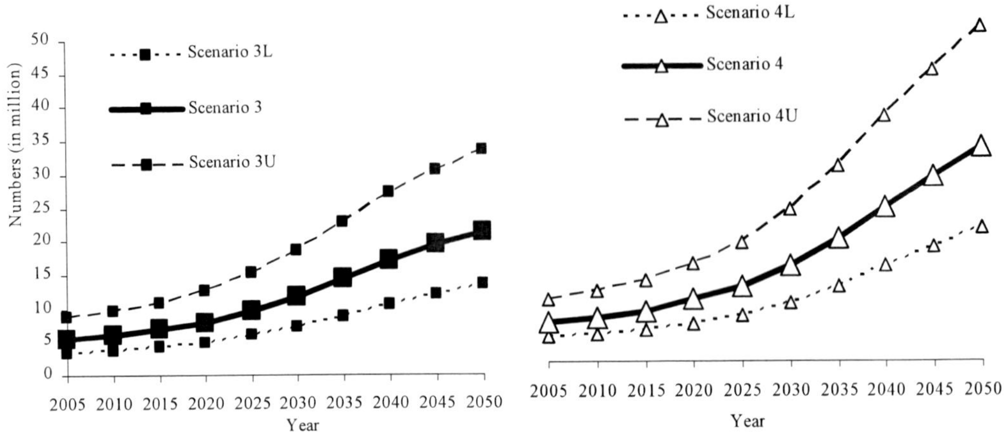

Figure 6. Projected elders who need long-term care services by scenarios and its 95% low and upper confidence intervals, 2005-2050, China

4.3. Insecurity of Economic Status of Future Elders

While projections of future long-term care needs must be used with caution, it is nearly impossible to predict the nature, size, and scope of the future supply of long-term care services. Services will not only depend on demand but upon affordability and willingness to pay. It has been reported that most of today's workers- and hence tomorrow's retirees- do not have sufficient economic resources to cover long-term care, or have no pension or healthcare coverage at all (Jackson & Howe 2004; Takayama 2002). As indicated above, although a unified old age insurance system for urban workers comprised of a social pool of funds and personal accounts has been in practice for more than ten years, the coverage was less than 60% in 2006 (see www.china.com). More importantly, the system suffers from a deficit equaling 10% of benefit costs that must be compensated for by government subsidies (Jackson & Howe 2004). The worst reality perhaps is that there is no pension system or retirement wage for rural seniors. Even though since 2004, rural couples who complied with the government's birth control policy are rewarded with a minimum of 600 Yuan per person per year after age 60 from state government (Information Office of the State Council of the People's Republic of China 2004), this compensation may not be sufficient.

4.4. Increased Health Expenses

Skyrocketing increases in health expenses have lessened long-term care affordability for future elder generations. In 1990, Chinese households paid for just 36% of health-care expenses out-of-pocket, a figure that climbed to 58% in 2002 (Jackson & Howe 2004). According to the Second National Health Service Survey in 1998, 87% of the rural population had no health benefits and paid all medical costs themselves (Ministry of Health of China 1999:18). Currently, only 50% urban elders can access free public medical services; as a result, 3% of this population has purchased commercial medical care. The corresponding numbers for rural elders are 3% and 0.1% (CNRCA 2003: 264-265). As a consequence, when a rural elder is ill his/her family may not be able to pay for needed medications or hospital care and the elder may have to go without treatment. According to the CLHLS in 2002, 65% of the rural elderly aged 65 and over who did not seek medication cited excessive cost and inability to pay as their primary reasons for not seeking treatment. This figure climbed to 80% among low income families. This increasing trend is accompanied by increased fees for formal long-term care services. For example, the monthly cost for hiring someone to cook meals in-home increased from RMB 200 *Yuan* in the early 1990s to 700 *Yuan* in 2005 in Huangzhou City (http://gd.southern.com)[9]. The average monthly expenditure for non-"Three-No" elders in institutional care facilities in Shanghai increased from RBM 2,400 *Yuan* in 1999 to 2,950 *Yuan* in 2002, a yearly increase of nearly 7% (Wang & Sun 2003). These increased expenses have resulted in huge disparities of access to long-term care between the poor and the rich. For the first time since economic reform healthcare has been a more important issue than employment among urban residents (Dong 2003:224).

4.5. Reduced Informal Caregivers

The aforementioned long-term care system problems could be exacerbated by demographic transitions, such as an increase in nuclear families, a reduction in family size due to the delay of marriage and the rising number of single-parent households. Problems may also be aggravated by socioeconomic development which encourages women to transition from the home and caregiving to outside employment (Joseph & Phillips 1999). It is estimated that the average number of children will decline from 3.0 at present to 1.3 in 2025 among urban elderly women and from 3.7 to 2.2 among rural elderly women in the same period (Qiao 2000). Even worse, nearly one-fourth of these older Chinese will have no living son on whom to rely for sustenance (Riley 2004). Meanwhile in the cities, as Western "individualistic" values gain in popularity, urban elders have lost their traditional decision-making power in the family. Multigenerational families, though still the norm, are already less common than a decade ago (Zeng & Wang 2003). The situation in rural areas will be likely further worsened by more rapid population aging due to out-migration (Zeng & George 2000). Further, while it is the son who bears responsibility for caring for his aged parents in Chinese culture, it is the daughter-in-law who actually does the caring. The high abnormal sex ratio at birth (more than 110 male births for every 100 female births) has lasted more than a decade .The missing brides of today will eventually result in the missing caregivers of tomorrow. Family care for elderly people in the future will become increasingly problematic (Zhang 2003).

4.6. Low Development of Home- and Community-Based Services

Although the emergence of home- and community-based long-term care has been a major achievement in urban China, the actual services offered and use have been relatively low. A nationwide administrative network down to the grassroots has been established since the

---

[9] http://gd/southern.com/bysx/bm/20050901001.htm

1950s, yet the network is overwhelmed by regulatory, managerial, organizational, and economic tasks, and thus it is unable to organize or provide the needed social services. In sum, the development of home- and community-based services in China is still in its infancy.

In addition, the family is overloaded with long-term care responsibilities that are imposed on them as the sole source of senior care due to the inadequacy of institutional and residential services. As noted earlier, social services account for less than 10% of all caregiving and unmet and undermet needs are substantial. Further, no formal (coordinated/established) social service referral system (i.e., individuals with chronic disabilities shifting among physicians, hospitals, nursing homes, and their own homes) has been developed in China, which is predominantly due to the underdevelopment of the profession of social work (Chen 1996). The absence of a management information system across times, places, and professions, and a patient database that spans times and places is another obstacle to the integration of acute and long-term care. Payments for these services are increasing and largely come from private and out-of-pocket expenses. Although some government money is available, eligibility is restricted. Some research reports that the role of non-governmental organizations (NGOs) in developing home- and community-based long-term care services is limited (Li 2007).The low development of home- and community-based services is mainly attributed to the paucity of community resources and the absence of major family support services. Even in existing home- and community- care programs, the quality of long-term care services is often problematic (Wu et al. 2005), which is related to the low quality of providers as indicated below. Thus, seniors have been prohibited from obtaining adequate services when they need a higher level or lower level of care, putting them in jeopardy.

4.7. Shortage of Trained Professional and Paraprofessional Providers

One of most neglected barriers in providing long-term care is the lack of a quality team of long-term care providers. Lack of knowledge, information, and training among long-term care providers is common (Wu et al. 2005).

The future demand for, and supply of, paraprofessional long-term care workers should be of major concern to policymakers, providers, and potential consumers. In Western nations, paraprofessional workers provide 80% of the direct care in nursing homes and over 90% of the formal direct services at home (Atchley 1996). According to the Study Group for Nursing Demand of Ministry of Health of China (2003), China has a shortage of more than 200 thousand trained doctors and nurses each year to provide service to older patients.

Other marked issues in the long-term care system in China are the differences in access to facilities and long-term care services between urban and rural residents, across geographic regions, and among elders with different SES. These inequities may get worse when urbanization, migration, and capitalization accelerate in the coming decades.

In summary, unlike some developed nations, China's long-term care system is facing numerous challenges in terms of sustainability of affordability, establishment and improvement of the provision system. These challenges are accompanied by changes in the demographic structure and social norms of the family, and thus are not problems merely rising from the natural aging of the population.

5. Policy Implications

As noted earlier, a number of factors are likely to shape the demand for long-term care: changes in demographics, the health and functional status of future seniors, affordability of care for future seniors, the availability of family and other "informal" caregivers, and the availability of institutional care and home- and community-based services. The most important issues are perhaps how to establish a well-organized service system and how to improve the affordability of services.

5.1. Implementing Old Age Insurance

One major determinant of the market for long-term care is the extent to which future generations of elderly people will be able to afford these services. Therefore, addressing and ensuring elders' financial security would be the first priority in establishing or improving the long-term care system. There has been a consistent effort by the Chinese government since the late 1970s when the family planning program was launched to emphasize that girls can support parents in their old age. For example, one successful family planning program helped families without sons learn to become financially better off. However, such innovative schemes are still very rare. As indicated previously, long-term care expenses in China are mainly covered by medical insurance, retirement income, or family support. Therefore, one possible solution to improve elders' financial capacity would be to pay for their long-term care services and to provide old age insurance for all parents regardless of whether they have sons or daughters. The only important way to correct the growing excess sex ratio and female infant and child deaths is to provide proper social provisions, or the implementation of old age insurance for rural couples, especially for couples without a son. Indeed, we believe that an old age insurance program and thus long-term care system will relieve the fear and anxieties of those with daughters only. It will guarantees an alternative to a son's support, which will eventually remove the excess sex ratio at birth and excessive early female deaths, which in turn will enhance population security, one of the hottest topics in the recent literature (Zheng 2003; Cincotta, Engelman, & Anastasion 2003; Esty et al. 1998; Hudson &d Den Boer 2004).

This is not a sufficient solution, however. As long as daughters continue to be entirely absorbed into their husband's home and cannot contribute to their natal parents' welfare, son preference (and the excess sex ratio and female infant and child deaths) will continue to persist even with elevation of female education and employment opportunities (Das Gupta et al. 2003). The sex ratio at birth is rising in urban areas probably due to excessive old age security concerns. Absence of a system to provide old age security for the parents of female children will lead to social strains or eventually violence (Hejazi & Shum 2002). Therefore, we propose implementation of long-term care insurance in rural China, accompanied by promotion of the of uxorilocal marriage form in which a couple resides with the wife's parents after marriage, if necessary. Actions should be taken to make it socially acceptable for daughters to help their parents and uxorilocal marriage. Actually, a recent empirical study using a Chinese rural county data in Hubei Province where uxorilocal marriage is common supports this proposal (Li, Feldman, & Jin 2004). In addition, according to the CLHLS data, all other conditions being equal, old parents who have living daughter(s) have better health and a higher survivorship than those who do not have living daughter(s) (Zeng & Gu 2007).

5.2. Developing Home- and Community-based Quality Care Programs

Equipped with the above evidence of population aging and reduced informal caregivers, we argue that there will be a shift, to a greater or lesser extent, from family care to home- and community-based care. This shift should not substitute the former with the latter, rather the two forms of care should supplement each other. Home- and community-based care could offer extra opportunities and autonomy for those who prefer to use social services, and the development of such home- and community-based care is also in line with senior preference (Zhang & Wang 2001).

So far, the state has provided guidelines but has not committed to investing a significant amount of resources to welfare delivery at the neighborhood level. Without such an investment, it is unlikely that such a formal social services network would be established. Elders have tremendous variations in service needs. Therefore, an assessment for long-term care needs must be more specific and responsive to the situation of the particular elder and their caregivers by concentrating on the family situation. In formulating comprehensive community care policies, decision makers should take the personal services, income, health care, housing, and other social services available to the family as well as the role of the commercial sectors into consideration. In the meantime, more attention from policymakers is required to ensure that the elderly population receives a high quality of care that is affordable to them and society.

5.3. Developing Respite Care and Continuing Care Retirement Communities

Proving caregiving to elderly parents often has a disruptive impact on family life and on other members of the family. As we will continue to rely on the unpaid informal family caregiver to provide the bulk of long-term care to the elderly, policymakers may pursue modest approaches to support informal care. A respite care program should be promoted to provide support to those family caregivers who are overloaded with long-term care responsibilities. Like in some European countries, governments or employers should pay employees on leave when they are providing long-term care. In the alternative, employers should offer extra subsidies to pay for hired services so that all caregivers can exercise their right to choose employment in addition to fulfilling their family obligations, as proposed by WHO (2004). The role of NGOs in establishing and improving long-term care should be also enhanced. In the housing market, a relevant housing policy should be established to encourage children to live with their old parents, in combination with an effort to improve housing conditions in the community.

Institutional care should be advanced as supplementary care for elders in China to narrow the gap in unmet needs. Multi-functional institutional care facilities such as continuing care retirement communities should be promoted to include various services to meet the differing needs of elderly people. Further, families in service formulation and evaluation should be recognized and emphasized.

5.4. Improving Skills of Providers

The demand for trained professional and paraprofessional long-term care workers will increase dramatically in the future. Therefore, professional training and intervention need to be emphasized. Care management techniques, general medicine, rehabilitation, and community nursing focusing on eldercare need should be disseminated among formal care providers so as to enable them to better provide quality services to each elderly client. Financial incentives and other benefits (including career promotion and housing) should be given to people seeking careers in geriatrics so as to recruit and retain people with quality skills (Fang 2007).

Provisions for specialized training and support for informal caregivers can enhance family solidarity and minimize the vulnerability of older people in need of care, especially in a cultural context like China. Therefore, the develoment and enhancement of existing formal community education institutions, respite care services, and support groups should be used to support informal family caregivers. Policymakers must work with the public and private sectors to offer training to unpaid "informal" caregivers and to individuals with disabilities who want to manage their own care.

5.5. Enhancing Integration and Improving Equitable Access

It is well-recognized that reliance on government subsidies alone will be insufficient to develop and run a long-term care network. Over the past decade, a network of various kinds of gerontological facilities has been gradually developing in urban China but greater coordination is required. Therefore, public funding, sponsorship and general fundraising are being strongly advocated, and private investment in the long-term care market should be encouraged. New policy mandates must be carefully shaped in order to avoid fragmentation of care provisions and to address service gaps. It is important to pursue a national consensus to stimulate collaboration and partnerships between the private and public sectors, and to clarify the roles and responsibilities of the private and public sectors. Another dimension of integration is to establish a complete system including need assessment, process monitoring, and performance evaluation.

Further, China should adopt a strategy in establishing its long-term care system that has been adopted in most of other countries to cover a greater number of its citizens rather than to provide more intensive services for a smaller group. Difficulties in access to long-term care services for elders in low socioeconomic groups, or their exclusion therefrom could result in a crisis or the collapse of the long-term care system. Developing a waiver program for poor elders would be wothwhile. Special programs that are appropriate to rural areas and localities are also warranted. In other words, promoting equity in access to long-term care services and expanding coverage of those services should be one of the most urgent issues with existing resources.

6. CONCLUSION

This chapter provides relatively rich information in formulating strategic plans to meet the mounting challenges of the future of the long-term care system in China. The uniqueness of this chapter lies in the exploration of the key factors that are associated with long-term care needs, service use, care cost, and unmet/under needs and in addressing the future possible trends and challenges of long-term care using nationwide datasets. We find that about 5-6% (or about 5.7 million) of the Chinese elderly needed long-term care in 2005 if need was defined as a status in which a person has been disabled in any of six of activities of daily living for more than ninety days. That figure will reach 27 million in 2050 given the same age-sex-specific prevalence rates. Yearly long-term care expenditures reached 21 billion *Yuan* in 2005, accounting for 2.7% of total health expenditures. The proportion of unmet and undermet needs was nearly 60%. In other words, there were 3.5 million Chinese elders who needed long-term care services but could not access them. This number could climb to 16 million in 2050 given the same age-sex-specific rate. Our results revealed that more than 80% of long-term care services were provided by family and more than 50% of costs were paid for by family. We further find that older age is associated with increased long-term care needs and elderly men have a lower long-term care need, a lower use of social services, and lower spending on long-term care as compared to elderly women. Elders with higher SES tend to have a higher long-term care need and use more long-term care services. Those living in poor economic conditions are less likely to use social services but they are more likely to experience unmet and undermet needs mainly due to limited resources. Those with limited family caregiving resources are more likely to use social services but are also more likely to have unmet/under needs.

Given rapid population aging, reduced family size, lower affordability, increasing medical expenses, and shortage of professional personnel, our findings are useful for policymakers to identify at-risk older persons who need long-term care. In particular, our results/analyses suggest the need to develop or expand home- and community-based care, provide greater support for vulnerable and disadvantaged elders, and provide more financing options for long-term care services, which will not only facilitate the establishment/improvement of the Chinese long-term care system and reduce unmet and undermet needs, but will improve human and demographic security in the future, as well.

ACKNOWLEDGEMENTS

The primary dataset used in this chapter is from the fourth wave of the Chinese Longitudinal Healthy Longevity Survey (CLHLS) in 2005, which was funded by the National Institute on Aging (R01 AG023627-01, PI: Zeng Yi), and the China Natural Science Foundation, China Social Science Foundation, UNFPA, and Hong Kong Research Grant Council. This chapter was reviewed by Prof. Priscilla (Lilly) Allen at Louisiana State University and Prof. Bei Wu at West Virginia University.

REFERENCES

Andersen, R.M. (1995). Revisiting the behavioral model and access to medical care: Does it matter? *Journal of Health and Social Behavior*, 36, 1–10.

Arnsberger, P. Fox, P. Zhang, X., & Gui, S. (2000). Population aging and the need for long-term care: A comparison of the United States and the People's Republic of China. *Journal of Cross-cultural Gerontology*, 15, 207-227.

Atchley, R.C. (1996). *Frontline Workers in Long-term Care: Recruitment, Retention, and Turnover Issues in An Era of Rapid Growth*. Oxford, OH: Scripps Gerontology Center.

Byung-Kwang Yo, BK., Bhattacharya, J., McDonald, K.M., & Garber, A.M. (2004). Impacts of informal caregiver availability on long-term care expenditures in OECD countries. *Health Services Research*, 39(6p2), 1971-1992.

Chadiha, L.A., Proctor, E.K., Morrow-Howell, N., Darkwa, O.K., & Dore, P. (1995). Posthospital home care for African-American and white elderly. *The Gerontologist*, 35, 233–239.

Chen, S. (1996). *Social Policy of the Economic State and Community care in Chinese Culture*. Brookfield, USA: Ashgate Publishing Company.

Chen, G., Du, P. & Chen, Y. (2001). Thoughts on the service reserve project in aged care. *Population and Economics*, 6, 67-73. (in Chinese)

China National Research Center on Aging (CNRCA) (2003). *Data Analysis on the Sampling Survey of the Aged Population in Urban/rural China*. Beijing: Standards Press of China.

Cincotta, R.P., Engelman, R. & Anastasion, D. (2003). *The Security Demographic: Population and Civil Conflict After the Cold War*. Population Action International. http://www.populationaction.org/resources/publications/archive.htm.

Crimmins, E.M., Hayward, M.D. & Saito, Y. (1996). Differentials in active life expectancy in the older population of the United States. *Journal of Gerontology: Social Sciences,* 51B(3), S111-S120.

Croll, E. (2000). *Endangered Daughters Discrimination and Development in Asia*. London: Routledge.

Das Gupta, M., Jiang, Z., Li, B., Xie, Z., Chung, W., & Hwa-Ok, B. (2003). Why is son preference so persistent in East and South Asia? A cross-country study of China, India and the republic of Korea. *The Journal of Development Studies*, 40(2), 153–187.

Ding, Y. & Ye, Z. (2001). Attitudes towards old age care at non-family settings and its associates among urban residents. *Population Journal*, 2, 12-27. (in Chinese).

Dong, W. (2003). Healthcare-financing reforms in transitional society: A Shanghai experience. *Journal of Health, Population, and Nutrition*, 21(3), 223-234.

Esty, D.C., Goldstone, J.A., Gurr, T.G., Harff, B., Levy, M., Dabelko, G.D., Surko, P.T., & Unger, A.N. (1998). *State Failure Task Force Report: Phase II Findings*. Science Applications International Corporation. Mclean, VA.

Fang, Z.Z. (2007). Potential of China in global nurse migration. *Health Service Research*, 42(3p2), 1419-1428.

Federal Interagency Forum on Aging Related Statistics (FIFARS) (2004). *Older Americans 2004: Key Indicators of Well-being*. Federal Interagency Forum on Aging-Related Statistics. Washington, D. C.: U.S. Government Print-Office. November.

Finlayson, M. (2002). Changes predicting long-term care use among the oldest-old. *Gerontologist*, 42, 443–453.

Gibson, M.J., Gregory, S.R. & Pandya, S.M. (2003).*Long-term Care in Developed Nations: A Brief Overview.* American Association of Retirement Persons. Washington, D.C. http://research.aarp.org/health/2003_13_ltc_dv.pdf. Accessed Nov. 11, 2006.

Gibson, M.J., & Verma, S. K. (2006). *Just Getting by: Unmet Need for Personal Assistance Services Among Persons 50 or Older with Disabilities.* American Association of Retirement Persons Public Policy Institute, Washington, D.C.

Gornick, M.E., Eggers, P.W. & Riley, G.F. (2001). Understanding Disparities in the Use of Medicare Services. *Yale Journal of Health Policy, Law and Ethics*, 1, 133-158.

Grundy, E. & Glaser, K. (2000). Socio-demographic Differences in the Onset and Progression of Disability in Early Old Age: A Longitudinal Study. *Age and Ageing*, 29, 149–157.

Gu, D. (2004). Healthy ageing in China: A summary report of the conference on Chinese Healthy Ageing and Socioeconomics: International Perspectives. *Chinese Cross Currents,* 1(4), 97-121.

Gu, D. (2008). General data assessment of the Chinese Longitudinal Healthy Longevity Survey in 2002. In Y. Zeng, D. L. Poston, D.A. Vlosky, & D. Gu. (eds.). *Healthy Longevity in China: Demographic, Socioeconomic, and Psychological Dimensions* (pp.39-59). Dordrecht, The Netherlands: Springer Publisher.

Gu, D., Dupre, M.E. & Liu, G. (2007). Characteristics of the institutionalized and community-residing oldest-old in China. *Social Science & Medicine*, 64, 871-883.

Gu, D. & Dupre, M.E. (2008). Assessment of reliability of mortality and morbidity in the 1998-2002 CLHLS waves. In Y. Zeng, D. L. Poston, D.A. Vlosky, & D. Gu. (eds.). *Healthy Longevity in China: Demographic, Socioeconomic, and Psychological Dimensions* (pp.99-115). Dordrecht, The Netherlands: Springer Publisher.

Gu, D., Wang, Z., & Zeng, Y. (2005). *Care Needs and Costs at the National Level for the United States 1989-1999.* Report No. 5. SBIR Phase I project "Demographic Tool and Database for Household Forecasting". Submitted to the National Institute on Aging. 2005 July. Duke University, Durham, NC. USA.

Gu, D. & Xu, Q. (2007). Socioeconomic effects on dynamics of task-specific ADL functioning at the oldest-old Ages. *Journal of Cross-cultural Gerontology, 27(1),* 61-81.

Gu, D. & Zeng, Y. (2004). Sociodemographic effects on the onset and recovery of ADL disability among Chinese oldest-old. *Demographic Research, 11,* 1-44.

Hejazi, W. & Shum, P. (2002). East Asia's aging populations: Pension reform and its implications. In A.E. Safarian and W. Dobson (Eds). *East Asia in transition: Economic and security challenges*. Toronto: University of Toronto Press.

Hua, F. & Di, X. (2003). Case study: China. In J. Brodsky, J. Habib, & M. Hirschfeld (Eds.). *Long-term care in developing countries: Ten case-studies* (pp25-68). Geneva: World Health Organization.

House, J. S., Landis, K. R. & Umberson, D. (1988). Social relationships and health. *Science,* 241, 540-545.

Hudson, V.W. & Den Boer, A. (2004). Bare Branches: *The security implications of Asia's surplus male population.* Cambridge, MA: MIT Press.

Ikels, C. (1993). Settling accounts: the intergenerational contract in an age of reform. In D. Davis, and S. Harrell (eds.), *Chinese Families in the Post-Mao Era*. Berkeley: University of California Press.

Information Office of the State Council of the People's Republic of China. (2004). *China's Social Security and Its Policy*. Information Office of the State Council of the People's Republic of China, Beijing.

Institute of Medicine (1986), *Improving the Quality of Nursing Homes*. Washington D.C.: National Academy Press.

Jackson, B. & Doty, P. (1997). *Unmet and undermet need for functional assistance among the U.S. disabled elderly*. Paper presented at the annual meeting of the Gerontological Society of America, Cincinnati, OH.

Jackson, R. & Howe, N. (2004). *The Graying of the Middle Kingdom: The Demographics and Economics of Retirements Policy in China*. Center for Strategic & International Studies and Prudential Foundation. http://www.csis.org/media/csis/pubs/grayingkingdom.pdf.

Joseph A.E. & Phillips D.R. (1999). Ageing in rural China: Impacts of increasing diversity in family and community resources. *Journal of Cross-Cultural Gerontology*, 14, 153–168.

Jenkins, C. L. (2001). Resource Effects on Access to Long-term Care for Frail Older People. *Journal of Aging and Social Policy*,13(4), 35-54.

Karlsson, M., Mayhew, L., Plumb, R., & Rickayzen, B. (2004). *An International Comparison of Long-term Care Arrangements*. Department of Economics, European University Institute, Florence, Italy.

Katz, S., Kabeto, J.M. & K.M. Langa. (2000). Gender disparities in receipt of home care of elderly people with disability in the United States. *Journal of the American Medical Association*, 284(23), 3022-3027.

Kemper, P. (1992). The use of formal and informal home care by the disabled elderly. *Health Services Research*, 27, 421-451.

Kennedy, J. (2001). Unmet and undermet need for activities of daily living and instrumental activities of daily living assistance among adults with disabilities: Estimates from the 1994 and 1995 disability follow-sack surveys. *Medical Care*, 39(12), 1305-1312.

Land, K.C., Guralnik, J.M., & Blazer, D.G. (1994). Estimating increment-decrement life tables with multiple covariates from panel Data: The case of active life expectancy. *Demography*, 31(2), 297-319.

Lane, D. (1996). The Gorbachev revolution: The role of the political elite in regime disintegration. *Political Studies*, 44, 4-23.

Li, J. (2007). Non-governmental organization is a crucial component of the socialized elder care system. *Reality Only*, 6, 84-88. (in Chinese)

Li, L. (1999). Family insurance or social insurance options for China's social security reform. *International Journal of Economic Development*, 1(4), 431-450.

Li, S., Feldman, M.W., & Jin, X. (2004). Children, marriage form, and family support for the elderly in contemporary rural China: The case of Songzi. *Research on Aging, 26(3),* 352-384.

Liu, S. & Mackellar, L. (2001). *Key issues of aging and social security in China*. Interim report IR-01-004/January, International Institute for Applied System Analysis. Laxenburg, Austria.

Liu, K., Manton, K.G. & Aragon, C. (2000). Changes in home care use by disabled elderly persons: 1982-1994. *The Journals of Gerontology: Social Sciences*, 55B (4), S245-S253.

Liu, X., Xu, L., & Wang, S. (1996). Reforming China's 50000 township hospitals-effectiveness, challenges and opportunities. *Health Policy*, 38, 13-29.

Logan, J.R. & Spitze, G. (1994). Informal Support and the Use of Formal Services by Older Americans. *Journal of Gerontology: Social Sciences*, 49: S25-S34.

Lok, S.H. (1995). Market Reforms and China's Health Care System. *Social Science and Medicine*, 41(8),1065-1072.

Manton, K.G., Gu, X. & Lamb, V. (2006). Change in Chronic Disability From 1982 to 2004/2005 as Measured by Long-Term Changes in Function and Health in the Elderly Population. *Proceedings of the National Academy of Sciences*, 103(48), 18734-18739.

Ministry of Civil Affairs. (2005). *China Civil Affairs' Statistical Yearbook.* Beijing: China Statistics Press.

Ministry of Health, China. (1999). *The Second National Health Service Survey.* http://www.moh.gov.cn. [accessed on August 15, 2007]

Ministry of Health of China. (2005). *China Health Statistics Yearbook.* http://www.moh.gov.cn. [accessed on August 18, 2007]

Morrow-Howell, N., Proctor, E. & Rozario, P. (2001). How Much Is Enough: Perspectives of Care Recipients and Professionals on the Sufficiency of In-home Care. *The Gerontologist*, 41, 723–732.

Mui, A.C. & Bumette, D. (1994). Long-term Care Services Used by Frail Elders: Is Ethnicity a Factor?" *The Gerontologist* 34, 190-198.

Myers, G.C., Lamb, V.L. & Agree, E.M. (2003). Patterns of Disability Change Associated With the Eepidemiological Transition. In J-M. Robine, C. Jagger, C.D. Mathers, E. M. Crimmins, and R. M. Suzman (Eds.). *Determining Health Expectancies* (Pp. 59-74). West Sussex, England: John Wiley & Sons Ltd.

Nation Bureau of Statistics of China. (2004). *China statistical yearbook.* Beijing: China Statistics Press.

National Bureau of Statistics of China. (2006). *China statistical yearbook.* Beijing: China Statistics Press.

Norton, E.C. (2000). Long-term care. In A. J. Culyer, & J. P. Newhouse (ed.), *Handbook of health economics. Volume 1B* (pp 955-994). Amsterdam: Elsevier.

Qiao, X. (2001). *Aging Issues and Policy Choices in Rural China.* Paper presented at the International Union for the Scientific Study of Population's 24th General Population Conference (Salvador, Brazil; August 20-24, 2001.

Riley, N.E. (2004). China's Population: New Trends and Challenges, *Population Bulletin*, 59(2), Population Reference Bureau, 2004 June.

Robine, J.M. & Michel, J.P. (2004). Looking forward to a general theory on population. *Journal of Gerontology: Medical Sciences*, 59(A), 590-597.

Rautio, N., Adamson, J., Heikkinen, E., & Ebrahim, S. (2006). Association of socioeconomic position and disability among older women in Britain and Jyväskylä, Finland. *Archives of Gerontology and Geriatrics*, 42, 141-155.

Schwab, T.C., Leung, K.M. Gelb, E., Meng, Y-Y., &d Cohen, J. (2003). Home-and community-based alternatives to nursing home: Services and costs to maintain nursing home eligible individuals at home. *Journal of Aging and Health*, 15(2), 353-370.

Sha, Y. (2007). China's social security system: Present status and issues. *Aging Population in Asia: Experience of Japan, Thailand and China* (pp39-56). Seminar Report on the

Parallel Session at the 8th Annual Global Development Conference. January 17, 2007, Beijing, China.

Shanghai Civil Affairs (2002). Shanghai: How does the platform of the community work? *Community*, 10(19), 55-56. (in Chinese).

Shi, L. (1993). Health care in China: A rural-urban comparison after the socioeconomic reforms. *Bulletin of World Health Organization*, 71(6), 723-736.

Soldo, B.J., Wolf, D.A. & Agree, E.A. (1990). Family, Households, and Care Arrangements of Frail Older Women: A Structural Analysis. *Journal of Gerontology: Social Sciences*, 45: S238-S249.

Stata Corp. *Stata Version 10.01*. Stata Corp LP. College Station, Texas.

Stone, R.I. (2000). *Long-term Care for the Elderly with Disabilities: Current Policy, Emerging Trends, and Implications for the Twenty-first Century*. New York: Milbank Memorial Fund.

Stuck, A.E., Walthert, J.M., Nikolaus, T., Bula, C. J., Hohmann, C., & Beck, J. C. (1999). Risk factors for functional status decline in community-living elderly people: A systematic literature review. *Social Science & Medicine*, 48, 445-469.

Study Group (MOH) for Nursing Demand. (2003). *Study of Chinese Nursing Human Resource Status and Suggestions on Strengthening Training Programs for Nursing Professionals in Shortage*. Ministry of Health (MOH, China), Special report 2003. Available at http://www.tech.net.cn/y-jxgg/ zysd/6238.shtml. [accessed on September 15, 2007]

Takayama, N. (2002). *Pension Reform in the PRC: Incentives, Governance, and Policy Options*. Paper presented at the Asian Development Bank Institute's 5th Anniversary Conference, Tokyo; December 5-6.

Thorborg, M. (2005). Where have all the young girls gone? Fatal discrimination of daughters- A regional comparison. *China Perspectives*, 75(2), 2-10.

Tomlinson, R. (1997). Health care in China is highly inequitable. *British Medical Journal*, 315, 835.

United Nations Population Division (2007). *World Population Prospects: The 2006 Revision* Population Database. http://esa.un.org/unpp/. [accessed on September 16, 2007]

Wang, G. & Sun, H. (2003). Nursing home dpending among the dischargers in Shanghai. *Journal of Community Healthcare*, 2(2), 93-96. (in Chinese).

Wang, H., Gu, D. & Dupre, M.E. (2008). Factors associated with enrollment, satisfaction, and sustainability of the New Cooperative Medical Scheme program in six study areas in rural Beijing. *Health Policy*, 85, 32-44..

Wang, H., Yip, W., Zhang, L., Wang, L., & Hsiao, W. (2005). Community-based health insurance in poor rural China: The distribution of net benefits. *Health Policy and Planning*, 20(6), 366-374.

Williams, J., Lyons, B. & Rowland, D. (1997). Unmet long-term care needs of elderly people in community: A review of the literature. *Home Health Care Services Quarterly*, 16(1/2), 93-119.

Winship, C. & Radbill, L. (1994). Sampling weights and regression analysis. *Sociological Methods and Research*, 23, 230-257.

World Health Organization (WHO) (2000). *Towards an International Consensus on Policy for Long-term Care of the Ageing*. http://www.milbank.org/000712oms.pdf. [accessed August 18 2007]

Wu, B., Carter, M.W., Goins, R.T., & Cheng, C. (2005). Emerging services for community-based long-term care in urban China: A systematic analysis of Shanghai's community-based agencies. *Journal of Aging and Social Policy*, 17(4), 37-60.

Wu, B., & Xu, Q. (2007). The community-based long-term care in urban setting: The case of Shanghai. *Population Research*, 3, 61-70. (in Chinese)

Wu, X., Wei, Y., Li, Z., Fu, A. & Chow, A. (2000), *The Demography of Aging in China and Its Implications for Old Age Pension*. http://www.actuaries.ca/meetings/aging/Chow.pdf [accessed August 18, 2007].

Zeng, Y. & George, L.K. (2000). Family dynamics of 63 million (in 1990) to more than 330 million (in 2050) elders in China. *Demographic Research*, (2), article No. 5.

Zeng, Y. & Gu, D. (2007). *Having a daughter may likely be beneficial at old ages-- Lessons learned from the Chinese Longitudinal Healthy Longevity Study*. Paper presented at the International Seminar on Aging in Developing Countries: Building Bridges for Integrated Research Agendas organized by the International Union for Scientific Studies of Population, Santiago, Chile, April 23-24, 2007.

Zeng, Y. & Gu, D. (2008). Reliability of age reporting among the Chinese oldest-old in the CLHLS data sets. In Y. Zeng, D.L. Poston, D.A. Vlosky, & D. Gu. (Eds.). *Healthy Longevity in China: Demographic, Socioeconomic, and Psychological Dimensions* (pp.61-78). Dordrecht, The Netherlands: Springer Publisher.

Zeng, Y. & Wang, Z. (2003). Dynamics of family and elderly living arrangements in China: New lessons learned from the 2000 Census. *The China Review*, 3(2), 95-119.

Zhan, H. J., Liu, G. & Bai, H. (2006). Recent development in Chinese institutional elder care: Changing concepts and attitudes. *The Journal of Aging and Social Policy*, 18(2), 85–108.

Zhan, H.J. & Montgomery, R.J.V. (2003). Gender and elder care in China: The influence of filial piety and structural constraints. *Gender and Society*, 17(2), 209-229.

Zhang, J. (2003). China's ageing, risk of the elderly and accounting for aged care. *Managerial Finance*, 29(5/6), 97-110.

Zhang, J. (2006). Long-term care for the aged: Critical issues and challenges to China's sustainable development *World Review of Entrepreneurship, Management and Sustainable Development*, 2(1/2), 126-143.

Zhang, X.M. & Lv, J.Q. (2001). The state of institutionalization in Shanghai and its policy strategy. *Housing Technology*, 8, 28-30. (in Chinese).

Zhang, Z. & Wang, N. (2001). Comparative studies on health and healthcare of the elderly in the xities: Cases from Tianjin and Shanghai. *Market and Demographic Analysis*, 7(4), 56-61. (in Chinese)

Zheng, S.Y. (2003). Establishing China's Strike Law. *Strategy and Management*, 3, 108-116 (in Chinese).

Zoubanov, A. (2000). *Population Aging and Population Declines: Government Views and Policies*. Population Division. United Nations. New York. http://www.un.org/esa/population/publications/popdecline/Zoubanov.pdf. [accessed August 18 2007]

In: Social Sciences in Health Care and Medicine ISBN: 978-1-60456-286-6
Editors: J. B. Garner, T. C. Christiansen, pp. 85-115

Chapter 3

THE SURVEILLANCE GAZE: A NEW PARADIGM FOR LONG-TERM CARE OF OLDER PEOPLE IN THE UK NATIONAL HEALTH SERVICE (NHS)

Susan Pickard
National Institute of Health Research
School for Primary Care Research
University of Manchester
Manchester M13 9PL, UK

ABSTRACT

Based on a recent evaluation, this chapter presents an account of the latest model of UK National Health Service (NHS)-led long-term care of older people. It reviews key aspects of the model which include a new role for primary care in anticipatory or preventive medicine for older people; mechanisms for co-ordinating health and social care; relationships between primary care practitioners and secondary care professionals; and the impact on older people's hospital admissions and length of stay. The chapter embeds this review in a historical account of theoretical, policy and service approaches to long-term care which enables the elements of continuity and change contained within the model to be picked up. This in turn permits the conclusion that the particular significance of this latest model in both theoretical and policy terms lies in the framing of illness in old age within the 'risk' paradigm that has come increasingly to characterize late modern society.

INTRODUCTION

When NHS-led case management was piloted in England in 2003-5, and shortly afterwards implemented nationwide, it represented a new departure for the NHS and its responsibility towards those older people with complex health needs requiring intermittent medical and/or nursing care. In this chapter the latter group will be referred to as the 'intermediates', a term first used in the 1950s (Lewis, 2001) and described by the Ministry of

Health as those older people "who waver between sickness and health and the 'border-line' case" (Ministry of Health, 1952, p16). In order to assess the place of NHS-led case management in the history of long-term care in the UK this chapter will examine theory, policy and service approaches towards the intermediates since the inception of the NHS in 1948 and before, where relevant. In doing so, the analysis will permit us to assess the degree of continuity and change contained in the most recent approach to long-term care and to suggest some conclusions about social and medical approaches to older age, about the relationship between health and social care and, more broadly, the impact of key aspects of high or late modernity (Giddens, 1991) on the experience of being old in the twenty-first century.

The chapter will be set out as follows. First we will outline a historical overview of approaches towards old age reflected both in policy approaches and wider social attitudes in which they were embedded. Then we will similarly trace the evolution of sociological theories of old age and ageing again placing them in historical context alongside policy developments. Next we will turn to an examination of a boundary struggle of particular relevance in framing the experience of old age in the UK: that of the struggle between hospitals and community-based Local Authorities over who should have responsibility for the intermediates. After this we will focus on the two professional groupings on either side of this struggle and look firstly at the attitude of the medical profession to long-term care and then at the approach of social care professionals, including also in our account a description of the crucial role played by informal carers in plugging the gaps between these two professional groupings. Finally we will return to the most recent policy and service initiative around care of the intermediates – the community matron model inaugurated in 2005. We will assess the implications of the model in terms of the new role for primary care with regard to the intermediates; the health and social care boundary; and the role of hospitals. We will conclude by assessing the elements of continuity and change respectively contained within the model with reference to our historical account and the significance of elements of change in respect to future policy towards older people.

Historical Overview of Approaches towards Old Age

The idea of 'the elderly' as a separate category in the population of western countries emerged at the end of the nineteenth century (Katz, 1996). Provision for old age was not at first differentiated from provision for sickness. It was only towards the end of the nineteenth century that the friendly societies and trades unions found themselves obliged to rule that sickness benefit should be ended at the age of 65 and replaced by an old age pension. However, old age remained undifferentiated from poverty in a very real sense (and, as we shall see, the old age pension was certainly not a vehicle to raise an individual out of poverty). By the age of 75, almost one in three in the Edwardian age was a pauper and this persisted well into the twentieth century; Lowe and colleague's community surveys of older people in the 1950s unearthed a huge amount of poverty among older people whereby of the 306 dwellings they assessed, 7% had no internal water supply, 72% had no bath and 80% no indoor sanitation (Lowe and McKeown, 1950). Meanwhile, older people too frail or poor and lacking family prepared to look after them continued to enter the workhouse (renamed public assistance institutions, or PAIs following the Local Government Act of 1929). In order that it not be thought of as a 'soft' option, however, the workhouse was based on the principle of 'less eligibility' which meant that conditions within workhouses were designed to be worse than the worse conditions one would experience in poverty in the community. This was intended to deter people from entering it unless they had no alternative; moreover the harshness of both its founding philosophy and its regime was based on a moral condemnation of the poor, which associated poverty with moral turpitude. Family duties were reiterated in the Poor Law of 1930 which reaffirmed in section 14 Elizabethan principles of family responsibility namely that:

> "It should be the duty of the father, grandfather, mother, grandmother, husband or child, of a poor, old, blind, lame or impotent person, or other poor person, not able to work, if possessed of sufficient means, to relieve and maintain that person."

Conditions were appalling in workhouse infirmaries; there was "no casualty provision, no trained nursing staff, no drugs and no surgical facilities" (Barton and Mulley, 2003, p 229). Following a campaign led by the editor of the Lancet, conditions finally improved and laws were passed to safeguard inmates' wellbeing. However, a two-tier service developed with voluntary hospitals of high status at the top tier who were reluctant to admit elderly people; care of older people took place in poor law infirmaries on the bottom tier where facilities were inferior and staffing levels poor.

There was a softening of attitude towards older people following the war, nevertheless, since it was believed that older people and especially those among them with health and social care needs had suffered disproportionately. Titmuss (1976) summarized the particular privations they experienced as: the war disrupted informal support networks; the establishment of the Emergency Medical Services (EMS) further reduced the number of hospital beds available to older people; older people in PAIs and Poor Law infirmaries at most risk of bombing raids were often not moved; elderly people in the large cities were the group hardest hit by bomb damage to their homes; when evacuation schemes for older people were finally established, this was prompted by a desire to reduce pressure and improve morale in air-raid shelters. This change in policy attitudes underpinned the post-war settlement, and the welfare institutions, greatest among them being the founding of the NHS, was intended to be a 'reward' for the national effort made in the war, just as universal suffrage had been a reward for participation in the First World War (and in both cases represented concessions intended to forestall dangerous social unrest and guarantee social and political stability: see Perkin, 1989). However, despite the shift during the welfare era, which lasted from the 1940s to the early 1970s, older people continued to be a low priority in social policy terms, an appraisal which was presented as 'natural'. As Beveridge wrote: "It is dangerous to be in any way lavish to old age until adequate provision has been made for all other vital needs such as the prevention of disease and the adequate nutrition of the young" (1942: paragraph 236) and many other scholarly assessments of this policy subsequently have been unquestioning of these priorities (eg Denham, 1994). This merely represented a continuation of past priorities: older people had not been amongst the groups chosen before the war as a focus for health improvements, which included efforts to improve child or maternal health and to eradicate infectious disease (Iliffe and Drennan, 2000).

However, overall this period was characterized by a Kantian belief in unlimited progress and social and moral improvement which, although unevenly distributed through the population, nevertheless impacted on older people too resulting in the 'modernization of ageing' due largely to optimism in the rapid developments in medicine and its success in eradicating deadly diseases. This led to an increasing 'medicalization' both of society in general and of old age in particular. In practice, this approach involved viewing the ageing process as one of decay and decline which could be, if not cured, then alleviated by the techniques and pharmaceutical regimes of biomedical science (Estes and Binney, 1989). As Phillipson points out (1998), this is reflected in the fact that by the 1970s one in five older people were taking three or more medicines daily and one in ten was taking upwards of four different medications.

Conceptions of old people's place in society shifted in line with an emphasis on social rights and 'social citizenship' with entitlements accruing from the status of citizen (Marshall, 1950). This was underpinned by the notion of an intergenerational contract, reinforced through the shared wartime experience, with old age the final stage in an 'institutional life-cycle' established through mandatory retirement and framed by welfare institutions including the NHS, residential and institutional care and state pensions. Pensions legislation in 1908 and 1925 began the association of the onset of old age with the start of retirement. However, in debates during the second reading of the Pension Bill in 1925 Chamberlain admitted the amount proposed was "obviously insufficient by itself to provide a grown man or woman with the necessities for life" (quoted in Fennell, Phillipson and Evers, 1988, p207) and reasons underlying their introduction were as much connected with the desire to increase the throughput of workers through industrial jobs and boost the ability of younger workers to find employment as they were about 'recognising' the contribution and loyalty of older workers.

The early 1970s to the late 1980s, was a transitional time during which the worldwide economic downturn ushered in the beginnings of a crisis of legitimization of the welfare state (Habermas, 1976), which has uneasily endured through the next period, in which we are currently situated, known variously as high or late modernity, post-industrialism or sometimes post-modernity: the era of "advanced liberalism". The ongoing need to secure legitimization for the welfare state has resulted in the piecemeal and to some extent clandestine dismantling/restructuring of the institutions of ageing, particularly the notion of retirement and of publicly-funded pensions, a process which has continued apace as the advent of mass unemployment and premature retirement has destabilized the institution of retirement. At the same time, with the cutting of the thread connecting work and retirement, the 'retirement wage' began to be questioned (Phillipson, 1998) and the interests of workers and pensioners were no longer considered to coincide. The final deathblow of the collective right to a state-funded pension appeared to come to an end in 1997 when the government refused to restore the link between working income and pensions and began officially to advocate the use of second pensions involving the private sector, aiming for a future situation in which private pensions will make up 60% of all pension provision. Indeed, following the previous Conservative government's lead, New Labour has utilized the Private Finance Initiative (PFI) to encourage private investment in the infrastructure and management of a wide range of health and social care facilities (Estes and Phillipson, 2002). The challenges presented by an 'ageing population' have often been used to explain these developments and indeed during this period for the very first time the European population contains as many people over 60 as it does children under 15, and as Gilleard and Higgs (2000) point out, societies of this type of age structure have no precedent. Alongside the rationalizing agenda of neo-liberal governments and a changing economic climate, there has thus been this rise of a kind of 'apocalyptic demography' comprising fears of being 'overwhelmed' by the demands of the ageing population which has further resulted in a questioning of the intergenerational contract which underpins the social contract. However, the 'facts' of demography have always tended to serve a political agenda. As far back as 1957 the Boucher Report was worrying about the changed demographic context: in 1901 only 1 in 25 people were over 65 but by 1954 this was 1 in 9. Though these same figures could be interpreted as progress directly linked with advances in medical as well as public health regimes they were yet seemingly never welcomed as a 'triumph' in policy terms. We can also see the continuity in policy priorities which remain underpinned by the same 'burden of ageing' approach as found in the Beveridge Report. Thus in 1998 Hicks, in his OECD report wrote that spending money on pensions and health care for older people "would be at the expense of higher priorities, such as investment to improve the opportunities of poor children or unemployed youth" (quoted in Estes and Phillipson, 2002, no page number given).

Sociological Theories of Old Age and Ageing during these Eras

As we will see, sociological ideas about old age in each of these three periods – those of pre-war, welfare and high modernity - are closely related to the political and economic backdrops which frame them. Thus, the classic works of sociology – by Marx, Weber, Durkheim and others – which appeared in the first pre-NHS period say very little about old age which was, in political and economic terms, similarly 'invisible' and, as we have seen, not clearly distinguished from sickness and poverty.

The second era, the 1940s to the 1970s, was dominated by liberal-pluralist, or consensus, theories which in sociology appeared as functionalism. The functionalist understanding of ageing is as a time of inevitable physical and mental decline and disengagement from productive society, and is dominated by two rival theories, disengagement and activity theories respectively, both positing alternative ways in which older people should normatively adjust to old age and retirement so as to assure minimal fallout for the rest of society (Phillipson, 1998).

By contrast, the 'social creation of dependency' , or 'structured dependency' thesis, also known as the 'political economy' approach in the US, and having its roots in Marxism, arose in reaction to these functionalist approaches and, crucially, appeared during the crisis of welfare, that is, when the institutions that underpinned the welfare state were themselves being critically scrutinised. Associated particularly with Alan Walker (1981), Peter Townsend (1981) and Chris Phillipson (1982) in the UK and Carroll Estes (1979) in the US, the basic thrust of the approach questions the 'naturalness' of the experience of old age and is concerned to display its political origins and social structuring. It also questions the dominant ideas of biomedicine that perceive old age as a time of increasing senescence, and posits instead that it is socially rather than biologically constructed. Structural dependency theorists see welfare institutions, whilst on the one hand intended to enhance the welfare of older people, as simultaneously creating dependency and powerlessness. For example, mandatory retirement means that old people require the old age pensions they are entitled to draw but at the same time are further marginalized and disempowered by the fact that pensions are set at rates considerably below average earnings. At the same time retirement itself has encouraged the view that past a certain age an individual's social worth is diminished and it implicitly advances the 'burden of ageing' thesis whilst such instruments as the 'age-dependency ratio' – which expresses a ratio between those over pension age and younger adults - explicitly advance it.

During the current period of high or late modernity, criticism of the structured dependency thesis have begun to appear. They are criticisms that such an approach is over-deterministic and fails to take into account the role of agency, and a general questioning of the centrality of economic class analysis in explaining the experience of ageing. Ironically, it is claimed, the focus on the created powerlessness of older people works to reinforce that very image of powerlessness itself, especially with its inbuilt expectation that the state alone is capable of improving - through higher pensions for example – the condition of older people, rather than individual agency (Gilleard and Higgs, 2000). A more fundamental issue is that the very institutions that created the dependency and powerlessness that formed the object of criticism of structural dependency theorists are in the process of breaking up and thus the theory has seemed consequently to lose its major purpose. However, far from applauding the demise of these dependency-creating institutions the structural dependency theorists have begun to discern further problems associated with this. For them the 'crisis in the welfare state' has become a 'crisis of identity in old age' as they recognized that the institutions which had once framed the experiences of older people, once removed, did not necessarily lead to liberation and empowerment but to the uncertainty and anxiety of change and a further, if qualitatively different, 'disempowerment'. The central argument of Phillipson's book 'Reconstructing Old Age' (1998) is to highlight the 'historic turning point' which has now been reached in discussions of the place and meaning of old age in society. As he writes: "The combined impact of the changes has been to place in doubt the meaning and purpose of growing old" (1998, p 3) which fundamentally entails a change in the notion both of the state and of the citizenship model associated with it from one of 'collective security and integration' (Gilleard and Higgs, 2000, p92) to one based on agency involving the abolishing of the very category of 'pensioner'. In this framework, leading philosopher of New Labour, Tony Giddens, goes so far – and some would say too far – as to say that ageing itself is a 'choice':

> "Ageing used to be more passive than it is now: the ageing body was simply something that had to be accepted. In the more active, reflexive society, ageing has become much more of an open process, on a physical as well as a psychic level" (Giddens, 1998, p119).

The result has been a shift in perspective from structural dependency theorists. They can no longer maintain their model of citizenship that started "from a welfarist belief in the centrality of mass social benefits" (Gilleard and Higgs, 2000, p17) given the change in the nature of politics: thus structural dependency has become 'critical gerontology', shifting from a primary focus on macro economic and political issues – though this has continued with a critique of the neo-liberal agenda of globalization (eg see Estes and Phillipson, 2002) - to also incorporate a focus on the micro and integrating the 'moral economy' (Minkler and Estes, 1991) and other cultural perspectives (eg Cole, 1992).

Other theoretical perspectives, however, seem more naturally constructed to address the specific issues associated with late modernity and the governance of 'advanced liberalism', many of them drawing on the ideas of Michel Foucault. The central aim of Gilleard and Higgs' book sums up the context for a new theoretical focus which it describes as being about "the erosion of this unitary 'ages of life' culture'" by a belief that "human agency can be exercised over how ageing will be expressed and experienced" (2000, p 2)with a key role played by reflexivity (Giddens, 1991) and self-determination meaning that identity is also determined by consumption and life-style choice rather than only by labour, social and economic class or even community and national identity. This reflexive project, moreover, brings a new set of existential problems which Bauman expresses thus:

> "In our postmodern times, the boundaries which tend to be simultaneously most strongly desired and most acutely missed are those of a rightful and secure place in society, of a space unquestionably one's own, where one can play one's roles in a game in which the rules do not change overnight" (1992, p26)

-even where those places and those rules were previously perceived to be restrictive and demanding of conformity. The dissolving role of the nationstate in determining policies for its citizens, the absorption of the UK into the greater EU, the onset of mass immigration and globalization, have all produced a disorientating effect and a loosening of the ties of community and familiarity which made the social contract underlying the welfare state tenable in the first place.

Moreover, the belief in 'progress' has diminished or is perceived to bring ambiguous results and the shortcomings of the positivist medical and scientific approach which Beck lists as "nuclear, chemical, genetic and ecological mega-hazards" (1992, p101-2) ultimately threaten not just the existence of human beings but of the planet itself. Interestingly, the ageing of populations has coincided with the working through of the modernist project, so that the greying of the population and the demise of the progress idea resonate together with an almost poetic harmony and one with somber and melancholy tints. As Cole has described, particularly for the case of old age in the US:

> "Awareness that the national population was ageing blended silently into fears of nuclear holocaust, environmental deterioration, military and economic decline, social conflict and cultural decadence, youthful optimism and belief in limitless progress appeared increasingly incongruous in a society confronting limits on all sides" (1992, pp233-4).

However, whilst the excess and deficiencies of positivist science produce risks, it also compensates for them through calculation and political regulation. This is part of the new definition of power. In line with cultural fragmentation, and the breakdown of collectivist welfare notions, advanced liberal society is characterized by the 'hollowed-out state' (Rhodes, 1997) whereby its 'frontiers' have been rolled back and there has been a deregulation at the macro-level but at the same time state power has been dispersed throughout the social body. The effect is that the shrinking state has in fact increased in potency, alongside supranational agencies that lie beyond the traditional nation states. Estes and Phillipson (2002) have pointed out that global institutions, such as the World Bank, international NGOs and the World Trade Organization, are increasingly determining agendas in social policy, in the direction of states providing increasingly residual welfare services and an increase in the role of private institutions. Thus behind New Labour's endorsement of private pensions stands the World Bank Report 'Averting the Old Age Crisis' (1994) with its advocacy of private pension plans in a multi-pillar pension system. In addition, one of the most potent tools of the new 'governmentality' is also one of the most subtle: that of the 'technologies of the self' leading to 'normalization' and 'responsibilization' whereby individuals adjust their own values and self-perceptions according to norms inculcated by government policies, largely through 'experts' of various kinds, and all of which are designed to minimize risk.

In fact, a key feature of the functioning of modern regimes is the increased surveillance which has been increasingly used to investigate and regulate the body of individuals and populations. This 'panopticism' (see Foucault, 1975) has been used to impose order and efficiency and increasingly to control risk. Experts do this by classifying and intervening in the lives of those who are perceived to diverge from the norm, presenting thereby either a present or future 'risk.'

Foucauldian-inspired approaches to social gerontology such as that by Katz (1996) focus on the processes by which 'the elderly' were created as a target for social policy and medical and social care experts and constructed and reconstructed over the course of the twentieth century by different public policies which required them "to adjust to the reification of age into convenient social categories" (Walker, 1999, p362). As Katz says: "To be old merely requires that one ages; however, to be part of a population of elderly persons requires that one be absorbed into a specific discourse of differentiation" (1996, p. 51). He demonstrates how geriatrics and gerontology first emerged as a disciplinary formation dominated by a medical model, employing statistics, medical sciences and demography, which equated old age with illness, decline and senescence of body and mind. From this, 'classification practices' created 'the elderly' as objects of knowledge on the basis of chronology, and 'dividing practices' further sub-divided the retired, the sick, the senile, those in need of health and/or social care, not just obeying the rules of science but also with an eye to the marking up of professional territories as we will see later in the chapter when looking at definitions of 'chronic sick'. Thirdly, self-subjectification technologies resulted in older people internalising these notions of themselves as frail, dependent, powerless and burdensome to others.

Within a regime of surveillance associated with risk, as far as older people are concerned, "targeting and risk assessment replace the institutions of the collective welfare state" (Gilleard and Higgs, 2000, p23). However, the clinical gaze has from the inception of the founding of 'geriatric' medicine had problems in distinguishing between the normal and the pathological (eg Armstrong, 1981; Morley, 2004) and the construction of the biomedical discourse meant that from the founding of the NHS it was with acute illness, amenable to 'cure' that medicine concerned itself whilst chronic illness – and thus most of the illness appearing in old age - requiring 'cure' rather than 'care' lay outside this boundary and fell to the remit of social care. Increasingly the clinical gaze has turned to surveillance, and the emphasis shifted to preventing illness and to the moral imperative to be well. This results in what Gilleard and Hughes (2000) call the 'fragmenting' of the ageing population into those capable of successfully marshalling the technologies of the self and those who are not so capable, and therefore place themselves 'at risk': thus the private pension holders are separated from older people relying on state benefits and the healthy old are set apart from the intermediates. It is to attitudes towards the latter 'fourth agers' that we turn next.

Long-Term Care of Older People: Health or Social Care?

In this section, we will look at the struggle between different groups of professionals to define long-term care of older people as either health or social care, a political and disciplinary dispute that had a significant impact on services, and continues to do so. After describing the various developments in this process over the sixty years since the creation of the NHS, we will focus in on medical attitudes towards old age and the emerging specialism of geriatric medicine and on the idea of 'community care' led by social care agencies. Finally we will look at the range and nature of informal care-giving during this period. Throughout the discussion, the important part played by both explicit and implicit social theories and ideas about older people as discussed in the preceding section will become apparent. As Walker points out (1999), when policy makers propose practical solutions to social problems, they are based on beliefs about the nature and causation of the problem. Sometimes these beliefs are made explicit, usually not, but we can trace clearly how the struggle to define long-term care as health or social care was underpinned by the liberal-pluralist consensus about the 'burden of ageing' thesis. We can also see how disciplinary struggles within medicine and between medicine and social care partly in themselves created the very problems then associated 'inherently' with ageing – bed blocking constituting a very prominent example of this, the distinction between acute and chronic care another.

The way in which the health/social boundary has been defined has shifted over time, but the following narrative will reveal much in the way of continuity (although with some important changes). In fact, the first point to note is that the ambiguous and contested boundary between health and social care pre-dated 1948[1]. Thereafter, attempts to define the boundary following the inception of the NHS, particularly in relation to institutional care, were made when, following the Rucker Report, the 1948 National Assistance Act gave Local Authorities responsibility for the provision of residential homes for older people; the chronic sick meanwhile would be cared for in hospitals rather than in these homes, which under the Poor Law had provided generally inadequate nursing and medical care. Ministry officials declared that LAs should be responsible for those in "need of care and attention, (But) not constant medical and nursing attention", while hospitals should take responsibility for "those in need of constant medical attention and those who are incapacitated by a medical disorder". (PRO MH80/47, undated memorandum on the abolition of the Poor Law).

As we have seen, prior to the setting up of the NHS, elderly people had to resort to either poor law or municipal hospitals where the standards of medical and nursing care for this group was often low. Thus access to care in NHS hospitals that was free at the point of delivery was highly regarded by patients and something that politicians did not wish to be seen to dilute. As Bridgen and Lewis point out: "In the early 1950s, the problem of elderly people gaining admission to hospital was as politically sensitive as the issue of hospital discharge is today" (1999, p12). Nevertheless, since the late 1950s policy has consistently edged towards limiting the role of the hospital. However, at the same time, the definitions as to what sort of need merited what kind of institutional care was not changed until the mid-1990s, when the particularly narrow role of hospitals was finally acknowledged, with a statement that only medical care or nursing care of a specialist nature should be provided by

[1] NB: there were several changes in nomenclature: the Ministry of Health existed until 1968; the Department of Health and Social Security (DHSS) until 1988; the Department of health (DH) thereafter.

the NHS. This officially recognized a situation that had prevailed in practice for several decades: in short, for many years leading to this point, the fact that both health and Local Authorities endeavoured to avoid responsibility for a growing 'intermediate' group of people who were in need of nursing and/or medical attention on a very regular but not constant basis. During this time, the funding for and expansion of domiciliary care was not seen as a priority and the only statutory provision that was generally available to the elderly as an alternative to hospital care was Local Authority residential accommodation (and not of the 'hotel' kind envisaged by Bevan and Rucker).

In practice, from the late 1950s, central government tacitly supported the view of the Ministry's hospital division and medical department, as well as that of many hospital doctors, that the number of geriatric beds should be limited. This joined policy makers concerned about costs, with doctors reluctant to treat chronic conditions, particularly of the elderly, which contained a large social component, in a common cause.

Bridgen and Lewis have shown that while central government was determined to reduce the number of geriatric hospital beds, it was not prepared to acknowledge that this would reduce the role of the hospitals in the continuing care of the elderly. To admit that the role of the hospitals was being reduced would have also been to admit that the Local Authorities would have to do more, which carried financial implications for them. They suggest that the internal contradictions of such a covert policy to shift more responsibility for the care of elderly people to the Local Authorities caused severe problems for service delivery. The obvious solution would have been to have expanded domiciliary care at this time. That this did not happen was down not only to the desire to limit expenses by the central government, but also partly the result of the Local Authorities' approach: they believed that an increase in domiciliary services would only help hospitals delay admission or speed up discharge of frail elderly people. Moreover, the County Councils Association (CCA) pointed out that good community care was not cheap to deliver. Thus it complained:

> "It is not accepted that it is universally agreed that the primary aim of services for the elderly is to help them remain in their own homes as long as possible. This doctrine can result in elderly people being kept at home at very considerable expense, by the provision of nursing, domestic help, night service and so on when their needs would be far better met by admission to hospital" (CCA, 1961: quoted in Bridgen and Lewis, 1999).

Denham (2004) views the evidence somewhat differently from Bridgen and Lewis. He points out that policy makers believed that a lowered bed norm was justified - and did not, by implication, necessarily mean more responsibilities for social care - by the potential of geriatrics to affect fast throughput. Indeed, the Boucher Report of 1957 stated its view that no correlation could be demonstrated between the number of chronic sick beds and the adequacy of the service provided. In subsequent years, moreover, although the number of geriatric beds remained constant, patient throughput increased. Even so, it must be added that progress in geriatric medicine was uneven throughout the country and depended on many local factors. Not all branches of the medical profession agreed that the low bed norm was an ideal state of affairs particularly with the increase in an ageing population. The British Medical Association (BMA) in 1976 called for an 'urgent' revision of geriatric bed norms. It is also fair to say that early intervention – the key to successful rehabilitation in old age, as defined by geriatricians themselves – depended on sufficient beds being available and that too low a number would certainly be counterproductive from the point of view of geriatric medicine should anything go wrong (such as a flu pandemic) causing the unit to fall behind.

In reality, the system was under pressure from the very earliest years. The first complaints came from GPs about the difficulties they were experiencing in securing old people access to hospital beds. As early as June 1949, the BMA reported that the GP service was coming under strain, largely because hospitals were refusing to admit elderly people. The Local Medical Committee for London in 1951 reported that a number of old people had died during 1951 because hospitals had not granted them admission (Bridgen and Lewis, 1999).

The Ministry took the view that the health/social care boundary was not a problem in and of itself. Rather, there was simply a need for increased provision on both sides of the boundary. There was a consensus within the medical profession that Local Authority homes and domiciliary services should be expected to take responsibility for elderly people with far greater degrees of infirmity than had hitherto been the case. The BMA's key report on geriatrics, published in 1955, and resulting from a committee set up in1953 to debate and research the matter, emphasised that admission to hospital should be a temporary interlude and the basic principle should be that the care of the elderly should be centred on the home and the GP. The report reiterated that, in respect of geriatric care, hospitals should increasingly focus their attention on acute treatment and rehabilitation.

In any case, the 1957 Boucher Committee meeting reported that the level of hospital provision was generally sufficient and that any problems were due to the inefficient use and distribution of beds. This conclusion resulted in a significant tightening in the role of hospitals. A bed norm was laid down in the government circulars that followed the publication of the Report in 1957 to 1.2 beds per thousand.

What made this difficult was the fact that hospitals were still expected to care for the long-term sick, despite the low bed norm. Thus the circulars that proceeded on from the Report formally confirmed the responsibility of hospitals for continuing care but there was no concomitant agreement that the responsibilities of Local Authorities for making provision for more infirm people in terms of residential and domiciliary care should be increased. This lowered geriatric bed norm was confirmed in the 'Hospital Plan for England and Wales' (Cmnd. 1604) in 1962 and the publication the following year of "Health and Welfare: the development of community care' (Cmnd. 1973). In fact, the aim was that the norm might be modified downwards and meanwhile it represented a 'maximum... for the purpose of reducing excesses above (it), not supplying deficiencies below' (PRO MH99/21 (1961), quoted in Bridgen and Lewis, 1999). It was the Ministry's faith in rehabilitation and active treatment that crucially underpinned this norm (Denham, 2004).

In this tightly-balanced system, correct allocation of beds was obviously key to its functioning. Indeed, the 'bed-blocking' controversy climbed to the top of the policy agenda in the late 1960s and early 1970s whereby hospitals claimed that older people were occupying hospital beds on social rather than medical grounds. Hall and Bytheway, who object to the term and prefer to use 'misplacement', concluded that the problem's significance "is that it represents certain beliefs about the purpose of hospitals" (1982, p 1989). It also, of course, represents certain beliefs about old age and its relative priority, or lack of it, in society. At the same time, Local Authorities claimed their own version of bed blocking with the inappropriate use of residential care by sick older people and thus the circulars became the basis of bargaining over individual cases between health and social services in which 'the swap' developed whereby many hospitals refused to accept a referral from a residential home unless that home would reciprocate (Means, 2001).

The government put its faith in the ability of the health and social care to work out their problems on the ground, such as through 'the swap'. Formal mechanisms for joint planning were introduced as part of the NHS reorganization of 1974. However, the limited nature of this reform reflected the fact that ultimately the Department still believed that 'goodwill' between the two sets of authorities was the best guarantee of co-operation. No attempt was made by the DHSS to redefine the responsibilities of the health and LAs. Thus despite the emphasis on planning during this time, the situation remained the same as it had been for the previous 25 years.

After the advent of Mrs Thatcher's government to power in 1979, the new government indicated its desire to fundamentally alter the nature of community care policy as early as 1981 saying it would not be regarded just as 'care in the community' but 'care by the community' and accompanied this by a reduction in government expenditure on Personal Social Services in an attempt to reduce them to residual organizations. Meanwhile the family would take up the slack with the role of Social Services being to back up the assistance given by family, private and voluntary support. A loophole in new regulations on supplementary benefit which allowed residents of private residential and nursing homes to claim full board and lodging charges plus an amount to cover personal expenses resulted in a social security budget which spiraled out of control and perverse incentives for older people to enter residential homes, despite the proclaimed policy of community care, and partly as a result of the lack of community-based alternatives.

The 1990 NHS Act and Community Care Act, arising from the Griffiths' review, was an attempt to rectify this situation. Local Authorities were now designated as the 'lead agencies' for community care. In fact, NHS officers regarded it as 'good grounds for getting rid of their long-term care responsibilities as soon as possible' (Lewis and Glennester, 1996, p16). Moreover, the Act created a new distinction between 'health' and 'social care' in which social care would be means-tested in contrast to health care which remained free at the point of access. Social care was henceforth defined to include all aspects of personal care and domestic tasks necessary for all aspects of daily living (see Department of Health (DH), 1989), thereby simultaneously transforming the definition of nursing care as synonymous with 'specialist care' and the Social Worker was transformed into the care manager, managing a tight budget.

Actually, as Means has pointed out (2001), the roots of this issue extend much deeper than is generally supposed in contemporary times and was contained, though never acted upon, in the Rucker Report. This report, incorporated into the National Assistance Act of 1948 recommended that home equity should be used to help fund the costs of residential-based social care. Financial issues arising from the placement of older people in poor law care for social reasons or in poor law infirmaries for health reasons also carried a financial implication in that the former lost their pensions whilst the latter retained them (Means, 2001).

Eventually the Department of Health had to publicly accept that the 1990 Act had led to a reduction in the responsibility of hospitals for long-term care with the immediate catalyst being a 1994 report by the Health Service Commissioner following the case of a brain-damaged patient for whom the LA had refused to accept responsibility. In response to widespread publicity created by this case, the Department of Health released new guidance on

NHS responsibilities, its first detailed statement on this matter for almost forty years. Whilst 'continuing in-patient care' was identified as one of the range of services which the NHS should provide, eligibility criteria were set out for this service and specified the need for patients of 'specialist' nurse or 'specialist health care equipment' or 'specialist medical or nursing supervision'. This represented a significant restriction of the NHS' role with the emphasis on 'specialist' care a new departure and indicated – in line with the definitions of personal care - that basic nursing care for chronically ill patients was no longer to be regarded as part of a 'comprehensive' NHS. In reality this was no more than a retrospective acknowledgement of a situation that had been developing steadily since the mid -1950s.

Thus, the outcome of these boundary struggles for long-term care of older people are clear. Echoing Titmuss' (1968) view that community care should not be thought of as inherently 'better', Lynham writes: "the difference between 1940 and 1994 is that whereas the chronic sick were "warehoused" in hospital, the frail and disabled now are "warehoused" in the community" (1995, p10), and subject to inadequate treatment, inadequate rehabilitation and an inadequate multi-disciplinary approach. Bridgen and Lewis also suggest that an enduring legacy of this professional, administrative and financial struggle of relevance to contemporary policy makers was in terms of the development of services for older people themselves: "Because the true nature of the struggle was never openly acknowledged, so the question 'what kind of care?' never reached the top of the agenda," they write (1999 p 120). Instead, the struggle was defined by professionals on either side of the boundary and came to centre on the nature and extent of their own disciplinary expertise, and also by Ministers, operating within a 'burden of ageing' paradigm, who were particularly keen to limit the amount of government expenditure in general and on older people in particular. Constraining the role of hospitals was intended to do this but when Local Authority care proved to be a more expensive option than was originally anticipated and particularly when in the 1980s the social security budget spiraled out of control the answer, it was believed, would be to shift the cost onto the older person and their family themselves.

More recently, hope of rectifying the situation lay with the Royal Commission on Long-term Care appointed in 1997 with an aim, among other things, to consider whether a clear distinction between health and social care could be made. In its report, it proposed to separate living and housing costs from personal care and recommended that personal care should be free, depending on an assessment of need and not on a means test. Living and housing costs would remain subject to a means test. However, as Land (2001) points out: "The government… rejected the Majority Commissioners' proposals on personal care and the line between health and personal care remains (p52).

Underlying this struggle, as well as government priorities and a rationalizing agenda, are the distinct theories and professional practices associated with two expert fields: that of medicine and social care. We will examine each of these in turn.

Attitude of the Medical Profession to Long-Term Care of Older People

Geriatrics as a science was born in the workhouse and the stigma of these origins lingered in the minds of both older people and the medical profession long after the demise of the workhouse. The development of British geriatrics came as a result of the interest of Dr Marjory Warren, to whom was given a former Poor Law Infirmary, and from the 714 chronically ill and mostly elderly patients in her care, she created the first geriatric unit in the UK. As a result of her work, she reduced the number of chronic beds to 240 with a turnover three times the previous rate, and cleared beds for the use of other consultants; she advocated the use of separate geriatric assessment units within general hospitals to better care for older chronically sick patients. As a result of her pioneering work, she showed that early examination, investigation and treatment could achieve considerable results with elderly patients who might previously have been considered incurable. Patients should be taken into hospital early, where multi-disciplinary teams including physiotherapy and occupational therapy (OT) would be made available; prompt treatment of this kind would enable many elderly people to return quickly to their own homes or Local Authority residential accommodation. Only the most severely sick would have to be cared for in hospital chronic sick wards (see Warren, 1943).

It is possible to trace how the evolution of 'classification' practices went hand-in-hand with the growth of this particular kind of geriatric expertise. To begin with, before the advent of geriatric medicine, there was no interest in anything other than the broadest classification, starting with Charcot's 'Clinical Lectures on the Diseases of Old Age' (1882) which confined itself to a detailed description of an extensive range of diseases. Classification was first attempted when it began to be understood that many 'chronic sick' medical patients were treatable and in turn medical expertise developed to treat them and categorized them for this task, in a circular process of increased expertise and increased classification. Nevertheless at this stage most general physicians ignored chronic sickness in old age for a variety of reasons including its lack of interest as compared to acute illness and the social-utility idea that there was no point in rehabilitating people with only a few years left (Denham, 2004).

Marjory Warren's was the first attempt to apply a systematic classification to patients so as to treat them more effectively – she classed patients into five groups (ambulatory, continent bed-ridden, incontinent women, senile but untroublesome and those with senile dementia: see, eg, Matthews, 1984), and her success in this stimulated others to follow and adapt her methods. These included Lord Amulree, who was appointed to the first geriatric consultant post at a London Teaching Hospital; Joseph Sheldon, who pioneered community geriatric medicine, and emphasized the importance of social and environmental factors in an older person's health status; and Lionel Cosin, who developed the first purpose-built geriatric day hospital. All agreed on the goals of early intervention, rehabilitation and discharge and all developed their own systems of classification which were often quite crude and pragmatic: for example, Trevor Howell's classification delineated the incurable, those treatable but not curable and those curable.

The imprecise and contestable nature of the term 'chronic sick' is apparent from earliest days: the Chief Medical Officer in 1934 viewed the term as a loose one which was interpreted differently in different areas of the county (Ministry of Health, 1934) and the truth of this is revealed in the way that, whilst 'chronic sick' was usually taken to mean those aged 65 and over, during the war it was extended to encompass babies with pneumonia, acute bronchitis in young men and women with influenza. Unfortunately, in practical terms, once a label of 'chronic sick' had been given to a patient, they were effectively 'written off' (Denham, 1994).

Despite the success of Warren and her followers, there were nevertheless several major obstacles to the establishment of the sub-specialty of geriatric medicine. First was resistance on the part of general physicians in particular for whom, as we have noted, the association with the workhouse was never forgotten. Thus geriatric medicine was disparaged as a "second-rate specialty, looking after third-rate patients in fourth-rate facilities" (Lye, 1982, p129). Complex relationships with general physicians led to several different accommodations with them in the form of three standard models: age-based, needs-based and integrated. Related to this, during the mid to late 1970s geriatricians and other doctors debated the merits and demerits of the following options for geriatric medicine: to abandon the specialty altogether; the make it an age-related specialty as with paediatrics; to foster integration with general medicine; or to retain the traditional, or needs-based, model, whereby geriatricians take selected referrals from other consultants, with a view to rehabilitation or placement in long-term care.

Arguments for abandoning the specialty altogether (eg Leonard, 1976) were often advanced by general physicians who saw an ambiguous boundary between their specialty and that of geriatrics and considered themselves to be under threat by this discipline, especially where it continued to attract more funding than their specialty. Their points reduced to two (Williamson, 1979): that geriatrics was no true specialty, since it was associated with no methodology or techniques of its own; moreover it was not practically viable owing to its consistent failure to attract staff to geriatric units, partly a result of the inability to attract medical students in the first place.

The age related specialty position, advocated by people like R.W. Stout (1979) claimed that this would eliminate problems of ownership of elderly people; enhance the standing of the geriatrician; and provide greater opportunities for study and research. In addition, it has been suggested that it would enhance continuity of care which is disrupted when patients are transferred between acute, rehabilitation and long-stay beds and which is less likely to occur in acute wards where the holistic approach, favoured by geriatric medicine, is less prominent (Harrison, 1992).

As regards the middle position, a working party of the Royal College of Physicians proposed a closer relationship between geriatric medicine and general medicine (Clarke et al, 1977). Described by some as 'the middle way' (Williamson, 1979), proponents favoured integration with hospital general medicine and with general practice but sometimes (eg Williamson, 1979) warned against the potential loss of doctors with an exclusive commitment to the specialty and a dilution by those who had 'an interest' in it. This approach seems to be the most popular model in contemporary times. However, as Barton and Mulley point out: "The debate for and against integration has continued and remains largely unresolved" (2003, p233).

Second, in terms of the obstacles afflicting the establishment of the specialty was the inability of the Ministry of Health to compel district hospitals to establish geriatric units, despite their support for them and their optimistic belief that they could significantly reduce the use of beds by elderly people. From 1953 Ministry of Health Circulars expressed the desire to see a geriatric unit established in every health district; however even as late as 1978 42 health districts in England still lacked geriatric beds (Denham, 2004). This was because, at the end of everything, the Ministry could only cajole but not coerce the Health Authorities, as Denham points out. The result of the lack of central direction, and the development of geriatrics at scattered centres of excellence around the country, meant that the difference between the highest and lowest standards in geriatric care was also notable.

Speaking of those places around the country that had less enthusiastically embraced the approach of geriatrics, The Hospital Advisory Service (HAS) in a 1971 report suggested that a substantial number of elderly people who were assigned as 'disposal problems' or 'bed blockers' suffered from 'complicated medical' conditions, "many of which could be dealt with if a total approach to patient care [ie rehabilitation and active treatment] had been applied at the time of admission" (p6). The issue of bed blocking, then, is a symbol not only of the disparaging and dismissive attitudes of society in general, including that of biomedical science, to the condition of older people, and the struggle to determine boundaries with social care, but also of the conflict between geriatricians and other physicians. However, if we examine the issue carefully, we can see that the 'blocked bed', as well as being highly contestable as a concept is not at all what it appears. As Denham points out, units with more beds tended to be less efficient than those with less; in addition, older patients invariably preferred day hospitals to in-patient beds. W.L Graham (1951) concluded as a result of research carried out between 1950 and 1951 that bed blocking was a fallacy, a finding backed up at the time by other data (eg Amulree, 1955). There was some resistance to leaving long-stay beds by older people and their families for a variety of reasons such as having no alternative accommodation. Moreover, the manipulations to which waiting lists were subjected and the inaccuracies they contained – lists choked with people who had died and moved away or recovered or who did not even know they were on them - meant that they in turn did not serve as accurate indicators of unmet need (Denham, 1994) again calling into question the very notion that beds were unduly 'blocked'. Again, the difficulty in defining who classed as 'chronic sick' is itself bound up with the problems encountered in correct placement, both in beds and on waiting lists.

Unsurprisingly in a sub-specialty covering such a contested area, geriatricians continued to struggle with each other and with other doctors not only over organizational issues but also over issues that traversed organizational and epistemological boundaries such as the search for the normal versus the pathological in ageing together with the search for predictors of ill health in old age. The distinction between acute and chronic medicine also proved contentious. Stout believed it to be 'totally inappropriate' in the case of older people in particular to draw a distinction between acute and chronic illness and to have separate services for each (1979). As he explains, while chronic illness often starts with an acute episode, and relief of acute illness may in reality mean relieving an episode in a recurring process, in old age "if the acute illness does not itself produce chronic disability it often occurs against the background of disability from some other cause" (1979, p139).

Nevertheless, geriatrics not only survived but thrived by the turn of the century. From a total of four geriatricians in 1947, this had risen to over 300 by 1973 and 676 in 1995 to 1, 092 in 2006, the largest sub-specialty represented in the Royal College of Physicians. Assessing the achievements of geriatric medicine, Barton and Mulley (2003) identify several innovations pertaining to the sub-specialty which include the following themes: awareness of atypical and non-specific presentation of acute illness in old age; a whole person approach to older people with co-morbidity and complex disability; interdisciplinary team working and comprehensive geriatric assessment; the central importance of rehabilitation; recognition of caregivers' stress and the need for respite care.

Williamson saw geriatric medicine as having passed through three phases. The first phase includes the realization that the acute hospital environment was inimical to elderly patients; the second represents a move towards the community and away from institutional care. The third phase, in which geriatric medicine still finds itself, has been characterized by the development of Preventive Geriatric Care. Developed largely in Scotland, it "arose from the realization that old people often suffered from multiple disabilities which tended to present as a result of crises" (1979, p145) and focused on primary-care led detection and identification of high-risk older people. Let us examine this further.

Anticipatory Care of Older People in General Practice

As we have seen, the development of geriatrics during the twentieth century showed that successful rehabilitation is dependent on early admission which in turn is dependent on early detection. Williams (1986) assessed that, although direct evidence as to the extent of General Practitioners (GPs)' visiting old people in their homes was limited, the evidence pointed to an impression of patchy and variable visiting patterns that have if anything decreased over the course of the century. Inspired by the successes of geriatric hospital medicine, the focus in general practice turned to finding a role for the GP to complement that of the hospital geriatrician (Iliffe and Drennan, 2000). This has taken the form of an attempt to develop methods for routine surveillance and anticipatory care which in older people can take one or more of four forms – primary prevention; secondary prevention; tertiary prevention or case management; and health education for self care – and which is more likely to succeed in tertiary prevention. A survey of GPs in 1983 showed that only 10% were actually undertaking screening of older patients (Williams, 1983) and this partly reflected the ambivalence about the effectiveness of its methods, at least in terms of case finding amongst the population in general. Annual comprehensive geriatric assessments of patients aged 75 years and over were built into the 1990 GP contract but they failed to make a significant impact on the health of older people partly because of the lack of evidence base for these checks and the absence of any training programme for staff involved in these checks (Iliffe, 2001).

Reviewing a range of screening and surveillance methods in primary care, Kennie (1993) concludes that the benefits from comprehensive screening are doubtful resulting in slight but ultimately inconclusive improvements in morbidity and mortality. The effect on quality of life is marginal; no effect has been shown on functional status and while rates of institutionalization may be reduced, use of hospital may increase. Alternatively screening can focus on 'at risk' groups rather than on the elderly population in general and whilst benefits have been attested to in certain groups such as patients with congestive heart failure (Rich et al, 1995), this example of success is not generalizable to the extent that in other cases 'at risk groups' did not seem to have an excess of morbidity when compared with other older people and thus did not prove to be an accurate predictor of future illness (Iliffe and Drennan, 2000).

Iliffe and Drennan (2000) warn of the use of 'evidence-based guidelines' in primary care for older people; they also point out some concerns they have with another arm of the preventive strategy, that of self-care. Identifying five types of knowledge needed for effective self-care – namely diagnostic skills, treatment skills, chronic illness management, health promotion and knowing how to access services – they ask "is it ethical to impose an agenda of self-reliance on patients whose perceptions of need and support may be much different and much simpler?" (2001, p. 31)

Clearly the role of prevention in primary care as well as good management (and possibly, though contentiously of self-care) of conditions that have been identified is crucial, particularly in solving the issue of 'bed blocking' and the role of hospitals. We will return to this subject later. However, one of the problems here is that whilst understanding and solving social problems afflicting older people is also vital in the process of avoiding hospital admission, relationships between general practice and social services – also key in this process - were throughout this time particularly challenging and faced both organizational and cultural obstacles. Let us now turn to 'community care' and what is meant by it.

Community Care and Older People

The Local Authority Social Services Act of 1970 created Social Services Departments (LASSDs) "to meet the social needs of individuals, families and communities" (Seebohm Report, 1968, p. 96). Up to then, welfare had been under the control of the Ministry of Health; after this point LASSDs were responsible for residential homes for older people, home help services, meals, aids, adaptations and so on. In 1974 when the NHS underwent its first major reorganization with the Health Services Reorganization Act, home nursing was transferred from control of Local Authorities to the Health Authorities (HAs).

As we have noted, in talking about boundaries it is important to recognize differences not only in terms of financial implications but also in professional cultures and approaches to ageing. To that extent, the positive impact of the contribution of social care should not be underestimated, not only in keeping people out of hospital in the first place but in influencing attitudes towards both long-term care and of older people in general. Twigg (1997) has drawn attention to the countervailing ideas to the medical model, that posited the importance of the social in the overall welfare, including the health, of the individual. Thus, during the 1960s, the new certificate in Social Work courses "conveyed the significance of the needs of the elderly, the social and emotional effects of growing old, seeing that old people are people first, but recognising that they are also old, and that this can make a difference" (Jones, 1963, p6: quoted in Means and Smith (1985)). This focus on the collective, or structural, experience of ageing, by implication resists the 'medicalization' of life's problems, a trend which has been welcomed by disabled and older people themselves (eg Morris, 1991) and which challenges the more paternalistic culture of dependency associated with hospitals and medicine generally, wherein older people are treated as 'cases'. The flipside, however has been that the focus on the person's whole life has too easily leant itself to overtones of a moralising or normative nature with social workers seeking not to address the structural reasons for their problems but rather to 'normalize' them thereby rendering them more pliant or 'governable' (Rose, 1999).

Another important aspect of the qualitative nature of long-term care for older people derives from its domestic setting which is associated with two important factors determining the older person's experience of receiving care. Firstly, the home is private territory which gives the older person more power or control, at least over the environment, and his or her capacity to both manage in it as well as impose a sense of order over its routines. Secondly it is the locus of family life. It is the arena of lay expertise, autonomy, leisure and freedom from employment demands, which offers an alternative framework to professional values.

Two significant policy implications arise from this. Firstly, in its association with the domestic setting, social care has a weaker legitimacy; all welfare systems retain some sense of social care as an area of personal responsibility (Twigg, 1997) and thus it is more difficult to counterpose pressures to charge for it. This is indeed the experience of the UK where increasingly Local Authorities have had to charge the full economic rate for services to the better off (not necessarily the rich), as determined by stringent means testing. Thus in practice the boundary dispute has meant that the responsibility for funding long-term care, for many years, has been shifted covertly onto the older people themselves and their families (Henwood, 1992). Secondly, the importance of informal care-givers in propping up this system is vast and has been recognised as such in contemporary legislation: we will look at the history of their contribution in the section following on from this one.

As we have already described above, perverse incentives in the 1980s led to a vast increase in the use of residential care with public expenditure on private residential care soaring from £10 million in 1979 to the quite astonishing figure of £1872 million by 1991 (Laing and Buisson, 1979). Reform via the vehicle of the 1989 White Paper gave new responsibilities to the Social Worker, the aim being to encourage the provision of services so that people who would previously have been institutionalized could now remain in the community. The Act also introduced a new framework for delivering community care for adults with disabilities (including older people) in the form of assessment and case management (now called care management, partly to distinguish it from NHS-based case management), clearly stating a cost-cutting rationale: "Case management provides an effective method of targeting resources and planning services to meet specific needs of individual clients" (Paras 3.3.2 and 3.3.3.).

The care management model originated in North America during the 1970s and 1980s out of concern with service fragmentation and cost-containment in long-term care (Zawadski and Eng, 1988) but was introduced into England by the Department of Health (DH) largely through the research findings of the Personal Social Services Research Unit at the University of Kent (Means and Smith, 1994) and their evaluation of care management pilot projects in Kent and Gateshead (see Challis et al, 1995; Challis and Davies, 1986). Both of the latter projects were aimed at frail elderly people at risk of entering residential or nursing home care and Challis (1989) proposed the following set of core tasks for care management: case finding and screening; assessment; care planning and monitoring; review. Case finding was particularly complex and required both the use of guidelines and application of professional discretion (Challis et al, 1995). Elsewhere in the country, multifarious models were emerging, distinguished by such factors as whether or not care managers themselves provided care or simply acted as brokers, the nature of accountabilities, the degree of control over resources, the agency in which the care manager was based, the extent to which agencies were able to pool resources. The Audit Commission's 1992 report identified seven typologies; in all these types, however, informal carers played a prominent role.

The multiplicity of models if anything increased following the implementation of the NHS and Community Care Act whose lack of detailed guidance contributed further to this wide variation in interpretation (Challis et al, 2007). These differences remain in care management models today. Although care management advocates the use of health staff to work as care managers where appropriate, Weiner et al (2003)'s recent survey of care management arrangements indicate that health staff involvement is in practice relatively limited, except in the case of older people with mental health problems, where Community Psychiatric Nurses are often involved. The focus of these staff in addition is generally on assessment rather than long-term care management. Moreover, the lack of resources means that they are focused on those with the most pressing needs, thereby reducing the possibility of preventive and rehabilitative work accordingly (Iliffe and Drennan, 2001) as social care is associated with a more reactive approach.

INFORMAL CARE OF OLDER PEOPLE WITH COMPLEX HEALTH PROBLEMS

From the outset – whether at the time of the Poor Law, the heyday of residential care or following the introduction of a mixed economy of welfare - care in the community has largely meant care 'by' the community, in fact wives and daughters. Introducing care management in1989 the White Paper recognized the continuing place of carers in making this possible: "the great bulk of community care is provided by friends, family and neighbours." Older people with complex health problems have always been supported in the community by family and detailed information about this fact has been available for many years (eg Sheldon, 1948; Townsend, 1957; Shanas et al, 1968). Many of the carers of older people have always been themselves older and with increasing longevity this is likely to be even more the case (see STG, 1996).

For many years, an important argument against the funding by government of the development of domiciliary services was the 'moral panic' claims that this would displace the 'natural' duties of family to undertake caring activities. Alternative arguments emphasized that without such development, family members might give up altogether under the severe strain thereby casting total responsibility for sick older people onto the state (eg. Moroney, 1976).With the change in the structure of the family – located geographically further apart, with daughters more likely to work outside the home – combined with the increasing longevity of older people, this acquired a particular urgency. These arguments were eventually convincing enough for governments to declare a new commitment to help informal care-givers. The NHS and Community Care Act (1990) affirmed the pivotal role of carers in terms professing an official appreciation while the Carers (Recognition and Services) Act, 1995 established the principle of assessing the particular needs of information, advice and practical support. The Carers and Disabled Children Act (2000) gave carers new rights to assessment and service independently of the person they look after, indicating that carers are considered integral to the way services are provided for older people. Finally, the Carers (Equal Opportunities) Act, 2004 facilitated cooperation between authorities in relation to the provision of services that are relevant to carers. Nevertheless, such support remains normative in the sense that it is intended to make it possible for informal carers to continue in their caring role and there is no question that they be substituted by formal services.

General Household Survey (GHS) data and other research (eg Pickard and Glendinning, 2000; 2002) carried out since this policy has indicated that much of what carers, many of them older themselves, carried out for relatives and friends comprises health care tasks, some of which have blurred with nursing roles. 53% of family carers assist with personal care activities, 46% give medication, 46% give physical help and 79% have to supervise the care-recipient (Green, 1988). Carers also undertake health care procedures across a whole range from giving medication and changing dressings to renal dialysis, colostomy and stoma care and parenteral feeding (Pickard et al, 2003) with or without the aid of health care professionals. They are therefore key allies in the work done by both health and social care professionals, both in the hospital – making it possible to discharge older people in the first place – and out in the community where they work alongside and with health professionals, with the latter having been criticized by researchers for treating them as 'resources' rather than experts (eg Nolan et al, 1995). As it is likely that carers will continue to play an important role in long-term care for older people, for the foreseeable future, it will be important to find ways of working with them in ways that will support them most effectively in their role. After all without them it is unlikely that either the NHS or Social Services would be able to cope with the long-term care needs of older people at all within the current resource constraints.

NHS-Led Case Management of Older People

Policy Background

The foundations of case management of older people were lain with The NHS Plan of 2000 (DH, 2000) which proposed new money to meet the needs of the intermediates and to develop new roles for health professionals to better serve these needs. We can see from our review how this commitment is exceptional in terms of the history of long-term care of older people, constituting the first time that the NHS had explicitly acknowledged its own inadequacies in this respect *and* taken responsibility to ameliorate them by increasing the scope of its role. The reason for this commitment was, however, not unusual at all: bed blocking had returned to the to the top of the policy agenda again at this time because the reduction in beds for older people (by 38% between 1983 and the mid-1990s) combined with a new pledge by the incoming government to reduce waiting times for NHS hospitals' admission for all categories of patient was unsustainable without some direct intervention into long-term care (3% of patients over 65 accounted for 35% of hospital admissions (Hutt et al, 2004).). This was compatible with the priority placed on chronic disease management, much of it inspired by examples from the USA: the aim of both chronic disease management generally and long-term care of older people in particular was to be reduction of hospital bed use.

Subsequently case management was developed through later publications including the NHS Improvement Plan (DH, 2004), the new General Medical Services Contract (April, 2004), Supporting People with Long-term Conditions (DH, 2005a) and others (eg, DH, 2005b). In terms of older people specifically, case management was also consistent with the aims of the National Service Framework for Older People which was published in 2001 (DH, 2001) as part of a raft of guidelines which set national standards and defined service models for specific patient groups. Among other things, this initiative promoted provision of person-centred care and the promotion of older people's independence and dignity whilst receiving services.

The Evercare model, adapted from a US prototype was piloted in 2003-4 to test the efficacy of case management in reducing the number of unplanned hospital admissions; subsequently its principles were introduced nationally, with license given for local conditions and variants. The NHS Improvement Plan promised recruitment of 3,000 community matrons using case-management to care for around 250,000 patients with complex needs (DH, 2004) and who were to provide "clinical intervention as well as care co-ordination" (DH, 2005a, p16) to vulnerable, very high intensity patients at greatest risk of admissions to hospital, which, it had already been noted, was a group largely composed of older people.

The Model

Based on the 'Kaiser Permanente Triangle' case management is aimed at 'level three' patients, or those suffering from chronic complex co-morbidities (DH, 2005a). The basic five principles of the case management are: definition of a target population; individual assessment and care planning; regular monitoring of patients and care group; ad-hoc interventions when incipient deterioration is found; exit or discharge from case management. Department of Health guidance (DH 2005a) advised that "Evercare is one model of case management" and that "Health and social care organizations should adopt the principles of case management set out in this document rather than any particular model" (DH, 2005a, p14). Since its introduction, variations across models have developed in terms of different use of pre-defined protocols; use of different instruments to predict risk and manage patient care; different health professionals – usually nurses but sometimes pharmacists - taking on the case management role; different approaches to monitoring and using information systems; differences in when and whether patients are discharged. With these provisos, then, the five elements of case management will now be discussed in more detail, taking descriptive data from an evaluation of the Evercare model and some selected variants carried out by a team based at Manchester, York and Sheffield Universities, of which the author was a member, from 2003-6 (see Boaden et al, 2006 for more details of methodology and remit)[2].

The model, essentially a model for tertiary prevention, was composed of the five elements described above and involved ongoing refinement of methods for, inter alia, discovering at risk groups; classifying patients according to their risk potential; carrying out more or less intensive surveillance of patients according to perceived risk; and making decisions about when and whether sufficient stability had been attained for the patient and their carer to be able to self-manage successfully and thus be discharged from the case management load. None of these elements were unproblematic and over the course of the evaluation were subject to significant modification, as we see below.

i. Identifying the Target Group

Sites initially selected patients on the basis of the patients' age (over 65 years old) and two or more emergency admissions in the previous year. However, as time progressed, and in non-Evercare sites, the selection criteria varied between sites, often including subjective qualitative judgments made by clinicians about patients' suitability for case management, and including meeting one or more of the following supplementary criteria, as the clinician (usually the GP) saw fit (and which could be broadened or narrowed, depending on capacity): exacerbation or decompensation of chronic illness within the past 90 days; two or more falls in the past two months; recent bereavement (death of spouse or family member in past 6 months) and at risk of medical decline; cognitively impaired; living alone; medically unstable; and requirement for high intensity social service package.

ii. Classification

Patients were assessed using structured assessment tools and a physical examination. The specialist nurse, or community matron acting as case manager, would then agree an

[2] The evaluation was funded by the Department of Health through core funding of National Primay Care Research and Development Centre

individualized care plan with the patient, their GP and other staff, a plan which was modified over time in accordance to the perceived requirements of the patient.

iii. Risk Surveillance

This involved regular monitoring of patients depending on risk classification. In addition, patients were able to maintain regular contact with case managers by mobile phone and to call for reassurance or immediate access to a specialist opinion. Primary Care Trust [3](PCT)-level monitoring of patients was very difficult, however, owing to the poor availability of data and information systems so meaningful data was only collected for individuals rather than the general population of older people, as had been originally intended.

iv. Intervention

Ad hoc intervention took place when incipient deterioration was found. Case managers reported many examples in which they had altered medication to avoid adverse reactions, co-ordinated care to reduce fragmentation among services, improved patient functional status, improved quality of life, avoided hospital admissions and referred patients to a range of other services, including social care, where necessary (where barriers to joint working proved challenging at times, considerably slowing down the process).

v. Exit/Discharge

Although in the original model patients were intended to stay on the case manager's caseload for life this was subsequently modified to discharging patients who were deemed stable and no longer 'at risk', although they could self-refer back if their condition changed.

Assessment of the Case Management Approach to Long-Term Care

We will examine four key aspects of this model: implications for primary care; the impact on the boundary between health and social care; relations between primary care and hospital care; effectiveness of the model in keeping older people out of hospital.

a) A New Role for Anticipatory Methods in Primary Care

The introduction of case management has created a new specialist community nursing role for older people very much distinguished from other nursing roles in being proactive, rather than reactive, and utilizing surveillance techniques in order to anticipate potential future health care problems in high-risk groups. Unlike the 75 years and over comprehensive geriatric assessment approach, it targets specific 'at risk' individuals on the GPs' list and aims to be holistic and centred on the individual's own 'norm'. It involves carers in the process and aims to teach self-management skills with an emphasis on self-care that will ultimately make the role of the case manager unnecessary.

---

[3] Since 2002, PCTs, which cover all parts of England and receive budgets directly from the DH, havae taken control of local healthcare, both purchasing and providing

b) Co-Ordination of Health with Social Care

Collaboration with social care staff proved problematic owing to separate and onerous bureaucratic procedures, heightened by the need to cross rigid boundaries. Case managers were not authorised to directly access equipment and in some sites even the most basic items such as commodes and toilet seats raisers required an Occupational Therapy (OT) assessment which could take up to a year. Delays were reported in referrals for Social Workers (SWs) and case managers also noted that social workers did not always comprehend nurse definitions of 'urgent' contributing to delays in social care – a well-noted difference in professional cultures. However, collaborative relationships between health and social care professionals sometimes facilitated the crossing of this bureaucratic divide; case managers sometimes succeeded in obtaining urgent social worker assessments by telephoning Social Services staff and informing them a hospital admission was otherwise imminent. Thus, many patients and carer comments show a high level of satisfaction with the case manager's role in the rapid installation of showers, stair lifts, safety rails and the quick delivery of basic home care equipment and their advocacy on the behalf of the patient and carer with local authorities to have environmental hazards such as uneven footpaths rectified were identified as a very valued role.

Indeed, case managers had to deal to such an extent with 'non-medical' problems that they found themselves taking on a large portion of 'social care' including psycho-social care and in particular the allaying of anxiety but also defined in terms of the kind of engagement this involved with patients and carers. The latter described their nurse as 'like your friend' or 'like a daughter' and community matrons also played a separate but equally important role in supporting carers in their own right with carers often expressing how she had 'taken the pressure off', helped to ease their stress and anxiety and helped them cope with the practical and emotional demands of informal care-giving. Along the same lines, community matrons noted that their advanced physical examination and assessment skills were utilised less as their case-loads stabilised, with a shift towards giving social support. While some disliked this, feeling that they were thereby being turned into 'social workers', others placed a positive emphasis on the 'whole-person' approach, which distinguished them both from other kinds of specialist nurses and from GPs and thought the contrast with the 'medical model' highly valuable and worth preserving and building on.

There was also, however, a structured aspect to health and social care collaboration built into the model. Guidance by the Department of Health indicates that patients should be stepped down, according to their needs. Thus, along with Level Three patients there are Level Two patients, frail and in need of care input but not judged at immediate risk of institutional admission. Level Two patients, the guidance (2005a) says will be cared for by multi-professional teams based in primary or community care employing disease specific care management. Both will, where appropriate, require input from social care agencies. The Level One patient is deemed capable of self-management. Patients at different levels are distinguished by treatment approaches, the case management being 'anticipatory' and the care management 'responsive'. However, the evaluation found no evidence of any 'step down' approach to case management, patients being discharged from the case manager's list without referral to another agency. Again, this indicates problems in effecting a 'joined-up' approach between health and social care, and a structural emphasis on collaboration in practice will require this co-operation on the ground if a joint approach is to exist in reality.

c) *Relationships Between Community Matrons and Secondary Care Providers*

One somewhat surprising finding that emerged from the evaluation was the way that building and sustaining good relationships with secondary care clinicians proved on balance to be more problematic than the negotiation of social care boundaries. Once patients had been admitted into hospital, the community matron was often not contacted, as had been the intended plan of action, sometimes because the pressure of the obligatory four-hour target in Accident and Emergency (A&E) meant there was not sufficient time to do so. Whilst case managers were involved in discharge procedures they were unable to influence the length of stay, which remained determined by secondary care clinicians alone, who, moreover, displayed a poor awareness both of community-based services and of home environments, usually contributing to the delay. Indeed, the challenges involved in influencing hospital working practices proved to be so intractable that eventually reduction of length hospital stay was dropped from the set of stated aims of the model altogether.

d) *Impact on Hospital Admissions and Length of Stay*

This is the crux of the model and the key reason for its establishment. Many case managers and patients in the evaluation provided evidence of averted admissions, forestalled by perceptive and timely intervention. However, when controlled statistical analyses of hospital admissions data from the sites were carried out they detected no significant reduction in admission rates overall (Gravelle et al, 2006). This is consistent with the findings of other studies of case management (eg Elkan et al, 2001) and with what we know about the high probability of risk falling outside 'at risk' groups. Another possibility, again consistent with previous evidence, may lie in the surveillance process uncovering unmet need which then requires hospitalisation. Perhaps the key question is not, then, did the model unblock beds but: did the model save lives? Anecdotal data from descriptive accounts given by case managers, patients and carers alike suggest that indeed it did. But this, unfortunately, cannot easily be proven from statistical data.

Discussion

What then, can we say about the most recent provision for long-term care in the UK? Having set out earlier in the chapter the antecedents of policy and practice we can attempt here to make an assessment of its continuity and change with respect to what has come before. This will then enable a judgment to be reached concerning the underlying theoretical approach(es) contained in the model and that underlie professional attitudes and policy approaches; and finally we can suggest a tentative conclusion for its significance in terms of policies towards older people in late modern society.

The overall impression is that elements of continuity with what has come before are plentiful; they often appear in a somewhat tweaked version, however, in ways that introduce change almost 'by the back door'. For example, with the continued presence of the bed blocking motif the 'burden of ageing' thesis remains dominant among policy makers and perhaps medical professionals too; however the aim of reducing older people's use of *acute* beds distinguishes this from all previous approaches and suggests an ever narrowing role for hospitals in the care of older people. Community matrons have a 'specialist' role – and a more highly developed one than previous nurses - indicating a fundamental consistency with the expressed role of the NHS as stated in 1995. In the attempt to keep older people from over-utilizing hospital beds, the efficient working across professional and organizational boundaries remains as crucial as ever; as always, it throws up challenges relating to bureaucratic and cultural divides which can, nevertheless, be overcome in some cases by the establishing of good relationships between individual professionals on the front-line. However the lack of a co-ordinated approach between health and social care in practice has meant that a stepped approach, whereby the patient can pass from care of a health professional to care of a social worker when judged no longer at immediate risk, does not necessarily seem to be happening. But what leaps out as new in this boundary issue is the difficulty experienced by primary care nurses in working with secondary care nurses and doctors. This perhaps indicates that the distinction between 'care' and 'cure' and the difference in professional cultures associated with both is even less easy to override or negotiate than is the distinction between health and social care when both are located firmly in the community and thus exposed to a 'whole person' in their individual context. In addition, current UK policy surrounding the role of hospitals more generally is intended to make hospitals more acute than ever, with less complex care, previously situated in hospitals, moving out into the community wherever possible (DH, 2006). Thus policy towards older people is consistent here with policy concerning the future role of hospitals more generally.

As far as geriatric medicine is concerned, the current model represents the further development of classificatory techniques to distinguish, this time not the 'chronics' from the others, nor different degrees of chronics from each other, but those at risk of becoming ill. This more than ever blurs the distinction between acute and chronic illness; it also attracts biomedical science to examining the conditions of old age – perhaps to continue that debate about the normal versus the pathological in old age – and at another level altogether.

As far as the older person and their carer is concerned, what Foucault called 'technologies of the self' proceed apace. Thus, in the same way Denham's study (1994) described how older people were unwilling to leave their long-stay beds, patients in our study feared more than anything having to go to hospital. Their wishes, and the intentions of case managers and thence policy makers, are thus happily aligned. As one perceptive older gentleman pointed out:

> "I think she was asked to call on me with a view to keeping me out of hospital, which really works both ways, for the hospital and for the older people. Cos old people don't like going in hospital, it makes us feel frightened."

CONCLUSION

For those who may see community care as a solution to the problems of the US health care system, it is important to look at the problems associated with a large social care component to long-term care, as occur in the British NHS. There are clear benefits as we have seen but also issues including financial implications for the older person and a lack of medical care and rehabilitation which might be of benefit. The review has also demonstrated the somewhat artificial nature of issues presented as 'inherent' to the condition of ageing itself and revealed them as constructs arising from policy priorities and professional disputes both of which have had the effect of rendering questions of actual service composition secondary.

The particular significance of the latest UK NHS-led long-term care model is in the framing of illness in old age within the risk paradigm. There is a shift from viewing old age predominantly as a 'burden' on society and the economy in the light of the fact that the era of collective state responsibility for its older citizens appears to be drawing to an end. The focus is more on the risk they pose and their potential to become a residual burden by requiring care. Thus the surveillance gaze is replacing the gaze of welfare and we can expect to see in future more and more emphasis on self-care and on the 'morality' of managing one's own health and illness. In this sense, there is a very real argument to be made that, for some portion of the ageing population, old age and sickness (current, known or unnoticed, or future) are once again undistinguished. We can expect to see similar developments in health care systems based on insurance, including private insurance, also, as companies and managed care organizations seek to reduce their expenses. This model, after all, was based on one originating in the US, with these very aims.

The development of anticipatory or preventive medicine, then, as represented in its most sophisticated form yet by this model, is an essential element of the machinery of measuring and calculating risk in late modernity. As Gilleard and Higgs have noted, while it has great benefits it also has negative attributes which should not be overlooked as:

> "In Britain, and in other countries this has meant that surveillance (health screening) has become almost as mandatory at the age of 75 as retirement is at age 65, potentially transforming the older person's body into little more than an object of health-care discourse" (2000, p104).

REFERENCES

Amulree, L. (1955), Modern Hospital Treatment and the Pensioner, *Lancet*, 2: 572-575.

Armstrong, D. (1981) Pathological Life and Death: Medical Spatialisation and Geriatrics, *Social Science and Medicine*, 15A: 253-7.

Barton, A. and Mulley, G. (2003) History of the Development of Geriatric Medicine in the UK, *Journal of Postgraduate Medicine*, 79: 229-234.

Beck, U. (1992) *Risk Society: towards a new modernity*. London: Sage.

Beveridge Report (1942) *Social Insurance and Allied Services*, London: HMSO.

Boaden, R., Dusheiko, M., Gravelle, H. et al. (2006). *Evaluation of Evercare: Final Report.* Manchester: National Primary Care Research and Development Centre.

Boucher Report (1957) *Survey of Services Available to the Chronic Sick and Elderly 1954-55*, Reports on Public Health and Medical Subjects No. 98, London: HMSO.

Bridgen, P. and Lewis, J. (1999) *Elderly People and the Boundary between Health and Social Care 1946-1991*, London: Nuffield Trust.

British Medical Association (1955) *Appendix IX Report of the Geriatrics Joint Subcommittee of the British Medical Association. BMJ (supplement)*, 1: 181-190.

British Medical Association: Board of Science and Education (1976) *Care of the Elderly.* London: British Medical Association.

Challis, D. (1989) *Case management: problems and possibilities.* Unpublished paper given at Policy Studies Institute seminar on care management.

Challis, D., et al. (1995) *Care management and health care of older people.* Aldershot: Arena.

Challis, D., Hughes, J., Jacobs, S., et al. (2007) Are different forms of care-management for older people in England associated with variations in case-mix, service use and care-managers' use of time? *Ageing and Society*. 27, 25-48.

Charcot, J.M. (translated by Hunt, L.H.) (1882) *Clinical Lectures on the Diseases of Old Age.* London: Sampson Low, Marston and Searle and Rivington.

Clarke, S.C., Badenoch, J., Winner, D.A., et al. (1977) Medical Care of the Elderly, *Lancet,* 1:1092-5.

Cmnd 1973 (1963) *Health and Welfare: the development of community care.*

Cmnd. 1604 (1962) *A Hospital Plan for England and Wales.*

Cole, T.R (1992) *The Journey of Life: A cultural history of aging in America.* Cambridge: Cambridge University Press.

Denham, M. (2004) *The History of Geriatric Medicine and Hospital Care of the Elderly in England between 1929 and the 1970s* London: PhD, University College London.

Department of Health (1989) *Caring for People: Community Care in the Next Decade and Beyond,* London: HMSO.

Department of Health (2000) *NHS Plan*. London: HMSO.

Department of Health. (2001) *The National Service Framework for Older People.* London: HMSO.

Department of Health. (2004). *NHS Improvement Plan.* London: HMSO.

Department of Health. (2005(a)) *Supporting People with Long-term conditions: an NHS and Social Care Model to support local innovation and integration*. London: HMSO.

Department of Health. (2005(b)). Supporting People with Long-Term Conditions: Liberating the Talents of Nurses who Care for People with Long-Term conditions. London: HMSO.

Department of Health (2006) *Our Health, Our Care, Our Say*. London: HMSO.

Department of Health and Social Security (1971) *The Report of the Hospital Advisory Service,* London: HMSO.

Estes, C.L. (1979) *The Aging Enterprise*. San Francisco: Jossey Bass.

Estes, C.L. and Binney, E.A. (1989) The biomedicalization of aging: dangers and dilemmas. *The Gerontologist*, 29 (5): 587-596.

Estes, C.L. and Phillipson, C. (2002) The Globalization of Capital, the Welfare State and Old age Policy. *International Journal of Health Services*, 32(2):279-297.

Fennell, G., Phillipson, C. and Evers, H. (1988) *The Sociology of Old Age*, Milton Keynes: Open University Press.

Foucault, M. (1975). (translated 1979) *Discipline and Punish: The Birth of the Prison*. New York: Vintage Books.

Giddens, A. (1991). *Modernity and Self-identity: self and society in the late modern age.* Cambridge: Polity Press.

Giddens, A. (1998). *The Third Way*, Cambridge: Polity Press

Gilleard, C. and Higgs, P. (2000) *Cultures of ageing: self, citizen and the body*, Harlow: Prentice Hall.

Graham, W.L. (1951). Length of Stay of Elderly in Hospitals, *Lancet*, 2: 931-932

Gravelle, H., Dusheiko, M., Sheaff, R., et al. (2006). Impact of case management (Evercare) on frail elderly patients. 1. Controlled before and after analysis of quantitative outcome data. *British Medical Journal*, doi:10.1136/bmj.39020.413310.55 (published 15.11.2006).

Habermas, J. (1976). *Legitimation Crisis*. London: Heinemann.

Hall, D. and Bytheway, B. (1982) The Blocked Bed: Definition of the Problem. *Social Science and Medicine* 16: 1985-1991.

Harrison, J. (1992) *Geriatric Medicine in South Birmingham: 1992-1997 and beyond*. A report to the Chief Executive. Birmingham: South Birmingham Health Authority.

Henwood, M. (1992). Twilight Zone. *Health Services Journal* ,5 November, 28-30.

Hicks, P. (1998) *The policy challenge of aging populations*. OECD Observer 212..

Hutt, R, Rosen, R. and McCauley, J. (2004) *Case-managing long-term conditions: what impact does it have in the treatment of older people?* London: King's Fund.

Iliffe, S. and Drennan, V. (2000) *Primary Care for Older People*, Oxford: Oxford University Press.

Iliffe, S. and Lenihan, P. (2001) Promoting innovative primary care for older people in general practice using a community-oriented approach, *Primary Health Care Research and Development*, 2:71-9.

Jones, R.H. (1963) *Discussion of the need for more adequate teaching of Gerontology in the Training of Social Workers*. International Society of Gerontology Conference, Copenhagen, mimeo.

Katz, S. (1996) *Disciplining old age: the formation of gerontological knowledge*. Charlottesville and London: University of Virginia Press.

Kennie, D.C. (1993) *Preventive Care for Elderly People*. Cambridge: Cambridge University Press.

Laing and Buisson (1992) *Laing's Review of Private Health Care*, 1992. London: Laing and Buisson.

Land, H. (2001) Future expectations of care in old age. In Robinson, J (Ed) *Towards a New Social Compact for Care in Old age*, pp47-65. London: King's Fund.

Leonard, J.C. (1976) Can geriatrics survive? *British Medical Journal*, 1: 1335-1336

Lewis, J. (2001) Older People and the Health-Social Care Boundary in the UK: half a century of hidden policy conflict. *Social Policy and Administration*, 35 (4) 343-359.

Lewis, J. and Glennerster, H. (1996) *Implementing the new community care*, Buckingham: Open University Press.

Lowe, C.R and McKeown, T. (1950) The Care of the Chronic Sick. II Social and Demographic Data. *British Journal of Social Medicine*, 4:61-74.

Lye, M. (1982) Geriatric Medicine and Medical Unemployment, *Journal of the Royal College of Physicians of London*, 16: 129-131.

Lynham, R. (1995). *Currents in Geriatric Medicine in the United Kingdom*, Synopsis of a presentation given at the Wilhelm Woort Stiftung Symposium, Cologne 21 June.

Marshall, T.H. (1950) *Citizenship and Social Class and other essays*. Cambridge: Cambridge University Press.

Matthews, D. (1984) Dr Marjory Warren and the origin of British geriatrics, *Journal of the American Geriatrics Society*, 32: 253-8.

Means, R. (2001) Lessons from the history of long-term care for older people. In J.Robinson (Ed) *Towards a new social compact for care in old age*, pp9-27. London: King's Fund.

Means, R. and Smith, R..(1994) *Community Care: Policy and Practice*. London: Macmillan.

Ministry of Health (1934) *Annual Report of the Chief Medical Officer 1933*. London: HMSO.

Ministry of Health (1951) Emergency Admissions to Hospital. RHB, (51) 115; HMC, (51) 107. London: Ministry of Health.

Ministry of Health (1952). Report of the Ministry of Health Part 1 for Period 1st April 1950-31st December 1951. London: HMSO.

Minkler, M. and Estes, C. (1991) *Critical Perspectives on Ageing: the Political and Moral Economy of Growing Old.* (Eds.) New York: Baywood.

Morley, J.E. (2004) A Brief History of Geriatrics, *The Journals of Gerontology* Series A: Biological Sciences and Medical Sciences, 59:1132-1152.

Moroney, R. (1976) *The family and the state*. London: Longman.

Morris, J. (1991) *Pride Against Prejudice: transforming attitudes to disability*. London: Women's Press.

Perkin, H. (1989) The Rise of Professional Society: England since 1880, London: Routledge.

Phillipson, C. (1982) Capitalism and the Construction of Old Age: London: Macmillan.

Phillipson, C. (1998) *Reconstructing Old Age,* London: Sage.

Pickard, S., Jacob, S., and Kirk, S. (2003). Challenging Professional Roles: Lay Carers' Involvement in Health Care in the Community. *Health and Social Care in the Community*. 37 (1), 82-96.

Pickard, S., Shaw, S. and Glendinning, C. (2000). Health care professionals' support for older carers. *Ageing and Society*, 20: 725-744.

Pickard, S. and Glendinning, C. (2002). Comparing and contrasting the role of family carers and nurses in the domestic health care of frail older people. *Health and Social Care in the Community*, 10 (3): 144-150.

PRO MH99/21 (1961) *Memorandum on discussions with RHBs on bed norms*, 30 June 1961.

Rhodes, R.A.W. (1997) *Understanding Governance: Policy Networks, Governance, Reflexivity and Accountability*. Buckingham: Open University Press.

Rich, M.W., Beekham, V., Wittenberg, C., et al (1995) A multidisciplinary intervention to prevent the readmission of elderly patients with congestive heart failure, *New England Journal of Medicine*, 333: 1190-5.

Rose, N. (1999) *Powers of Freedom,* Cambridge: Cambridge University Press.

Shanas, E., Townsend, P., Wedderburn, D., et al. (1968) *Old People in Three Industrialised Societies*. London: Routledge and Kegan Paul.

Sheldon, J. (1948) *The Social Medicine of Old Age*, London: Oxford University Press.

Steering Committee on Future Health Scenarios (STG). (1996) *The Elderly in 2005: Health and Care. Updated Scenarios on Health and Aging 1990-2005.* Holland: Steering Committee on Future Health Scenarios.

Stout, R.W. Hospital Care of the Elderly: General or Geriatric Medicine? *Age and Ageing*, 3(8):137-140.

Titmuss, R. (1968) *Commitment to Welfare*. London: Allen and Unwin.

Titmuss, R (1976 edition) *Problems of Social Policy*, London: HMSO.

Townsend, P. (1957) *The family life of old people*. Harmondsworth: Penguin.

Townsend, P. (1981) The Structured Dependency of the Elderly: A creation of social policy in the twentieth century. *Ageing and Society* 1(1): 5-28.

Twigg, J. (1997) Deconstructing the 'social bath': help with bathing at home for older and disabled people. *Journal of Social Policy,* 26 (2): 211-232.

Walker, A. (1981) Towards a Political Economy of Old Age. *Ageing and Society*, 1: 73-94.

Walker, A. (1999) Public Policy and Theories of Aging: Constructing and Reconstuction Old Age. In V. Bengtson and W Schaie (Eds) *Handbook of Theories of Aging*, (pp361-378) New York: Springer.

Warren, M. (1943) Care of the Chronic Sick. British Medical Journal i:822-3

Weiner, K., Hughes, J., Challis, D., and Pedersen, I. (2003) Integrating Health and Social Care at the Micro Level: Health Care Professionals as Care Managers for Older People. *Social Policy and Administration*, 37 (5): 498-515.

Williams, E.I. (1986) The Evolution of Anticipatory Care for Elderly Patients in General Practice, *Family Practice*, 3 (1): 49-53.

Williams, E.I. (1983) The general practitioner and the disabled, *Journal of the Royal College of General Practice*, 33: 296-299.

Williamson, J. (1979) Notes on the Historical Development of Geriatric Medicine as a Specialty, *Age and Ageing*, 3, (8): 144-148.

World Bank (1994) *Averting the Old Age Crisis*, Oxford: Oxford University Press,

Zawadski and Eng (1988) Case management in capitated long-term care. *Health Care Financing Review Special Supplement.*

In: Social Sciences in Health Care and Medicine ISBN: 978-1-60456-286-6
Editors: J. B. Garner, T. C. Christiansen, pp. 117-138

Chapter 4

ADVANCES IN PRIORITY SETTING METHODS AND THE PROGRAMME BUDGETING AND MARGINAL ANALYSIS (PBMA) FRAMEWORK

***Stuart Peacock*[1, 2]*, Craig Mitton*[3,4]*, Cam Donaldson*[5,6] *and Angela Bate*[5]**

[1]Centre for Health Economics in Cancer, British Columbia Cancer Agency
[2]Department of Health Care and Epidemiology, University of British Columbia
[3]Faculty of Health and Social Development, University of British Columbia Okanagan
[4]Child and Family Research Institute of British Columbia
[5]Institute of Health and Society, Newcastle University
[6]Business School (Economics), Newcastle University

ABSTRACT

Programme budgeting and marginal analysis (PBMA) is as an explicit, robust, and practical tool to assist decision-makers in setting priorities in health care. The PBMA framework has been used in at least 70 health service organisations across the UK, Australia, and Canada over the last 25 years. In this chapter, we synthesise experiences from these countries in both developing the PBMA framework and implementing the results of PBMA exercises. In particular, we have found the methods used in PBMA are now less mechanistic than they have been in the past, recognising the need to balance pragmatic and ethical considerations with economic rationality. We identify and discuss international consistencies and controversies in the treatment of these considerations, as well as, international challenges in the application of the PBMA framework in local health service organisations. Finally, we describe a framework for pragmatic study design in PBMA studies, based on lessons learnt from the practical application of PBMA, including institutional and managerial challenges in health systems.

INTRODUCTION

Decisions concerning the allocation of health care resources (herein referred to as priority setting) are guided both explicitly and implicitly by local health service managers and clinicians. However, local health service organisations often lack knowledge of economic tools to aid the process of priority setting. In the context of making decisions over the use of scarce health care resources, economic tools have much to offer. From an economic perspective, there are some basic principles to which any priority setting framework should adhere: they should consider opportunity cost and 'the margin'. Programme budgeting and marginal analysis (PBMA) is one such economic tool that encompasses these principles and provides a framework to aid local decision-makers in setting health service priorities [1-3].

The intent of PBMA is to provide assistance to local decision-makers in directing resources in order to maximise benefits from health services. [4]. In doing so, PBMA considers both opportunity cost and resource shifts 'at the margin'. Most importantly, PBMA is the only priority setting framework that applies these economic principles where resource scarcity actually bites – at the local level. It is local managers and clinicians who have to bear the opportunity cost of resource reallocation decisions elsewhere in their budgets.

The PBMA framework has been used in health care for almost three decades, in at least 70 health authorities across the UK, Australia, and Canada [5]. Use of the framework in these countries has grown significantly since 1990 [6], and has been accompanied by a number of advances in the methods used in PBMA. Methods are now less mechanistic than they have been in the past, recognising the need to balance pragmatic and ethical considerations with economic rationality.

However, despite the widespread use of PBMA, comparative analysis of the application of PBMA in different contexts in the priority setting literature is limited. Conversely, the priority setting literature has given significant attention to other tools such as needs assessment, core services, health economic evaluation, and cost-per-Quality Adjusted Life Year (QALY) league tables. This is perhaps surprising as such approaches have been criticised on economic grounds [7-9] and have only enjoyed limited or moderate success in practice [10, 11]. In particular, local health service organisations - such as health authorities, health maintenance organisations, primary care trusts and hospitals - have had difficulty implementing evidence from economic appraisals [12, 13]. An important message from this literature is the need to be practical, and not to expect universal uptake of mechanistic approaches to priority setting [6]. The PBMA framework, we argue, provides decision-makers with an approach to health care priority setting that is both principled and pragmatic [3].

In this chapter we therefore focus specifically on PBMA, examining recent international advances in the methods used in PBMA studies and the lessons to be learnt for decision-makers and researchers. It is timely to take stock of both shared and individual lessons from different contexts, so that decision-makers and researchers can learn from each other's experiences. It is important to draw on these international experiences to: identify accomplishments and challenges in the application of PBMA; examine the relative merits of methodological advances and place them within the PBMA framework; and provide a focus for future research on priority setting.

The purpose of this chapter is to synthesise the international evidence on recent advances in PBMA methods, and the implementation of their results. More specifically, the chapter aims to: (i) identify international consistencies and controversies in the treatment of pragmatic and ethical considerations under the PBMA framework; (ii) identify international challenges in the application of PBMA for priority setting in local health service organisations; and (iii) describe a framework for pragmatic study design in PBMA studies, based on lessons learnt from the practical application of PBMA, including institutional and managerial challenges in health systems.

The chapter draws on evidence and our experiences from:

1) earlier review of the PBMA literature describing the outcomes of over 70 PBMA studies [5],
2) our experiences of conducting and evaluating approximately 35 such studies in the UK, Australia, and Canada (for examples see [14-19]), and
3) conducting over 100 priority setting workshops with decision-makers in the last 15 years.

Finally, it is also worth noting that we are not discussing PBMA as a framework for use in national bodies, such as the UK's National Institute for Health and Clinical Excellence (NICE) or Australia's Pharmaceutical Benefits Advisory Committee (PBAC). NICE and the PBAC can be characterised as conducting one-off, in-depth evaluations of single technologies before making recommendations to health service decision-makers as to whether such technologies should be adopted. Instead we are considering how cash-limited decision-makers manage competing claims on their resources, with national health technology guidance being one such claim among many.

Economic Principles

PBMA offers a pragmatic framework to aid health service decision-makers in setting priorities using the principles of opportunity cost, marginal analysis and maximising benefits from scarce resources [7]. These principles also provide the foundations for cost-effectiveness, cost-utility, and cost-benefit analysis, and, based on them, it is possible to design a priority setting process to aid decision-making about changes in resource allocation.

The principle of opportunity cost arises from the economic problem: resources for health services are scarce, and are insufficient to provide all health services that may provide benefits to society. Decision-makers therefore have to address a series of questions: how, when, where and what health services should be provided, and for whom? This involves deciding which services to provide, and which not to provide, recognising either implicitly or explicitly that providing one service may result in an alternative service not being provided due to resource scarcity. The benefit forgone from not providing the alternative service is the opportunity cost. PBMA recognises the need to carefully consider the costs and benefits of alternative health services, and their opportunity costs.

The principle of the margin refers to the next unit of benefit gained (or lost) or the next unit of resources invested (or disinvested). Thinking and acting 'at the margin' typically involves shifting resources from areas of low health gain per dollar spent to areas of higher health gain per dollar spent in order to improve benefit to the population as a whole. If the marginal benefit per dollar spent from programme A is greater than that for B, then resources should be taken from B and given to A. On the (reasonable) assumption of diminishing marginal benefit, whereby people are treated in order of magnitude of benefits to be gained, other things being equal, cutting back on B will increase the ratio of marginal benefits per dollar spent, whilst expanding A will diminish its equivalent ratio. Thus, the process of reallocation should continue until the ratios of marginal benefit to marginal cost for the programmes are equal. This will maximise total patient benefit derived from the two programmes combined.

The focus of PBMA is on incremental change rather than global reform in service delivery. However, the principle of maximising benefits from scarce resources for a given programme remains intact. In the first instance, PBMA seeks to maximise benefits from only those services that are 'at the programme margin' at a given point in time. If the framework is used as a longer term decision-making tool, different services may be identified to be 'at the programme margin' at different points in time. PBMA can then be used sequentially to address all services within a programme over a period of time, seeking to maximise benefits across the whole programme.

The PBMA Framework

A PBMA study can be broken down into the seven stages shown in Table 1, which are designed to provide a systematic and explicit framework for priority setting [1-3].

PBMA asks decision-makers to construct a programme budget (a map of how resources are currently spent) and then assists them in making recommendations for changing existing allocations of resources to services using marginal analysis. This type of priority setting process can be used to examine changes in services within a given programme (micro/within programme study design) [20, 21] or between programmes (macro/between programme study design) [22]. The exact choice and nature of the programme(s) to be examined will depend on the organisation, its objectives and existing budget areas. The programme structure should be manageable in the sense that programme areas are comprehensive but do not overlap (programmes should represent mutually exclusive sets of health services, and be collectively exhaustive of all services provided within a given budget). Resources allocated to the individual programmes may need to be identified, and the costs of providing the different services quantified. These costs are then incorporated with the activity information to produce the programme budget.

The advisory panel plays a central role in any PBMA study, and is typically made up 8-30 individuals from relevant clinical and non-clinical disciplines [1]. The panel is responsible for: determining locally relevant decision-making criteria; identifying service options for investment and disinvestment; evaluating those options by considering decision-making criteria, available evidence and local data; and making recommendations for resource allocation.

Table 1. Stages in a PBMA priority setting exercise

1.	**Determine the aim and scope of the priority setting exercise** Determine whether PBMA will be used to examine changes in services within a given programme (micro/within programme study design) or between programmes (macro/between programme study design).
2.	**Compile a "programme budget"** Resources and costs of programmes will need to be identified and quantified, which, when combined with activity information, becomes the programme budget.
3.	**Form a "marginal analysis" advisory panel** A panel of 8-30 people, made up of key stakeholders (managers, physicians, nurses, finance personnel, consumers, community representatives etc.) is formed to advise the priority setting process.
4.	**Determine locally relevant decision-making criteria** Elicited from the expertise of the advisory panel (e.g. maximising benefits, improving access and equity, reducing waiting times etc.), with reference to national, regional and local objectives, and specified objectives of the health system and the community.
5.	**Identify options for (a) service growth (b) resource release from gains in operational efficiencies (c) resource release from scaling back or ceasing some services** The programme budget, along with information on decision-making objectives, evidence on benefits from service, changes in local health care needs, and policy guidance, are used to highlight options for investment and disinvestment.
6.	**Evaluate investments and disinvestments** Evaluate in terms of costs and benefits and make recommendations for (a) funding growth areas with new resources (b) moving resources from 5 (b) and 5 (c) to 5 (a).
7.	**Validate results and reallocate resources** Re-examine and validate evidence and judgements used in the process and reallocate resources according to cost-benefit ratios and other decision-making criteria.

Options for investment and disinvestment are generated from data gathered in constructing the programme budget, along with information on decision-making objectives, evidence on the benefits of existing and potential new services, changes in local health care needs, and policy guidance [23]. This may include identifying services that can potentially be provided as effectively using fewer resources, as well as identifying services that should receive fewer resources because they may provide less benefit per dollar than one or more of the investments.

Investments and disinvestments are evaluated in terms of both their costs and benefits, where benefits may be expressed in effectiveness, utility or monetary terms. Published evidence on the benefits from services can be used (where available) to evaluate the investments/ disinvestments. Where published evidence is unavailable, expert opinion can be used to estimate benefits using decision analytic techniques [20,24]. If the principle of maximising benefits from scarce resources is being followed, resources should be reallocated from services with lowest ratios of benefit to cost to those services with the highest ratios of benefit to cost. Importantly, the implications of changes in the configuration of services in terms of other decision-making criteria (e.g., access, equity, waiting times etc.), in addition to costs and benefits, should be assessed. Defining these criteria is also useful when no evidence exists; so expert opinion can be used to inform judgements about the performance of investment and disinvestment options.

Recommendations for resource allocation are based on the evaluation of investments and disinvestments described above. The process can then be repeated over a period of time so that services which are more difficult to evaluate, or change, are progressively assessed. By sequentially repeating the process, the emphasis of PBMA is gradually to move towards the goal of maximising benefits for a given level of resources. In this way, use of the PBMA framework is relevant regardless of the total amount of resources available.

Of course, there are other approaches to priority setting. These include QALY league tables, defining core services and using needs assessment. However, these approaches have been criticised on grounds that they do not recognise fundamental economic principles such as opportunity cost and the margin, that they are too resource intensive for practical decision-making, or that they have failed to produce meaningful lists of services for funding [7, 8, 25, 26].

Another approach available to decision-makers is that of economic evaluation. Economic evaluation studies provide comparisons of two or more interventions or services on the basis of costs and benefits, using cost-effectiveness, cost-utility or cost-benefit analysis methodologies. These types of studies are an important tool but have some significant limitations for real world priority setting [27]. Economic evaluation studies have limited systemic generalisability as health care systems and relative costs differ between settings. They also have limited population generalisability as disease incidence and target populations differ between settings. Both factors will influence benefit-cost ratios in different local contexts. Further, in real world settings programmes may exhibit important interactions including joint costs of shared infrastructure and other economies of scale.

PBMA is distinct from these other approaches in that it considers a wider range of services, works within existing budget boundaries, and explicitly recognises the impact of organisational context on priority setting. Most importantly, PBMA is applied at the local level - where resource scarcity actually bites. Local managers and clinicians bear the opportunity cost of resource reallocation decisions elsewhere in their budgets. This is not accounted for in economic evaluation [8], but is accounted for in PBMA. However, economic evaluation and PBMA should be seen as complements rather than substitutes. PBMA provides a more holistic approach to priority setting at the local level, through its explicit consideration of opportunity costs, but information from the 'technical' economic evaluation literature is an important input into the PBMA process.

International Consistencies and Controversies

In this section, we first highlight international trends in the development of PBMA, and then discuss developments in the UK, Australia and Canada in more detail.

All PBMA studies share the common economic principles of opportunity cost, marginal analysis, and maximising benefits from scarce resources. PBMA studies have shown a high level of consistency in terms of adopting a health system study viewpoint, employing a micro/within programme study design, and using disease or client based programme frameworks. Differences have emerged in methods used to generate investments and disinvestments in service provision, including using stakeholder polling, published literature, and/or national health priorities. Similarly, differences have emerged in the methods used to evaluate services, including using published effectiveness literature, local effectiveness data, decision analysis of expert judgement, and disability adjusted life years. Recent methodological advances have focussed on some of the more challenging aspects of priority setting, including identifying options for service disinvestments, priority setting at the macro/between programme level, and aligning health economics with organisational values.

Perhaps the most significant advances in the PBMA framework have been in the treatment of pragmatic and ethical considerations. PBMA studies are increasingly recognising the need to address the complexities of organisational contexts and decision-making processes, which ultimately determine patterns of resource allocation. Pragmatic considerations include identifying key health service and community stakeholders, eliciting stakeholder values and preferences, establishing contextual barriers to change, and developing adequate implementation processes. Recent innovations have also extended methods to include equity weights in priority setting, to consider a wide range of managerial objectives within the utility function, and to place priority setting within wider ethical frameworks like Accountability for Reasonableness.

The United Kingdom

The first applications of PBMA in health care arose in the UK in the 1970s when used by the Department of Health and Social Security in England to set priorities for spending in the National Health Service (NHS) [28,29]. Interest in the framework seemed to wane in the 1980s and then enjoy a 'relative' renaissance during the 1990s. During this time, published studies revealed that both micro and macro-level exercises had been conducted across Grampian Health Board [30,31], Newcastle and North Tyneside Health Authority [32], Greater Glasgow Health Board [33], Tayside Health Board [23] and North Merseyside [34].

In recent years, NHS re-organisations have posed new challenges for priority setting in the UK. In England, local health service organisations (Primary Care Trusts or PCTs) charged with commissioning primary and secondary health services for their geographical populations, are faced with the difficulty of doing so whilst also implementing national guidelines (such as those issued by NICE), conforming to national targets, and accounting for local directives. More recently, policy direction has switched to promoting practice-based commissioning (GP level commissioning) [35]. The only constant in these re-organisations is the *absence* of guidance on how decision-makers, at whatever level, are to commission 'effectively' [36-38]. However, PBMA activity during this time (through several micro-level exercises) has demonstrated the usefulness of the principles of the framework, and the ability of decision-makers to adapt and apply the concepts [39-43].

Ongoing work focuses on using PBMA to align the principles of health economics with the core values of healthcare organisations. Specifically, qualitative research conducted with PCTs in the North of England is being used to develop PBMA as a management framework based both on economic and ethical principles which recognises scarcity, the complexity of health care and thus the need for pragmatism to be built into such priority setting processes [44]. A recent, and further, significant step forward in the UK has been the development of national-level programme budgeting data which can be used to examine spending by any PCT across 23 programme areas (mostly disease-based). PCTs' spending can be benchmarked against others with similar populations or in similar locations and can also be combined with data on health outcomes, enabling questions to be asked about spending relative to performance [45].

Australia

In Australia, use of PBMA arose in the early 1990s, primarily through the introduction of the framework by health economists in the Eastern and Southern States [46,47]. Since that time, both State and Federal levels of government have funded applications of PBMA in a wide range of contexts. In New South Wales, PBMA has successfully been used to aid priority setting in dental, asthma, family health, diabetes, and mental health services [48]. In South Australia, a significant PBMA programme was developed in both the acute hospital and community health settings, under the guidance of health economists from Sydney and Monash Universities (see [15] for references to individual studies). Applications ranged from indigenous health to injury prevention to surgical services. Similarly, a programme of work has been developed in Western Australia in recent years.

Australian applications have included a number of important developments for the PBMA framework. Several PBMA studies have taken advantage of detailed, patient level, clinical costing data collected under Australian Diagnosis Related Group (DRG) frameworks. Such data are routinely available, reducing time spent on the programme budget, and providing high quality cost information. Other studies have developed more rigorous methods to elicit and weight criteria used in decision-making, drawing on multi-attribute utility theory and decision analytic techniques [20,24]. Methods for evaluating PBMA studies have also been developed, focusing on evaluating both methodological rigor, and the ability of PBMA to achieve real changes in resource allocation in different organisational contexts [15]. Finally, a national PBMA study of priorities for reducing the burden of cancer has been the first to incorporate mortality and morbidity data across diverse programmes using disability adjusted life years [49]. This development highlights the complementary nature of effectiveness evidence (in this case measured by reduction in disease burden attributable to programmes) and PBMA.

Canada

In Canada, formal application of the framework to date has been limited to Alberta and British Columbia. In Alberta, since 1998, at least seven micro-level case studies within three regional health authorities have been carried out [50]. PBMA has also been applied at a macro-level, across all major service areas within one health authority in Alberta [22], with further work at a macro level ongoing in another health authority in British Columbia. The macro level activity in Alberta was an important addition to the literature; as such broad level marginal-value type re-allocations had not been previously reported. Whilst the initial work in these health regions was funded through research activity and directly involved university-based health economists, decision-makers within the regions have continued to use PBMA in further applications. It is thought that genuine gains can only be made through ongoing, systematic application of the PBMA approach, both within and across programmes.

Through the application of PBMA in Alberta and British Columbia, the intention is to: build on research around organisational challenges including issues of physician involvement and incentive systems; further develop means of evaluating the process from an ethical perspective [51]; and, examine alternative methods in measuring benefit such as discrete choice experiments [52]. Recent Canadian work, like research in the UK, has focussed on describing priority setting processes in health authorities and aligning health economics with organisational values. Qualitative survey methods have been used to identify a range of areas from improvement in such processes [17-19, 53]. These include the need for greater transparency and fairness in decision-making and the need to develop organisational cultures which support priority setting.

CHALLENGES AND ADVANCES IN METHODS

Recent experiences within the UK, Australia, and Canada have highlighted a range of considerations that need to be addressed if PBMA is to be applied successfully in practice. In particular, experiences have demonstrated the need to balance pragmatic and ethical considerations with sound economic methodology.

Advisory Panels

International experiences have highlighted the central role of the PBMA advisory panel. As specific evidence to inform local decisions will not always be present, an advisory panel is used in PBMA to weigh the options for service delivery through considering available evidence, but also relying on local data and expert opinion. Typically, the advisory panel is also charged with establishing decision-making criteria and identifying service investments and disinvestments. The advisory panel should receive training in the principles of priority setting. This is a necessary pre-requisite if the panel is to have ownership of the process and the results of the study. Should the panel feel that they do not understand the methods used, and the process by which resource allocation decisions were reached, the likelihood of results being implemented will drop significantly.

The advisory panel can be comprised of an array of individuals spanning relevant clinical and non-clinical disciplines. In some cases, if the question at hand is narrow in scope, the panel may be quite small, whereas in other cases potential re-allocation decisions may include many disciplines and thus broader representation will be required. Recent developments in PBMA have included inviting other key stakeholders, including service providers in related services (e.g. secondary care providers on prevention programmes) and consumer and community representatives, to join PBMA advisory panels. This reflects a growing awareness of the need to recognise inter-agency links in the provision of health care, which may act as a barrier to achieving real resource shifts.

There are many inputs into this type of priority setting process, including, but not limited to, evidence from the literature such as outcomes studies, economic evaluations or health technology assessments, quality reports, regional or state policies and guidelines, local utilisation data, informal input from staff, clinicians and members of the public, and reports from government health departments. As such, the advisory panel may want to pragmatically weigh out the investment and disinvestment options against the pre-defined criteria. The challenge comes in sifting through the wealth of available data and information and applying it in a systematic manner, with an explicit priority setting process; it is here that the real added-value of PBMA can be seen.

Community Participation and Values

Incorporating community opinions and values in PBMA raises several issues, including what methods should be used to elicit consumer preferences. One option is to have members of the public on the advisory panel. Whilst this may be challenging because of the difficulty of a small number of individuals being representative of the population at large, work in Ontario has shown that community stakeholders can play an integral and direct role in the decision-making process [54]. Important aspects of this might include defining appropriate criteria for decision-making based on community values and ensuring the needs of specific groups within the community are addressed (e.g. ensuring services for Indigenous populations are culturally appropriate). Service providers and decision-makers may be better placed to interpret evidence on the cost-effectiveness of services and make technical judgements about service delivery and patient outcomes.

In fact, recent work on public involvement in priority setting suggests that the public may best be used to develop the criteria or principles on which decision-making processes are based [55,56]. A pitfall is that this type of public consultation can be resource intensive. Another is that such principles can act only as a general guide, as each decision will involve trading the principles 'at the margin' thus requiring a level of detail which may never be achievable through public consultation. Thus, whilst it could be argued that the public should be involved, decision-makers may in the end choose to develop local criteria based on existing business planning documents within the organisation, or through consultation with the given health organisation's governance structure. It is important nonetheless to recognise that this still represents progress in how health service priorities are set.

Organisational Context and Behaviour

Perhaps the strongest challenge to PBMA, and likely to any explicit, evidence based approach to priority setting in health care, is that of organisational context and behaviour. Issues such as the need for organisational stability, the active involvement of high level champions, an organisational culture which is receptive to fostering change, and openness to learning are all critical factors for the use of PBMA as a practical decision-making aid [15]. Drawing on work from Canada and Australia, a depiction of the PBMA process set within the organisational context has been developed, which includes barriers and facilitators for the uptake of PBMA and follow-through of advisory panel recommendations (see [16]). Barriers for the uptake of PBMA may be interpreted as transactions costs in the priority setting process [57] and include: too many demands/time pressures placed on managers and information personnel; hidden agendas/vested interests; and, lack of trust between stakeholders. A first step to overcoming many of the barriers is to embark upon qualitative research specific to the context of priority setting in health care organisations. Such qualitative research can be based on open ended-interviews evaluating PBMA exercises [16] or on more detailed Participatory Action Research (or PAR) [44,53] which focuses on getting decision-makers and researchers to work together in order to develop better priority setting processes.

The trialling and application of new priority setting processes should only be undertaken during periods of relative organisational stability. For new decision-making tools to be developed, a stable planning environment is needed which allows key stakeholders to explore new methods and discuss their application. Organisational changes will reduce the willingness of key stakeholders to develop alternative approaches to health service planning. Stability in the planning environment is needed both within the relevant health authority and the provider(s) involved. This allows the strategic directions of the health authority and providers to be developed and clearly understood. During periods of major organisational instability and uncertainty it is likely prudent not to attempt the trialling of new priority setting techniques.

The application of new priority setting processes results in significant changes in decision-making culture, and potentially in the configuration of health services. Change management strategies should be developed to identify and address potential problems in the application of priority setting methods and their results. One of the key elements of a successful PBMA study is strong leadership from managers, which Jan terms 'credible commitment' [58], combined with enthusiasm from service providers. If strong management leadership is absent it is unlikely that a priority setting process will be successful [5]. One of the roles of managers is to negotiate the study through a series of changes in decision-making and planning cultures. Furthermore, managers have the responsibility for implementing changes in service provision and managing the associated potential for dislocation of services and staff.

Providers will only own the process if they are involved from the outset and the process is driven internally. This includes involving providers in initial discussions about appropriate priority setting processes for development, as much of the development of a priority setting process depends on information and expertise held by service providers. More importantly, the implementation of changes to service delivery becomes extremely difficult without provider acceptance and ownership of those changes. Indeed, setting PBMA within the organisational context, and viewing the framework as a management process that is based on economic principles (as opposed to a technically driven economic approach) is critical to the success of this type of priority setting process [1,3].

Integration of Funding and Priority Setting Mechanisms

Successful application of a priority setting process requires a degree of integration in funding and priority setting mechanisms. If priority setting processes conflict with funding mechanisms at the local or regional levels, or with budget setting mechanisms within provider organisations, it is unlikely that those processes will lead to changes in the allocation of resources. Before priority setting processes are trialled, careful consideration should be given to the broader health service resource allocation framework.

Population based funding models are most compatible with PBMA. PBMA is based on maximising benefits from available funds, whilst population based funding allocates resources on the basis of population needs. Assuming that population needs reflect the potential for a population to benefit from health services, the focus of population funding is consistent with economic principles for priority setting. Under this funding approach, health service organisations (which are responsible for providing health services for a defined population) receive funds based on the health care needs of their population. Health service organisations with greater population needs, and therefore greater potential to benefit from health services, get more funds. That is, this funding approach supports the notion of maximising benefits from health services. PBMA may then be used by organisations to set priorities within the funding envelope made available to them.

Case-mix, or throughput, funding has two main strengths in the context of priority setting. First, case-mix classification systems for health services are often well developed and are based on clinical parameters. Second, the construction of cost weights produces detailed cost information on a range of health services. PBMA can draw on case-mix information by using the DRG (or similar) classification system and the cost information used to construct cost weights. The major drawback with case-mix funding is that it places a significant emphasis on throughput rather than capacity to benefit and outcomes in health service planning. This may lead to planning strategies at the local, regional, and provider levels which are based mainly on throughput considerations, which may conflict with considerations of costs and benefits in priority setting models.

It is worth noting that funding mechanisms will also be determined by organisational context – through the organisation of responsibilities in the health system. Typically, the organisation of these responsibilities will be pre-determined, and will represent a set of organisational constraints on local decision-makers. Whilst local decision-makers seek to pursue local goals, they may be constrained by the pursuit of objectives at other levels of the health system. Organisational responsibilities go beyond the chosen funding model, re-emphasising the need to understand organisational context and behaviour if priority setting processes are to be successful.

Identifying Service Investments and Disinvestments

Another challenge that has arisen in the literature is that advisory panel members may be reluctant to produce specific suggestions for resource release due to the culture in health care of expecting more resources rather than having to make trade-off decisions and re-allocations [59]. Whilst an advisory panel may be quick to come up with areas for expansion, a much more difficult challenge is then identifying areas from which to obtain resources to fund priority areas [39, 60]. A number of methods have been proposed to address this issue, including drawing on clinical pathways models [15]. Research in Alberta involving the piloting of PBMA in a number of micro level case studies found the use of one-on-one interviews with advisory panel members to be useful in brainstorming areas for resource release, before bringing the group back together to make recommendations for change [50]. The main issue here is in alleviating potential social desirability bias in the group setting, and helping individuals to think about re-allocation as opposed to always relying on additional resources.

Our experience would indicate that, although the notion of scarcity is initially accepted, decision-makers have problems at the stage of identifying disinvestments so that some proposed investments can be correspondingly funded. There is a natural reluctance on the part of decision-makers to take from one area to fund service growth options in other areas. However, the very explicitness of PBMA can encourage identification of possible disinvestments. By working down a list of areas for investment to be funded by new monies, decision-makers eventually reach proposed investments that are on the cusp (or margin) of being funded, but will not be funded unless some disinvestments are made. Seeing explicitly what might not be funded can encourage decision-makers to start thinking more seriously about such disinvestments.

Decision-Making Criteria

A major, and recent, development in PBMA has been the explicit inclusion of decision-making criteria beyond cost-effectiveness. This development recognises the need for priority setting frameworks to capture the inherent complexity of health care decision-making, which is based on a diverse set of criteria (such as effectiveness, access, equity, waiting times etc.) [20, 24, 41, 61-63]. It is important that the criteria be explicitly defined, and that if possible, the criteria are given specific weights as it is unlikely that all criteria will have equal importance. Two key strengths of this approach are that the panel defines (or adopts) the decision-making criteria which are relevant to the context of the PBMA study and that judgements are explicit and based on shared understanding of the criteria. As a result, the panel has full ownership over the criteria with which its services are evaluated, and the approach is explicit and open for scrutiny, enabling issues to be discussed which may have previously been left unaddressed and implicit in decision-making.

There are a number of potential ways in which these criteria can be incorporated into PBMA. The most explicit approach has been to use decision analysis to construct multi-attribute utility models [20, 24]. These models combine criteria by eliciting the advisory panel's importance weights for each and constructing a utility function which is used to inform cost-effectiveness (or cost-value) ratios. The criteria identified by the advisory panel may be specific to the context of the study, and should be informed by both micro (local) and macro (regional or national) level objectives. Criteria should be carefully defined and described so that key principles of multi-attribute utility theory are adhered to i.e. criteria should be mutually exclusive (orthogonal) to avoid double counting, and collectively exhaustive to ensure all relevant aspects of the decision-makers' utility function are captured. Other preference elicitation techniques, such as willingness to pay and discrete choice experiments, can also be incorporated into the PBMA framework [52], though their use to date has been relatively limited.

A variant of this approach explored incorporating vertical equity and other criteria as 'second-stage decision filters' [49]. In this study, cost-benefit ratios for cancer services were constructed using disability adjusted life years. Vertical equity was measured in terms of gross health inequalities (excess mortality) for specific population groups. A second cost-benefit tariff was constructed for all investments and disinvestments, where ratios were weighted for excess mortality by population group. Service investments and disinvestments first had to clear the cost-benefit hurdle, and only then were they assessed relative to the equity-weighted cost-benefit hurdle.

Ethical Considerations

A process like PBMA, which is meant to operate within the complex environment faced by health care decision-makers, should also undergo some sort of evaluation. That is, irrespective of the final re-allocation recommendations made by an advisory panel, one may also be interested in whether the process itself was fair. An ethical framework for evaluating priority setting activity has been developed, and is referred to as 'Accountability for Reasonableness' [64]. Under this framework, a priority setting process is considered to be fair if it satisfies the four conditions required to demonstrate accountability for reasonableness. These conditions (see Table 2) relate to: 1) publicity (whether decisions are publicly accessible); 2) relevance (whether rationales for decisions can be agreed upon); 3) appeals (whether there is a mechanism for dispute resolution); and 4) enforcement (whether there is regulation to enforce the first three conditions).

Table 2. Conditions of the Accountability for Reasonableness framework

1.	**Ensure transparent communication of priority setting processes** Priority setting processes and decisions, and the rationales for those processes and decisions should be made accessible to managers, clinicians, patients, and the public.
2.	**Ensure relevance of priority setting processes** The rationale for priority setting processes and decisions should be based on principles, reasons, and evidence that managers, clinicians, patients, and the public can agree are relevant in deciding how to meet the diverse needs of the community given resource constraints.
3.	**Establish an appeals mechanism** An appeals mechanism should be established for challenge and dispute resolution regarding priority setting decisions, including the opportunity for revising decisions in light of further evidence or arguments.
4.	**Establish an enforcement mechanism** Voluntary or public regulation mechanisms should be established for the priority setting process to ensure that the first three conditions are met.

Specifically, one could envision the conducting of a PBMA exercise by a group of decision-makers, based on the four stages outlined above [51]. Following this, relevant stakeholders could be interviewed to examine the priority setting process in light of the four main conditions of Accountability for Reasonableness. The insight gained could then be fed back to directly impact future processes in the given organisation. Alternatively, the PBMA approach could be built from the outset with the ethical conditions listed above in mind. In these ways, not only are resources likely to be used in a manner which are most in line with the stated local criteria, but as well, the process itself can be made as fair as possible.

Importantly, the latter can lead to perceived credibility which will likely help to mitigate problems which may arise due to resources being shifted from one area into another.

Pragmatic Study Design for PBMA

PBMA is based on fundamental economic principles and addresses resource reallocation within or across programme areas to better meet local objectives. Whilst often unheralded, a pragmatic approach to priority setting is not only what managers seem to be looking for [65], but as well, PBMA can enable decisions to be made based on best evidence and local practice [66]. Further, decisions to fund or stop funding a service are not made once and for all, in all settings. Whilst this may be seen as a disadvantage, it actually allows local decision-makers to allocate available resources in the best way possible (i.e. at the margin), with reference to the opportunity cost of the decisions made.

It is held that through greater adherence to fundamental economic concepts and broader implementation of economic approaches like PBMA, health care organisations will move towards maximizing benefit, or better meeting other important criteria, for the available resources. That said, an important message for health economists is the need to be practical, and to not expect universal (or indeed any) uptake of mechanistic approaches to evaluation of options. In our view, PBMA provides decision-makers with an approach to health care priority setting that is both principled and pragmatic.

There are four pragmatic foundations for the successful design and implementation of priority setting tools [3], which are summarised in Table 3.

Table 3. Pragmatic foundations for successful priority setting

1. Establish the organisational objectives
- Multiple objectives (effectiveness, equity etc., trade-offs between objectives)
- Hierarchical objectives (micro level - provider, local; macro level - regional, national)
- Inter-temporal objectives (short-term, long-term)
2. Ensure there is organisational readiness
- Leadership and ownership (managers, providers, consumers, community)
- Timing and stability (organisational reforms)
- Institutional boundaries (budgetary, service fragmentation/integration)
- Incentive and sanction mechanisms (financial, managerial)
3. Establish an appropriate advisory panel structure
- Advisory panel composition (service managers/providers, consumers/community)
- Roles and responsibilities (values, decision-making criteria, evaluation of services)
- Training of key stakeholders (information provision/education)
- Community participation and values (values, decision-making criteria, specific needs)
4. Ensure that implementation of results is feasible
- Feasibility of resource reallocation (ability to reallocate resources, institutional boundaries)
- Desirability of resource reallocation (desire to reallocate resources, ownership)
- Funding and priority setting mechanisms (degree of integration/conflict)
- Ethical considerations (process fairness, Accountability for Reasonableness)

First, establish the organisational objectives. The objectives of the organisation should be ascertained at the outset of any priority setting study. It is important to know where the organisation is going and why. Establishing decision-makers objectives requires careful consideration of three interrelated issues. Firstly, decision-makers may have multiple objectives (e.g. effectiveness, equity, access, cultural appropriateness etc.). Second, objectives should reflect the local decision-making context, but also should be compatible with policies at higher levels of decision-making (hierarchical objectives). In the local context, providers/commissioners of health services may have a set of micro level objectives, whereas in the regional/national context there may be a set of macro level objectives. Third, organisations will have different short and long-term objectives (inter-temporal objectives), differences that may occur at all levels of the decision-making hierarchy.

Second, ensure there is organisational readiness. Strong management leadership is required to drive any priority setting process; if leadership is absent it is unlikely that a priority setting process will be successful. At the same time, ownership by key stakeholders is necessary, service managers/providers and community/consumer representatives. Priority setting studies should be undertaken in a context of relative organisational stability, with coherence in long-term strategies for planning across health services. Institutional boundaries, such as budget and service delivery boundaries should be clearly established. A key question is whether stated objectives are achievable within current institutional boundaries. If not, the objectives being considered should be revised, or institutional boundaries reformed (which may be impractical in the short term). Incentive and sanction mechanisms, including remuneration and funding mechanisms, should be identified, so that decision-makers' and service providers' potential responses to resource shifts can be explored.

Third, establish an appropriate advisory panel structure. The advisory panel should be comprised of an array of individuals spanning relevant clinical and non-clinical disciplines. Key stakeholders may include those directly involved in the programmes being considered (health care providers, managers, and consumer representatives) and those indirectly involved (collaborating/inter-related providers, policy-makers, finance/information personnel, and community representatives). The advisory panel should receive training in the principles of priority setting, a necessary pre-requisite if the key stakeholders are to have ownership of the process. Community stakeholders should play an integral part in the process (where possible), including defining appropriate criteria for decision-making based on community values and ensuring the needs of specific groups within the community are addressed (e.g. ensuring services for indigenous populations are culturally appropriate).

Fourth, ensure that implementation of results is feasible. Some services may be impractical options for change in the short term, often including services which require joint provision with other agencies. These options may be potential candidates for examination in the future, when the means to overcome institutional boundaries have been more fully explored. Implementation of PBMA results will only occur if a decision making culture which considers costs and outcomes has been established - decision-makers must have the 'stomach' for resource reallocation. Successful application of priority setting methods requires a degree of integration in funding and priority setting mechanisms. If priority setting mechanisms conflict with funding mechanisms at the local or regional levels, or with budget setting mechanisms within provider organisations, it is unlikely that priority setting methods will lead to changes in the allocation of resources. The priority setting process itself should be evaluated to determine whether it was fair, which may be achieved by using the Accountability for Reasonableness framework alongside PBMA.

Before undertaking a priority setting exercise, decision-makers and analysts should also address a number of questions in determining the potential usefulness of PBMA at the local level. How might the PBMA framework fit into the structure of health care financing and consequent levels of decision-making in the health care system? Is there a culture for use of such an approach? In addressing this question, one might reflect on how health care managers are trained, and whether there is a tendency towards evidence-based approaches to decision-making. How does the political climate influence the potential for using such frameworks? What is the quality of information in the health care system and can this be used (or adapted for use) in a PBMA-type framework? Do incentives and/or the current balance of power (or property rights) in the system mitigate against or in favour of the use of such a framework?

Conclusion

This chapter has sought to synthesise international evidence on recent advances in PBMA and the implementation of study results. Recent methodological advances have focussed on some of the most challenging technical aspects of the PBMA process, including: setting priorities between programmes using macro marginal analysis; identifying options for service disinvestments; evidence-based priority setting at the local level; and, eliciting decision-makers preferences. Perhaps the most significant advances in the PBMA framework have been in the treatment of pragmatic and ethical considerations, recognising the need to address the complexities of organisational context and decision-making processes. PBMA has increasingly sought to balance pragmatic and ethical considerations with the economic principles of opportunity cost and marginal analysis. There are several pragmatic foundations for the successful design and implementation of PBMA, including: developing a clear understanding of both organisational objectives and organisational context; establishing an appropriate advisory panel; and, ensuring that the implementation of study results is feasible. Notably, the foundations of understanding organisational objectives and context, and ensuring feasibility of implementation, should be central to all priority setting tools.

Of course, many challenges remain for the successful design and implementation of priority setting tools at the local level. These challenges present a rich agenda for future research, spanning health economics, health services research, bioethics, management science, political economy, and health policy. This includes examining: the information (transaction) costs for health service agencies and the opportunity cost of time for decision-makers of priority setting processes; the level and role of community participation in setting local priorities; the impact of alternative incentive structures and behaviours on identifying options for service investments and disinvestments; and, methods for valuing multiple decision-making criteria. Perhaps the most important area of future research lies in incorporating organisational context into economists' approaches to priority setting, whilst making economics an integral part of the management process.

Several final points can be made about PBMA. First, PBMA is intuitive. Many decision-makers already think in a manner as outlined above without even knowing that they are using a PBMA approach. The value-added of PBMA is in making the process more explicit and systematic. Second, PBMA can be thought of as a vehicle for drawing evidence into the decision-making process in health organisations, and as a means of applying input from the public. It could be said that PBMA recognises the non-rationality of decision-making in health care and accounts for it through enabling pragmatic decisions to be made. Third, PBMA does not provide a formulaic response to challenging health care decisions. Through a mix of evidence and local expert decision-making, explicit decisions are made in a manner thought to best meet the relevant criteria. Precisely because it is based on locally relevant inputs, and relies on local expert opinion, decisions made in one context will differ from those in another. Most importantly, whilst achieving the above, the PBMA process is based explicitly on the premise of having to make difficult choices amongst competing claims on scarce resources.

ACKNOWLEDGEMENTS

Stuart Peacock and Craig Mitton are Michael Smith Foundation for Health Research Scholars. Craig Mitton also holds a Canada Research Chair (Tier 2) in Health Care Priority Setting. Cam Donaldson holds the Health Foundation Chair in Health Economics. Angela Bate holds a Primary Care Researcher Development Award, funded by the Department of Health's National Coordinating Centre for Research Capacity Building. Research was undertaken whilst Stuart Peacock was a visiting health economist at Newcastle University funded by the Health Foundation and at the BC Cancer Agency funded by Canadian Institutes of Health Research grant no. 162964. The views expressed in this chapter are those of the authors, not the funding agencies.

REFERENCES

[1] Mitton, C. and Donaldson, C. (2004). *Priority Setting Toolkit: a Guide to the use of Economics in Healthcare Decision Making*. London: BMJ Books.

[2] Ruta, D., Mitton, C., Bate A., and Donaldson C. (2005). Program budgeting and marginal analysis: bridging the divide between doctors and managers. *British Medical Journal* 330:1501-3.

[3] Peacock, S., Ruta, D., Mitton, C., Donaldson C., Bate A., and Murtagh M. (2006). Using economics to set pragmatic and ethical priorities. *British Medical Journal* 332:482-485.

[4] Donaldson, C. and Mooney, G. (1991). Needs assessment, priority setting and contracts for health care: an economic view. *British Medical Journal* 303:1529-1530.

[5] Mitton, C. and Donaldson, C. (2001). Twenty-five years of programme budgeting and marginal analysis in the health sector, 1974-1999. *Journal of Health Services Research and Policy* 6(4):239-248.

[6] Mitton, C., Peacock, S., Donaldson, C., and Bate A. (2003). Using PBMA in Health Care Priority Setting: Description, Challenges and Experience. *Applied Health Economics and Policy* 2:121-134.

[7] Mooney, G., Gerard, K., Donaldson, C., and Farrar S. (1992). *Priority Setting in Purchasing: Some Practical Guidelines.* (Research paper number 6) Scotland: National Association of Health Authorities and Trusts.

[8] Birch, S. and Gafni, A. (1992). Cost-effectiveness ratios: in a league of their own. *Health Policy* 28:133-141.

[9] Donaldson, C., Mitton, C. and Currie, G. (2002). *Managing Medicare: the Pre-requisite to Spending or Reform.* Toronto: CD Howe Institute.

[10] Hoffmann, C. and von der Schulenburg, J.M.G. (On behalf of the EUROMET group). (2000). The influence of economic evaluation studies on decision making. A European survey. *Health Policy* 52:179-92.

[11] Williams, I. and Bryan, S. (2007). Understanding the limited impact of economic evaluation in health care resource allocation: A conceptual framework. *Health Policy* 80: 135-143.

[12] MacDonald, R. (2002). *Using Health Economics in Health Services: Rationing Rationally?* Houston: Open University Press.

[13] Barrett, A., Roques, T., Small, M., et al. (2006). How much will Herceptin really cost? *British Medical Journal* 333:1118-20.

[14] Donaldson, C. and Farrar, S. (1993). Needs assessment: developing an economic approach. *Health Policy* 25, 95-108.

[15] Peacock, S. (1998). *An Evaluation of Program Budgeting and Marginal Analysis Applied in South Australian Hospitals.* Melbourne: Centre for Health Program Evaluation, Monash University.

[16] Mitton, C. and Donaldson, C. (2003). Setting priorities and allocating resources in health regions: lessons from a project evaluating budgeting and marginal analysis (PBMA). *Health Policy* 64:335-348.

[17] Patten, S., Mitton, C. and Donaldson, C. (2005). From the trenches: views from decision-makers on health services priority setting. *Health Services Management Research* 18:100-8.

[18] Mitton, C., Patten, S., Donaldson, C., and Waldner H. (2005). Priority-setting in health authorities: moving beyond the barriers. The Calgary experience. *Healthcare Quarterly* 8: 49-55.

[19] Teng, F., Mitton, C. and Mackenzie, J. (2007). Priority setting in the provincial health services authority: a survey of key decision-makers. *BMC Health Services Research* 12; 7:84.

[20] Peacock, S., Richardson, J. and Carter, R. (1998). *Setting Priorities in South Australian Community Health II: marginal analysis of mental health services.* Melbourne: Centre for Health Program Evaluation, Monash University.

[21] Mooney, G. (2002). Priority setting in mental health services. *Applied Health Economics and Health Policy* 1(2):65-74.

[22] Mitton, C., Patten, S., Waldner, H., and Donaldson C. (2003). Priority setting in health authorities: a novel approach to a historical activity. *Social Science and Medicine* 57:1653-1663.

[23] Ruta, D., Donaldson, C. and Gilray, I. (1996). Economics, public health and health care purchasing: the Tayside experience of programme budgeting and marginal analysis. *Journal of Health Service Research and Policy* 1(4):185-193.

[24] Peacock, S., Richardson, J., Carter, R., and Edwards D. (2007). Priority setting in health care using multi-attribute utility theory and program budgeting and marginal analysis PBMA. *Social Science and Medicine* 64: 897-910.

[25] Mooney, G., Russell, E. and Weir, R. (1986). *Choices for Health Care: a Practical Introduction to the Economics of Health Provision.* London: Macmillan.

[26] Hurley, J., Birch, S., Stoddart, G., and Torrance G. (1997). Medical necessity, benefit and resource allocation in health care. *Journal of Health Services Research and Policy* 2:223-230.

[27] Hauck, K., Smith, P. and Goddard, M. (2003). *The economics of priority setting for health care: a literature review.* Washington: HNP Discussion Paper, The World Bank.

[28] Perrin, J.R., Bevan, G., Owen, J., and Copeman H.A. (1978). *A management of financial resources in the National Health Service.* (Research Report No 2) Royal Commission on the National Health Service (Ed.), London: HSMO.

[29] Bevan, G., Copeman, H.A., Perrin, J.R., and Rosser R.M. (1980). *Health Care: Priorities and Management.* London: Croon Helm.

[30] Ratcliffe, J., Donaldson, C. and Macphee, S. (1996). Programme budgeting and marginal analysis: a case study of maternity services. *Journal of Public Health Medicine* 18(2):175-182.

[31] Scott, A., Currie, N. and Donaldson, C. (1998). Evaluating innovation in general practice: a pragmatic framework using programme budgeting and marginal analysis. *Family Practice* 15(3): 216-222.

[32] Craig, N., Parkin, D. and Gerard, K. (1995). Clearing the fog on the Tyne: programme budgeting in Newcastle and North Tyneside Health Authority. *Health Policy* 33:107-125.

[33] Twaddle, S. and Walker, A. (1995). Programme budgeting and marginal analysis: application within programmes to assist purchasing in Greater Glasgow Health Board. *Health Policy* 33:91-105.

[34] Madden, L., Hussey, R., Mooney, G., and Church E. (1995). Public health and economics in tandem: programme budgeting, marginal analysis and priority setting in practice. *Health Policy* 33:161-168.

[35] Department of Health (UK). (2004). *Practice Based Commissioning*. London: Department of Health. http://www.dh.gov.uk/assetRoot/04/09/85/65/04098565.pdf.

[36] Robert, G. (2003). The United Kingdom in Ham C, Robert G (eds.) *Reasonable Rationing: International Experience of Priority Setting in Health Care*. Maidenhead: Open University Press.

[37] Smith, J., Mays, N., Dixon, J. et al. (2004). *A review of the effectiveness of primary care-led commissioning and its place in the NHS.* London: The Health Foundation.

[38] Health Committee. (2002). *Second Report of Session 2001-02 on the National Institute for Clinical Excellence. Vol. 1: Report and Proceedings of the committee (HC 515-I). 2002.* London: The Stationary Office.

[39] McIver, S., Baines, D., Ham, C., and McLeod H. (2000). *Setting Priorities and managing demand in the NHS.* Birmingham: Health Services Management Centre, University of Birmingham.

[40] Chappel, D., Bailey, J., Stacy, R., Rodgers H., and Thomson R. (2001). Implementation and evaluation of local-level priority setting for stroke. *Public Health* 115:21-29.

[41] Wilson, E.C.F., Rees, J. and Fordham, R.J. (2006). Developing a prioritization framework in an English Primary Care Trust. *Cost Effectiveness and Resource Allocation*; 4 3.

[42] Wilson, E., Sussex, J., Macleod, C., and Fordham R. (2007). Prioritizing health technologies in a Primary Care Trust. *Journal of Health Services Research and Policy* 12(2):80-5.

[43] Bate, A., Donaldson, C. and Ray, H. (2007). Resource Allocation in Orthopaedics: Economic Evaluation to Priority Setting. *Clinical Orthopaedics and Related Research* 457:49-56.

[44] Bate, A., Donaldson, C. and Murtagh, M. (2007). Managing to manage healthcare resources in the English NHS? What can health economics teach? What can health economics learn? *Health Policy*. Epub ahead of print.

[45] Department of Health (UK). (2007). National Programme Budget Project. http://www.dh.gov.uk/en/Policyandguidance/Organisationpolicy/Financeandplanning/Programmebudgeting/index.htm.

[46] Shiell, A., Hall, J., Jan, S., and Seymour J. (1993). *Advancing Health in NSW: Planning in an Economic Framework.* Sydney: CHERE.

[47] Viney, R., Haas, M. and Mooney, G. (1995). Program Budgeting and Marginal Analysis: a guide to resource allocation. *New South Wales Public Health Bulletin* 6(4):29-32.

[48] Mooney, G., Haas, M., Viney, R., and Cooper L. (1997). *Linking health outcomes to priority setting, planning and resource allocation.* Sydney: CHERE.

[49] Carter, R., Stone, C., Vos, T., Hocking J., Mihalopoulous C., Peacock S., and Crowley S. (2000). *Trial of Program Budgeting and Marginal Analysis (PBMA) to assist cancer control planning in Australia.* Melbourne: Centre for Health Program Evaluation, Monash University.

[50] Mitton, C. and Donaldson, C. (2002). *Priority Setting in health Care: from Research to Practice.* Alberta Heritage Foundation for Medical Research Health Technology Assessment Unit Working Series: Edmonton.

[51] Gibson, J.L., Mitton, C., Martin, D.K., Donaldson C., and Singer PA. (2006). Evaluating a PBMA-based priority setting process using "Accountability for reasonableness". *Journal of Health Services Research and Policy* 11: 32-37.

[52] Ryan, M., Kromm, S. and Mitton, C. (2004). Into the Margin: *Using discrete choice experiments to develop the PBMA framework.* Calgary, Alberta: Calgary Health Region.

[53] Patten, S., Mitton, C. and Donaldson, C. (2006). Using participatory action research to build a priority setting process in a Canadian Regional Health Authority. *Social Science and Medicine*, 63: 1121-34.

[54] Martin, D., Abelson, J. and Singer, P. (2002). Participation in health care priority-setting through the eyes of the participants. *Journal of Health Services Research and Policy* 7(4):222-229.

[55] Litva, A., Coast, J., Donovan, J., Eyles J., Shepherd M., Tacchi J., Abelson J., Morgan K. (2001). 'The public is too subjective': public involvement at different levels of health-care decision making. *Social Science and Medicine* 54:1825-37.

[56] Wiseman, V., Mooney, G., Berry, G., Tang K.C. (2003). Involving the general public in priority setting: experiences from Australia. *Social Science and Medicine* 56:1001-1012.

[57] Jan, S. (2000). Institutional considerations in priority setting: transactions costs perspective on PBMA. *Health Economics* 9: 631-641.

[58] Jan, S. (2003). A perspective on the analysis of credible commitment and myopia in health sector decision making. *Health Policy* 63:269-278.

[59] Brambleby, P. (1995). A survivor's guide to programme budgeting. *Health Policy* 33:127-145.

[60] Posnett, J. and Street, A. (1996). Programme budgeting and marginal analysis: An approach to priority setting in need of refinement. *Journal of Health Services Research and Policy* 1:147-153.

[61] Caulfield, T. (1996). Wishful thinking: defining 'medically necessary' in Canada. *Health Law Journal* 4:63-85.

[62] Ham, C. and Coulter, A. (2001). Explicit and implicit rationing: taking responsibility and avoiding blame for health care choices. *Journal of Health Services Research and Policy* 6(3):163-169.

[63] Baltussen, R. and Niessen, L. (2006). Priority setting of health interventions: the need for multi-criteria decision analysis. *Cost Effectiveness and Resource Allocation*; 4: 14.

[64] Daniels, N. and Sabin, J. (1998). The ethics of accountability in managed care reform. *Health Affairs* 17:50-64.

[65] Mitton, C. and Donaldson, C. (2002). Setting priorities in Canadian regional health authorities: A survey of key decision makers. *Health Policy* 60(1):39-58.

[66] Haas, M., Viney, R., Kristensen, E., Pain C., and Foulds K. (2001). Using program budgeting and marginal analysis to assist population based strategic planning for coronary heart disease. *Health Policy* 55:173-186.

In: Social Sciences in Health Care and Medicine ISBN: 978-1-60456-286-6
Editors: J. B. Garner, T. C. Christiansen, pp. 139-165

Chapter 5

SOCIOECONOMIC, LIFESTYLE, AND OCCUPATIONAL FACTORS ASSOCIATED WITH POOR SELF-RATED HEALTH IN WORKERS OF SMALL AND MEDIUM-SCALE MANUFACTURING BUSINESSES

Akinori Nakata*[1*]*, Masaya Takahashi*[2]*, Tomoko Ikeda*[3]*,
***Minoru Hojou*[4]**

[1]National Institute for Occupational Safety and Health, Cincinnati, Ohio, USA
[2]National Institute of Occupational Safety and Health, Japan, Kawasaki, Japan
[3] Department of Nursing, School of Health Sciences, Ibaraki Prefectural University of Health Sciences, Ibaraki, Japan.
[4] Ota Regional Occupational Health Center, Tokyo, Japan.

ABSTRACT

Self-rated health (SRH) has become an increasingly common measure used in population surveys because it has been proven to be a robust predictor of functional disability, mortality, morbidity, and health care use. The present study investigated the correlation of poor SRH in 2,205 randomly selected workers aged 16-83 years among 244 small- and medium-scale manufacturing enterprises (SMMEs) by means of a self-administered questionnaire. SRH was assessed with a question: How would you describe your health during the past 1-year period? Response options were 'very good', 'good', 'poor', and 'very poor.' Poor SRH was defined by rating the above question as 'poor' or 'very poor' (while good SRH was defined by 'good' or 'very good'). Overall, 33.4% of men and 32.1% of women rated their health as poor. Multivariable logistic regression analysis was carried out to estimate the risk of having poor (against good) SRH. The analysis revealed that female gender, poor household financial situation, higher educational attainment, current smoking, insomnia symptoms, depressive symptoms, poor health condition, and long work hours are associated with poor SRH. Several

* Corresponding author: Akinori Nakata, National Institute for Occupational Safety and Health, MS-C24, 4676 Columbia Parkway, Cincinnati, OH 45226, USA, Tel: 513-533-8628, Fax: 513-533-8596, E-mail: cji5@cdc.gov.

industry sectors such as papermaking, printing and chemical had a higher prevalence of poor SRH as compared to the textile industry. Gender-specific analysis did not show much difference in associated factors between men and women in this sample, but men in the highest group of BMI and women working under a shift/night schedule were gender-unique factors related to poor SRH. Although the results should be interpreted cautiously because of self-reporting and cross-sectional study design, we conclude that poor SRH is prevalent among workers in SMMEs, and is associated with a number of modifiable factors at individual and organizational level.

Keywords: self-rated health, working population, socioeconomic status, lifestyle, occupational factors, smoking, work hour, work schedule, work organization, financial situation, insomnia, depressive symptoms, small- and medium-scale enterprise, social epidemiology, occupational health.

INTRODUCTION

Self-rated health (SRH) or self-perceived health has become an increasingly common measure used in population surveys. It is often based on a simple question where people are asked to rate their current overall health, typically on a four or five-point scale ranging from "very good (excellent)" to "very poor." Despite its simplicity, responses to this question have proven to be a robust predictor of functional disability (Amos, Currie, Hunt, & Martin, 1990; Farmer & Ferraro, 1997; Idler & Kasl, 1995), mortality (Idler & Benyamini, 1997), morbidity (Farmer & Ferraro, 1997; Idler & Benyamini, 1997; Miilunpalo, Vuori, Oja, Pasanen, & Urponen, 1997; Weinberger, Darnell, Tierney, Martz, Hiner, Barker et al., 1986), and health care use (Mossey & Shapiro, 1982), even after adjusting for sociodemographic, behavioral, psychosocial, environmental, physician-observed health status, and/or health-related risk factors. SRH has also been indicated to be a stronger predictor of mortality than medical records or self-reported medical conditions among the elderly population (Mossey & Shapiro, 1982).

Previous studies have identified various factors associated with poor SRH. These include lower educational attainment (Honjo, Kawakami, Takeshima, Tachimori, Ono, Uda et al., 2006; von dem Knesebeck, Luschen, Cockerham, & Siegrist, 2003), lower socioeconomic status (Honjo et al., 2006; Laaksonen, Rahkonen, Martikainen, & Lahelma, 2005; Lindstrom, 2005), female gender (Kaleta, Makowiec-Dabrowska, Dziankowska-Zaborszczyk, & Jegier, 2006; McCullough & Laurenceau, 2004), ageing (Andersen, Christensen, & Frederiksen, 2007; Leinonen, Heikkinen, & Jylha, 2001), smoking (af Sillen, Nilsson, Mansson, & Nilsson, 2005; CDC, 1996; Froom, Melamed, Triber, Ratson, & Hermoni, 2004; Kaleta et al., 2006; Kaplan, Goldberg, Everson, Cohen, Salonen, Tuomilehto et al., 1996; Kawachi, Kennedy, & Glass, 1999; Kennedy, Kawachi, & Prothrow-Stith, 1996; Yen & Kaplan, 1999), heavy drinking (Okosun, Seale, Daniel, & Eriksen, 2005), obesity (Okosun, Choi, Matamoros, & Dever, 2001; Seidell, Bakx, Deurenberg, Burema, Hautvast, & Huygen, 1986), poor physical functioning (Lee & Shinkai, 2003; Martikainen, Lahelma, Marmot, Sekine, Nishi, & Kagamimori, 2004), and chronic disease (Idler, Russell, & Davis, 2000; Pijls, Feskens, & Kromhout, 1993).

However, factors identified as risks in these studies were often derived from geriatric or general population, which include the non-working population such as retired/unemployed people, students and homemakers. When the study population focused on occupationally active individuals specifically, analysis may provide different information because occupational and organizational variables are reported to modify SRH significantly. For example, workers in higher occupational class/prestige perceived their health better than in workers of lower class (Laaksonen et al., 2005; Lahelma, Martikainen, Laaksonen, & Aittomaki, 2004; Mustard, Vermeulen, & Lavis, 2003; von dem Knesebeck et al., 2003). Poor psychosocial work environment such as high stress at work (Hillen, Davies, Rudd, Kieselbach, & Wolfe, 2003; Pikhart, Bobak, Siegrist, Pajak, Rywik, Kyshegyi et al., 2001; Stavem, Hofoss, & Aasland, 2003), long working hours (Kopp, Stauder, Purebl, Janszky, & Skrabski, 2007), and shift or night work schedule (Karlson, Eek, Hansen, Garde, Osterberg, & Orbaek, 2006) are also connected to poor SRH. In addition, work conditions in small- and medium-scale enterprises (SMEs) are often worse that those in large-scale enterprises) (CDC, 1999; Ikeda, Nakata, Kobori, Hojo, & Sugishita, 2002; Nakata, Ikeda, Takahashi, Haratani, Hojou, Swanson et al., 2006b) because of poorer occupational health and safety activities (Furuki, Hirata, & Kage, 2006; Hirata, Kumagai, Tabuchi, Tainaka, Andoh, & Oda, 1999; Kumagai, Hirata, Tabuchi, Tainaka, Andoh, & Oda, 2000).

Therefore, this study was designed to identify the factors associated with poor SRH in workers of small- and medium-scale manufacturing enterprises (SMMEs). We included not only major and classical variables known to relate to SRH, but estimated some variables considered to be unique to SMEs.

SUBJECTS AND METHODS

Study Design and Subjects

The study design was cross-sectional and data were collected by a self-rating questionnaire from August to December 2002. Subjects were workers in SMMEs with 1 to 158 workers in Yashio city, Saitama prefecture, Japan. The city has the highest percentages of both manufacturing plants and people working in manufacturing in the prefecture. In this area, 1,813 small-and medium-scale manufacturing factories were listed in the 2000 edition of the city commercial directory. We randomly selected 329 factories from the directory, depending on the distribution of types of businesses in this city (n=3,514). We contacted each factory by telephone and requested participation in a questionnaire survey concerning "lifestyle and health." Of these, 248 factories agreed to participate in the survey and questionnaires were distributed during visits to each factory and were given to 2,591 full-time workers (participation rate 73.7%). Finally, responses were obtained from 2,302 workers from 244 factories, representing a response rate of 88.8% (Nakata, Ikeda, Takahashi, Haratani, Hojou, Fujioka et al., 2006a).

Items on the questionnaire concerned sociodemographic and socioeconomic factors, lifestyle, health condition, and occupational and organizational information. A total of 1,490 men and 715 women completed questions about sociodemography, lifestyle, health condition, and occupational factors (Table 1).

The Medical Ethical Committee of the University of Tokyo approved the study, and written informed consent was obtained from all participants.

Table 1. Descriptive statistics for demographics, lifestyles, and occupational characteristics of the study population

Characteristics	Men		Women		P^a
Number of subjects (%)	1,490	(67.6)	715	(32.4)	
Self-rated health					.287
Very good	187	(12.6)	73	(10.2)	
Good	805	(54.0)	412	(57.6)	
Poor	459	(30.8)	214	(29.9)	
Very poor	39	(2.6)	16	(2.2)	
Sociodemographic factors:					
Age group, years					<.001
16-29	233	(15.6)	131	(18.3)	
30-39	371	(24.9)	115	(16.1)	
40-49	254	(17.0)	111	(15.5)	
50-59	394	(26.4)	252	(35.2)	
60 and over	238	(16.0)	106	(14.8)	
Mean [SD]	44.9	[13.6]	45.5	[13.7]	.366
Marital status					<.001
Single	399	(26.8)	141	(19.7)	
Married	1,023	(68.7)	489	(68.4)	
Separeted/divorced	55	(3.7)	56	(7.8)	
Bereaved	13	(0.9)	29	(4.1)	
Socioeconomic factors:					
Highest education					<.001
Junior high school	370	(24.8)	154	(21.5)	
High school	662	(44.4)	389	(54.4)	
Vocational/college/university	458	(30.7)	172	(24.1)	
Household financial situation					.015
Very comfortable/comfortable	109	(7.3)	63	(8.8)	
Just getting by	685	(46.0)	365	(51.0)	
Finding it difficult/very difficult	696	(46.7)	287	(40.1)	

Characteristics	Men		Women		P^a
Behavioral factors:					<.001
Smoking history					
Never smoker	445	(29.9)	521	(72.9)	
Former smoker	172	(11.5)	36	(5.0)	
Current smoker	873	(58.6)	158	(22.1)	
Drinking habit (g ethanol/day)					<.001
Non-drinker (0.0)	372	(25.0)	402	(56.2)	
0.01 to 4.9	192	(12.9)	168	(23.5)	
5.0 to 14.9	337	(22.6)	101	(14.1)	
15.0 to 24.9	286	(19.2)	30	(4.2)	
25.0 or more	303	(20.3)	14	(2.0)	
Caffeine intake (cups of coffee or tea/day)					.028
Almost none	143	(9.6)	47	(6.6)	
1 to 2	680	(45.6)	326	(45.6)	
3 or more	667	(44.8)	342	(47.8)	
Physical/psychological health factors:					
Body mass index (kg/height $(m)^2$)					
Mean [SD]	23.2	[3.4]	22.1	[3.1]	<.001
Insomnia symptoms					.661
No	1,140	(76.5)	541	(75.7)	
Yes	350	(23.5)	174	(24.3)	
Depressive symptoms					.731
CES-D score < 16	910	(61.1)	443	(62.0)	
CES-D score ≥ 16	580	(38.9)	272	(38.0)	
Number of chronic disease currently under treatment					.201
None	1,108	(74.4)	550	(76.9)	
1	324	(21.7)	146	(20.4)	
2 or more	58	(3.9)	19	(2.7)	
Occupational factors:					
Job type					<.001
Sales/service	147	(9.9)	11	(1.5)	
Managerial/clerical	247	(16.6)	351	(49.1)	

Table 1. Continued

Characteristics	Men		Women		P^a
Technical	67	(4.5)	16	(2.2)	
Manufacturing	767	(51.5)	240	(33.6)	
Other	262	(17.6)	97	(13.6)	
Work schedule					.032
Non-shift/daytime	1,442	(96.8)	675	(94.4)	
Shift/night	48	(3.2)	40	(5.6)	
Regular work hours a day					<.001
Less than 8 hrs	795	(53.4)	570	(79.7)	
8 hrs or more	695	(46.6)	145	(20.3)	
Personal relationship with the company					<.001
An owner	252	(16.9)	80	(11.2)	
An owner's family member, sibling or relative	258	(17.3)	185	(25.9)	
A non-family or non-relative	980	(65.8)	450	(62.9)	
Industry sector					<.001
Textile	29	(1.9)	30	(4.2)	
Food	73	(4.9)	80	(11.2)	
Papermaking	101	(6.8)	56	(7.8)	
Printing	32	(2.1)	25	(3.5)	
Chemical	248	(16.6)	130	(18.2)	
Leather	26	(1.7)	25	(3.5)	
Metalworking	630	(42.3)	245	(34.3)	
Machinery	260	(17.4)	89	(12.4)	
Other	91	(6.1)	35	(4.9)	
Company size by number of workers					<.001
1 to 49	1,124	(75.4)	497	(69.5)	
50 to 99	253	(17.0)	134	(18.7)	
100 or more	113	(7.6)	84	(11.7)	

[a]p value derived from $\chi 2$ test for categorical variables and Student's t-test for continuous variables.
Note. SD, standard deviation; CES-D, Center for Epidemiologic Studies Depression Scale.

Measures

Self-Rated Health (SRH)

SRH was assessed with a question: How would you describe your health during the past 1-year period? Response options were 'very good', 'good', 'poor', and 'very poor.' We dichotomized SRH into 1) poor or very poor (suboptimal) health and 2) good or very good (optimal) health. Similar use of SRH is common in studies of this kind (Heidrich, Liese, Lowel, & Keil, 2002; Ho, Lam, Fielding, & Janus, 2003; Idler & Benyamini, 1997; Kawachi et al., 1999; Malmstrom, Sundquist, & Johansson, 1999; Svedberg, Lichtenstein, & Pedersen, 2001).

Sociodemographic and Socioeconomic Variables

Sociodemographic and socioeconomic variables were age in years, marital status, highest educational attainment, and perceived household financial situation. Marital status was classified into four categories: 1) single, 2) married, 3) separated/divorced, and 4) bereaved. Educational attainment was assessed as the highest level reached and classified into three categories: 1) junior high school (years of education; 9 years or less), 2) high school (years of education; 9 -12 years), and 3) vocational/college/university (years of education; 12 years or more). We assessed respondent's household financial situation by asking a following question: Overall, how would you rate your current household financial situation? Response options were 'very comfortable', 'comfortable', 'just getting by', 'finding it difficult', and 'finding it very difficult.' Responses were classified into three levels as 1) very comfortable/comfortable, 2) just getting by, and 3) finding it difficult/very difficult.

Lifestyle Variables

Lifestyle variables were smoking status, drinking habit, and daily caffeine intake. Smoking status was classified into three categories: 1) current smoker, 2) former smoker, and 3) lifetime never smoker. Drinking habit was estimated by asking the number of alcoholic drinks consumed a day, with one drink estimated as about 9 g of pure ethanol. The amount of ethanol consumed a day was computed and classified into five groups: 0.0 g/day (non-drinker), 0.01 to 4.9 g/day, 5.0 to 14.9 g/day, 15.0 to 24.9 g/day, 25.0 or more. Caffeine intake was estimated by asking number of cups of tea or coffee consumed a day and classified into three categories: 1) almost none, 2) 1 to 2 cups/day, and 3) 3 cups/day or more.

Health Related Variables

Health related variables were body mass index (BMI), number of chronic disease currently under treatment, insomnia symptoms, and depressive symptoms. BMI was calculated as weight in kilograms divided by the square of height in meters (self-reported) and was divided into quintiles. For chronic health condition, participants were asked if they were currently under treatment for any of the following diseases: hypertension, hyperlipidemia, diabetes mellitus, major depression, menopausal disorder, or other diseases. If the subjects reported 'other diseases,' they were asked to specify the condition. Subjects reported various diseases including cardiovascular disease, cancer, liver disease, renal disease, peptic ulcer, gastrointestinal diseases, neurological diseases, hyperthyroidism, prostatomegaly, rheumatism, musculoskeletal disorders, panic disorder, and allergy.

Insomnia symptoms were defined by either taking more than 30 minutes to fall asleep, awakening during sleep more than 3 times a week, or early morning awakening more than 3 times a week during the last 1-year period (Nakata, Haratani, Kawakami, Miki, Kurabayashi, & Shimizu, 2000; Nakata, Haratani, Takahashi, Kawakami, Arito, Kobayashi et al., 2004a; Nakata, Haratani, Takahashi, Kawakami, Arito, Kobayashi et al., 2004b; Nakata, Ikeda, Takahashi, Haratani, Fujioka, Fukui et al., 2005; Nakata et al., 2006b). The reliability of sleep questions used in this survey was assessed in our previous study (Nakata, Takahashi, Haratani, Ikeda, Hojou, Fujioka et al., *in press*). Briefly, test-retest over a 1-year period for above sleep questions were examined by Spearman's rank correlation coefficients and found that correlation coefficients were at least $r = .545$ with $p<.001$. The validity was estimated by calculating Spearman's rank correlation coefficients among demographic, lifestyle factors and sleep questions. The results revealed that all correlations were in the expected direction, and the sleep questions properly showed an almost zero correlation with a measure with which it was predicted to have no relationship.

Depressive symptoms were measured by a Japanese version (Shima, Shikano, Kitamura, & Asai, 1985) of the Center for Epidemiologic Studies Depression (CES-D) scale (Radloff, 1977). The 20-item depressive symptom scale measures the level of depressive symptoms experienced in the past week. The CES-D scale cut-off score is 16, which differentiates between those exhibiting high levels of depressive symptoms (score $\geq$ 16) from those with lower levels of such symptoms (score $<$ 16). The internal consistency of the CES-D scale for the study sample was 0.83 (Nakata, Takahashi, Ikeda, Haratani, Hojou, & Araki, 2007).

Occupational and Organizational Variables

Occupational and organizational variables were job type, industry sector, work schedule, respondents' personal relationship with the company, company size, and regular work hours a day. Job type was grouped into five categories: 1) sale/service, 2) managerial/clerical, 3) technical, 4) manufacturing, and 5) other. Since workers in SME engage in various jobs, we asked their main job. We identified 11 industry sectors in this survey (food, textile, woodwork, papermaking, printing, chemical, leather, metalworking, machinery, ceramic/stone/clay, and other) but were classified into nine groups because some sectors had a small sample size: 1) textile, 2) food, 3) papermaking, 4) printing, 5) chemical, 6) leather, 7) metalworking, 8) machinery, and 9) other. Work schedule was dichotomized into: 1) non-shift/daytime work and 2) night/shift work. Respondents' personal relationship with the company was estimated with the following question: What is your relationship with the owner of company where you work? Response options were 'a family member', 'a sibling', 'a relative', 'a non-family or a non-relative', and 'I myself is an owner.' We grouped respondents into three classes: 1) an owner, 2) an owner's family member, sibling or relative, and 3) a non-family/non-relative. Company size was assessed by total number of workers in each company and classified as follows: 1) 1-49 workers, 2) 50-99 workers, and 3) 100 or more workers. Work hours were asked by a following question: How many hours do you regularly work? Work hours were grouped into 1) less than 8 hours, and 2) 8 hours or more.

Statistical Analyses

Differences in sociodemographic and socioeconomic, lifestyle, health condition, and occupational variables between men and women were tested by the χ^2 test for categorical/nominal variables and Student's t-tests for continuous variables. We attempted to identify the associated factors underlying poor SRH using univariable and multivariable logistic regression analyses. Univariable analyses were performed to detect the relationship of poor SRH with each of the variables. For multivariable analyses, we entered all variables (as listed in Table 1) into the model. Because several previous studies have found a gender difference in judging and evaluating SRH (Benyamini, Idler, Leventhal, & Leventhal, 2000; Prager, Walter-Ginzburg, Blumstein, & Modan, 1999; Unden & Elofsson, 2006) and there were large differences in characteristics between men and women (Table 1), the odds ratios (ORs) and 95% confidence intervals (CIs) were calculated for men and women together, as well as for the men and women separately. The significance level for all statistical analyses was $p < 0.05$ (two-tailed test). All data were analyzed using the Statistical Package for the Social Sciences version 14.0 (SPSS Inc., Chicago, USA).

RESULTS

The characteristics of participants in the study are shown in Table 1. The average age of the study population was 45 for men and 46 for women, with about 2:1 proportions for men and women. Approximately two-thirds of men and women reported optimal SRH. More than two-thirds of participants were married. Men had higher educational attainment than women. About 47% of men and 40% of women rated their household financial situation as poor/very poor.

Overall, 58.6% of men and 22.1% of women were current smokers. Men tend to drink alcohol more than women but women tend to drink coffee/tea more than men. The average BMI was 23.2 for men and 22.1 for women. Prevalence of insomnia symptoms was 23.5% for men and 24.3% for women. Prevalence of high depressive symptoms was 38.9% for men and 38.0% for women. Both insomnia and depressive symptoms had no significant gender differences. Participants suffering from chronic condition were 25.6% for men and 23.1% for women.

More than 90% of study population worked in non-shift/daytime work schedule. Approximately 47% of men and 20% of women worked more than 8 hours a day. Overall, 17% of men and 11% of women reported that they were owners of company. More than half of men were working as manufacturing and about half of women were working as managerial/clerical work. More than two-thirds of study population was working in small businesses (as defined by less than 50 workers in the company).

Variables associated with poor SRH in total population are shown in Table 2. Univariable analyses showed that perceiving poor household financial situation, current smoking, insomnia symptoms, depressive symptoms, chronic disease, and long work hours are significant factors associated with poor SRH. However, multivariable analyses showed that female gender, higher educational attainment, and industry sector (papermaking, printing, and chemical as compared to textile) are additional factors associated with poor SRH.

Table 2. Variables associated with poor self-rated health among 2,205 workers in small- and medium-scale enterprises

Variables	n	Univariable OR (95%CI)	*p*	Multivariable OR (95%CI)	*p*
Gender			.558		.015
Men	1,490	1.00 (Reference)		1.00 (Reference)	
Women	715	0.95 (0.78-1.14)		1.56 (1.09-2.23)	
Age (in years)			.914		.652
16 to 29	364	1.11 (0.83-1.49)		1.35 (0.79-2.29)	
30 to 39	486	1.00 (Reference)		1.00 (Reference)	
40 to 49	365	1.03 (0.77-1.38)		1.24 (0.84-1.83)	
50 to 59	646	1.11 (0.86-1.43)		0.98 (0.66-1.47)	
60 and over	344	1.03 (0.76-1.38)		0.94 (0.62-1.42)	
Marital status			.119		.254
Single	540	1.89 (0.88-4.05)		3.33 (0.81-13.7)	
Married	1,512	1.60 (0.75-3.38)		2.67 (0.67-10.5)	
Separated/divorced	111	2.15 (0.93-4.99)		2.13 (0.48-9.55)	
Bereaved	42	1.00 (Reference)		1.00 (Reference)	
Highest educational level			.445		.043
Junior high school	524	1.00 (Reference)		1.00 (Reference)	
High school	1,051	1.16 (0.92-1.46)		1.53 (1.05-2.24)	
Vocational/college/university	630	1.14 (0.89-1.47)		1.71 (1.11-2.16)	
Household financial situation			<.001		.001
Very comfortable/comfortable	172	1.37 (0.96-1.95)		1.47 (0.92-2.36)	
Just getting by	1,050	1.00 (Reference)		1.00 (Reference)	
Finding it difficult/very difficult	983	1.95 (1.61-2.36)		1.67 (1.28-2.19)	
Smoking			.036		.012
Never smoker	966	1.00 (Reference)		1.00 (Reference)	
Former smoker	208	1.15 (0.83-1.58)		1.33 (0.83-2.11)	
Current smoker	1,031	1.28 (1.06-1.54)		1.58 (1.17-2.14)	
Drinking habit (g ethanol/day)			.718		.846
Non-drinker (0.0)	774	1.19 (0.90-1.58)		1.24 (0.81-1.90)	
0.01 to 4.9	360	1.03 (0.75-1.43)		1.11 (0.69-1.77)	
5.0 to 14.9	438	1.09 (0.80-1.49)		1.07 (0.69-1.77)	

Variables	n	Univariable OR (95%CI)	*p*	Multivariable OR (95%CI)	*p*
15.0 to 24.9	316	1.14 (0.82-1.60)		1.03 (0.65-1.63)	
25.0 or more	317	1.00 (Reference)		1.00 (Reference)	
Caffeine (cups/day)			.754		.924
Almost none	190	1.00 (Reference)		1.00 (Reference)	
1 to 2	1,006	1.12 (0.80-1.56)		1.11 (0.67-1.85)	
3 or more	1,009	1.07 (0.76-1.49)		1.10 (0.66-1.83)	
Body mass quintile			.153		.059
Lowest	444	1.31 (0.99-1.74)		1.00 (0.66-1.53)	
Low-moderate	449	1.03 (0.77-1.38)		1.14 (0.75-1.72)	
Moderate	430	1.09 (0.81-1.45)		1.39 (0.92-2.08)	
High-moderate	442	1.00 (Reference)		1.00 (Reference)	
Highest	440	1.32 (0.99-1.75)		1.65 (1.10-2.47)	
Insomnia symptoms[a]			<.001		<.001
No	1,681	1.00 (Reference)		1.00 (Reference)	
Yes	524	1.99 (1.62-2.43)		1.85 (1.38-2.48)	
Depressive symptoms			<.001		<.001
CES-D score < 16	1,353	1.00 (Reference)		1.00 (Reference)	
CES-D score ≥ 16	852	3.40 (2.78-4.16)		3.03 (2.34-3.91)	
Number of chronic disease currently under treatment			<.001		<.001
None	1,658	1.00 (Reference)		1.00 (Reference)	
1	470	2.23 (1.81-2.76)		2.48 (1.80-3.43)	
2 or more	77	3.13 (1.98-4.96)		3.27 (1.60-6.69)	
Job type			.399		.179
Sales/service	158	1.00 (Reference)		1.00 (Reference)	
Managerial/clerical	598	1.04 (0.70-1.55)		0.98 (0.57-1.69)	
Technical	83	1.43 (0.80-2.57)		1.48 (0.71-3.10)	
Manufacturing	1,007	1.25 (0.86-1.84)		1.44 (0.86-2.41)	
Other	359	1.19 (0.78-1.82)		1.22 (0.68-2.16)	
Work schedule			.172		.081
Non-shift/daytime	2,117	1.00 (Reference)		1.00 (Reference)	
Shift/night	88	1.37 (0.87-2.17)		1.92 (0.92-4.00)	
Regular work hours a day			<.001		.001
Less than 8 hrs	1,365	1.00 (Reference)		1.00 (Reference)	
8 hrs or more	840	1.41 (1.17-1.69)		1.60 (1.21-2.13)	

Table 2. Continued

Variables	n	Univariable OR (95%CI)	*p*	Multivariable OR (95%CI)	*p*
Personal relationship with the company			.148		.196
An owner	332	1.29 (0.95-1.75)		1.22 (0.75-1.99)	
An owner's family member, sibling or relative	443	1.00 (Reference)		1.00 (Reference)	
A non-family or non-relative	1,430	1.25 (0.99-1.58)		1.39 (0.97-1.99)	
Industry sector			.101		.005
Textile	59	1.00 (Reference)		1.00 (Reference)	
Food	153	1.56 (0.78-3.10)		1.89 (0.62-5.74)	
Papermaking	157	1.70 (0.95-4.63)		3.60 (1.22-10.6)	
Printing	57	2.10 (0.95-4.63)		4.19 (1.23-14.2)	
Chemical	378	1.89 (1.00-3.56)		3.09 (1.10-8.66)	
Leather	51	1.22 (0.52-2.89)		1.31 (0.31-5.49)	
Metalworking	875	1.36 (0.73-2.53)		1.77 (0.65-4.85)	
Machinery	349	1.55 (0.81-2.93)		1.84 (0.65-5.17)	
Other	126	2.05 (1.03-4.08)		2.94 (1.00-8.62)	
Company size by number of workers			.345		.416
1 to 49	1,621	1.19 (0.94-1.52)		1.18 (0.83-1.66)	
50 to 99	387	1.00 (Reference)		1.00 (Reference)	
100 or more	197	1.19 (0.83-1.72)		1.46 (0.81-2.62)	

OR, odds ratio; CI, confidence interval.

Variables associated with poor SRH in men and women are shown in Tables 3 and 4. Univariable analyses showed that poor household financial situation, insomnia symptoms, depressive symptoms, chronic disease, and long work hours are significant factors associated with poor SRH in men while poor household financial situation, insomnia symptoms, depressive symptoms, and chronic disease were associated in women. In men, in addition to above factors, the highest quintile of BMI and working in printing sector (as compared to textile sector) were related to poor SRH in multivariable analyses. In women, working under shift/night schedules was an additional factor that associated with poor SRH in multivariable analyses.

Table 3. Variables associated with poor self-rated health among 1,490 male workers in small- and medium-scale enterprises

Variables	n	Univariable OR (95%CI)	*p*	Multivariable OR (95%CI)	*p*
Age (in years)			.956		.737
16 to 29	233	1.09 (0.77-1.54)		0.82 (0.50-1.34)	
30 to 39	371	1.00 (Reference)		1.00 (Reference)	
40 to 49	254	1.00 (0.71-1.41)		1.00 (0.63-1.59)	
50 to 59	394	1.05 (0.78-1.42)		1.01 (0.63-1.61)	
60 and over	238	0.94 (0.66-1.34)		1.36 (0.73-2.55)	
Marital status			.195		-
Single	399	1.50 (0.39-5.74)		-	
Married	1,023	1.24 (0.33-4.70)		-	
Separated/divorced	55	2.02 (0.48-8.52)		-	
Bereaved	13	1.00 (Reference)		-	
Highest educational level			.068		.121
Junior high school	370	1.00 (Reference)		1.00 (Reference)	
High school	662	1.38 (1.04-1.83)		1.59 (1.00-2.51)	
Vocational/college/university	458	1.34 (0.99-1.82)		1.64 (0.97-2.77)	
Household financial situation			<.001		.011
Very comfortable/comfortable	109	1.48 (0.95-2.30)		1.59 (0.89-2.83)	
Just getting by	685	1.00 (Reference)		1.00 (Reference)	
Finding it difficult/very difficult	696	1.90 (1.51-2.40)		1.60 (1.15-2.21)	
Smoking			.488		.598
Never smoker	445	1.00 (Reference)		1.00 (Reference)	
Former smoker	172	1.09 (0.75-1.58)		1.17 (0.67-2.02)	
Current smoker	873	1.16 (0.91-1.48)		1.21 (0.84-1.74)	
Drinking habit (g ethanol/day)			.030		.463
Non-drinker (0.0)	372	1.55 (1.12-2.14)		1.37 (0.86-2.18)	
0.01 to 4.9	192	0.97 (0.65-1.44)		0.94 (0.54-1.62)	
5.0 to 14.9	337	1.08 (0.76-1.50)		0.94 (0.58-1.52)	
15.0 to 24.9	286	1.10 (0.78-1.56)		1.04 (0.65-1.69)	
25.0 or more	303	1.00 (Reference)		1.00 (Reference)	
Caffeine (cups/day)			.286		.281

Table 3. Continued

Variables	n	Univariable OR (95%CI)	*p*	Multivariable OR (95%CI)	*p*
Almost none	143	1.00 (Reference)		1.00 (Reference)	
1 to 2	680	1.38 (0.93-2.06)		1.65 (0.88-3.08)	
3 or more	667	1.30 (0.87-1.94)		1.62 (0.86-3.04)	
Body mass quintile			.079		.040
Lowest	299	1.48 (1.05-2.09)		1.17 (0.70-1.97)	
Low-moderate	301	1.04 (0.74-1.48)		1.42 (0.86-2.35)	
Moderate	291	1.07 (0.76-1.53)		1.62 (0.98-2.67)	
High-moderate	300	1.00 (Reference)		1.00 (Reference)	
Highest	299	1.37 (0.97-1.93)		2.05 (1.25-3.35)	
Insomnia symptoms			<.001		.005
No	1,140	1.00 (Reference)		1.00 (Reference)	
Yes	350	1.97 (1.53-2.52)		1.66 (1.16-2.38)	
Depressive symptoms			<.001		<.001
CES-D score < 16	910	1.00 (Reference)		1.00 (Reference)	
CES-D score ≥ 16	580	3.97 (3.11-5.08)		3.96 (2.88-5.44)	
Number of chronic disease currently under treatment			<.001		<.001
None	1,108	1.00 (Reference)		1.00 (Reference)	
1	324	1.99 (1.54-2.56)		2.25 (1.50-3.36)	
2 or more	58	2.26 (1.33-3.84)		2.74 (1.18-6.35)	
Job type			.713		.152
Sales/service	147	1.00 (Reference)		1.00 (Reference)	
Managerial/clerical	247	1.11 (0.70-1.76)		0.79 (0.43-1.45)	
Technical	67	1.57 (0.84-2.93)		1.54 (0.68-3.49)	
Manufacturing	767	1.19 (0.80-1.77)		1.37 (0.79-2.38)	
Other	262	1.16 (0.73-1.83)		1.20 (0.64-2.25)	
Work schedule			.517		.626
Non-shift/daytime	1,442	1.00 (Reference)		1.00 (Reference)	
Shift/night	48	1.23 (0.66-2.26)		1.29 (0.47-3.55)	
Regular work hours a day			.001		.005
Less than 8 hrs	795	1.00 (Reference)		1.00 (Reference)	
8 hrs or more	695	1.49 (1.18-1.88)		1.62 (1.16-2.27)	
Personal relationship with the company			.248		.284

Variables	n	Univariable OR (95%CI)	*p*	Multivariable OR (95%CI)	*p*
An owner	252	1.21 (0.83-1.77)		1.21 (0.68-2.18)	
An owner's family member, sibling or relative	285 -	1.00 (Reference)		1.00 (Reference)	
A non-family or non-relative	980	1.30 (0.96-1.76)		1.45 (0.90-2.33)	
Industry sector			.055		.014
Textile	29	1.00 (Reference)		1.00 (Reference)	
Food	73	1.71 (0.61-4.80)		1.63 (0.28-9.60)	
Papermaking	101	1.53 (0.56-4.16)		2.82 (0.51-15.7)	
Printing	32	2.45 (0.79-7.63)		9.46 (1.40-63.9)	
Chemical	248	2.47 (0.96-6.34)		3.12 (0.59-16.5)	
Leather	26	1.56 (0.45-5.33)		1.71 (0.23-12.9)	
Metalworking	630	1.47 (0.58-3.70)		1.61 (0.31-8.34)	
Machinery	260	1.93 (0.75-4.95)		1.95 (0.37-10.2)	
Other	91	2.10 (0.78-5.69)		2.69 (0.49-14.9)	
Company size by number of workers			.673		.532
1 to 49	1,124	1.12 (0.84-1.50)		1.05 (0.69-1.60)	
50 to 99	253	1.00 (Reference)		1.00 (Reference)	
100 or more	113	1.21 (0.76-1.93)		1.50 (0.72-3.12)	

OR, odds ratio; CI, confidence interval; -, Estimates could not be calculated.

Table 4. Variables associated with poor self-rated health among 715 female workers in small- and medium-scale enterprises

Variables	n	Univariable OR (95%CI)	*p*	Multivariable OR (95%CI)	*p*
Age (in years)			.818		.515
16 to 29	131	1.27 (0.73-2.19)		1.23 (0.47-3.23)	
30 to 39	115	1.00 (Reference)		1.00 (Reference)	
40 to 49	111	1.15 (0.65-2.03)		1.20 (0.49-2.94)	
50 to 59	252	1.34 (0.82-2.18)		2.04 (0.89-4.65)	
60 and over	106	1.28 (0.72-2.28)		1.79 (0.55-5.78)	
Marital status			.549		.686
Single	141	1.96 (0.75-5.15)		2.72 (0.44-17.0)	
Married	489	1.74 (0.70-4.37)		1.69 (0.34-8.48)	
Separated/divorced	56	2.03 (0.70-5.89)		1.79 (0.28-11.5)	

Table 4. Continued

Variables	n	Univariable OR (95%CI)	*p*	Multivariable OR (95%CI)	*p*
Bereaved	29	1.00 (Reference)		1.00 (Reference)	
Highest educational level			.530		.263
Junior high school	154	1.29 (0.81-2.08)		1.40 (0.63-3.10)	
High school	389	1.07 (0.72-1.58)		2.00 (0.83-4.79)	
Vocational/college/university	172	1.00 (Reference)		1.00 (Reference)	
Household financial situation			<.001		.188
Very comfortable/comfortable	63	1.23 (0.68-2.25)		1.33 (0.52-3.42)	
Just getting by	365	1.00 (Reference)		1.00 (Reference)	
Finding it difficult/very difficult	287	2.08 (1.49-2.92)		1.65 (0.97-2.79)	
Smoking			.013		.002
Never smoker	521	1.00 (Reference)		1.00 (Reference)	
Former smoker	36	1.21 (0.59-2.48)		2.75 (0.97-7.79)	
Current smoker	158	1.74 (1.20-2.51)		2.73 (1.49-5.00)	
Drinking habit (g ethanol/day)			.341		.704
Non-drinker (0.0)	402	1.00 (Reference)		1.00 (Reference)	
0.01 to 4.9	168	1.20 (0.82-1.77)		1.45 (0.78-2.67)	
5.0 to 14.9	101	1.30 (0.82-2.07)		1.34 (0.66-2.75)	
15.0 to 24.9	30	2.09 (0.96-4.53)		1.10 (0.33-3.65)	
25.0 or more	14	1.34 (0.44-4.08)		0.56 (0.09-3.68)	
Caffeine (cups/day)			.462		.151
Almost none	47	1.47 (0.79-2.76)		2.77 (0.99-7.74)	
1 to 2	326	1.00 (Reference)		1.00 (Reference)	
3 or more	342	1.00 (0.72-1.39)		1.14 (0.68-1.93)	
Body mass quintile			.445		.439
Lowest	145	1.54 (0.93-2.57)		1.58 (0.73-3.40)	
Low-moderate	148	1.00 (Reference)		1.00 (Reference)	
Moderate	139	1.18 (0.70-2.00)		2.04 (0.91-4.58)	
High-moderate	142	1.50 (0.90-2.50)		1.96 (0.89-4.32)	
Highest	141	1.28 (0.76-2.16)		1.61 (0.69-3.73)	
Insomnia symptoms[a]			<.001		.004
No	541	1.00 (Reference)		1.00 (Reference)	
Yes	174	2.08 (1.45-2.97)		2.43 (1.34-4.42)	
Depressive symptoms			<.001		.031

Variables	n	Univariable OR (95%CI)	*p*	Multivariable OR (95%CI)	*p*
CES-D score < 16	443	1.00 (Reference)		1.00 (Reference)	
CES-D score ≥ 16	272	2.48 (1.73-3.54)		1.75 (1.05-2.90)	
Number of chronic disease currently under treatment			<.001		<.001
None	550	1.00 (Reference)		1.00 (Reference)	
1	146	2.85 (1.95-4.15)		3.76 (2.00-7.08)	
2 or more	19	7.97 (2.82-22.5)		18.5 (2.90-117.6)	
Job type			.394		.558
Sales/service	11	1.00 (Reference)		1.00 (Reference)	
Managerial/clerical	351	1.43 (0.29-7.03)		6.79 (0.54-84.9)	
Technical	16	1.27 (0.18-8.89)		8.29 (0.48-144.1)	
Manufacturing	240	2.04 (0.41-10.1)		8.15 (0.64-103.4)	
Other	97	1.69 (0.33-8.67)		5.89 (0.46-76.2)	
Work schedule			.165		.032
Non-shift/daytime	675	1.00 (Reference)		1.00 (Reference)	
Shift/night	40	1.63 (0.82-3.25)		4.08 (1.13-14.8)	
Regular work hours a day			.089		.137
Less than 8 hrs	570	1.00 (Reference)		1.00 (Reference)	
8 hrs or more	145	1.40 (0.95-2.07)		1.60 (0.86-2.96)	
Personal relationship with the company			.385		.430
An owner	80	1.49 (0.85-2.60)		1.37 (0.42-4.45)	
An owner's family member, sibling or relative	185	1.00 (Reference)		1.00 (Reference)	
A non-family or non-relative	450	1.14 (0.78-1.66)		1.57 (0.80-3.07)	
Industry sector			.261		.169
Textile	30	1.25 (0.35-4.49)		1.11 (0.07-17.0)	
Food	80	1.80 (0.60-5.39)		2.78 (0.25-30.6)	
Papermaking	56	2.67 (0.86-8.25)		7.16 (0.59-87.0)	
Printing	25	2.40 (0.67-8.58)		2.21 (0.15-33.0)	
Chemical	130	1.62 (0.56-4.66)		3.50 (0.30-40.5)	
Leather	25	1.00 (Reference)		1.00 (Reference)	
Metalworking	245	1.67 (0.60-4.66)		2.42 (0.23-25.9)	
Machinery	89	1.18 (0.39-3.56)		1.54 (0.13-18.7)	
Other	35	2.77 (0.88-8.74)		4.29 (0.35-52.8)	

Table 4. Continued

Variables	n	Univariable OR (95%CI)	*p*	Multivariable OR (95%CI)	*p*
Company size by number of workers			.304		.937
1 to 49	497	1.39 (0.91-2.13)		0.98 (0.48-2.00)	
50 to 99	134	1.00 (Reference)		1.00 (Reference)	
100 or more	84	1.22 (0.67-2.22)		1.19 (0.39-3.64)	

OR, odds ratio; CI, confidence interval.

Discussion

A focus of the present study was to examine the correlates of poor SRH in workers of SMMEs. A wide range of factors was included in the model to identify the variables associated with poor SRH. The results suggested that about one-third of participants perceived their health as poor, with no statistical difference between men and women. Multivariable logistic regression analysis revealed that female gender, poor household financial situation, higher educational attainment, current smoking, insomnia symptoms, depressive symptoms, chronic condition, long work hours, and shift/night work schedule are factors independently associated with poor SRH. Some industry sectors (papermaking, printing, and chemical) had a higher prevalence of poor SRH than the textile industry (reference sector). Gender-specific analysis did no show a large difference in associated factors of poor SRH between men and women, but men in the highest group of BMI and women working under shift/night work schedule were found to be gender-specific factors related to poor SRH in this population. Although the results should be interpreted cautiously because of self-reporting and cross-sectional study design, we conclude that poor SRH is prevalent among workers in SMMEs, and is associated with a number of modifiable factors at individual and organizational level.

Socioeconomic Factors and SRH

In this study, perceived poor household financial situation was significantly associated with poor SRH. Participants finding household financial situation 'difficult' or 'very difficult' reported about 1.6 times increase in poor SRH as compared to participants reporting 'just getting by.' Many previous studies have found that people with economic difficulties (Laaksonen et al., 2005; Lindstrom, 2005), low household income (Honjo et al., 2006; Kaleta et al., 2006; Lahelma et al., 2004), and material deprivation (von dem Knesebeck et al., 2003) are related to poor SRH, which is supportive to the findings of our study. A recent study by Laaksonen et al. (2005) reported that women with 'frequent' and 'occasional' economic difficulties had ORs of respective 1.76 (95% CI 1.51, 2.05) and 1.31 (95% CI 1.13, 1.51) of poor SRH compared to women without economic difficulties in a middle-aged adults employed by the City of Helsinki (Laaksonen et al., 2005). Similarly, men with 'frequent' difficulties had OR of 1.65 (95% CI 1.23, 2.21) while men with 'occasional' difficulties had OR of 1.18 (95% CI 0.89, 1.56) of poor SRH compared to men without such difficulties. The results remained significant even after controlling for other socioeconomic indicators such as parental education, own education, childhood economic difficulties, occupational class, household income, and home ownership. The results also suggested that self-reported economic difficulties were more sensitive to SRH than gross household income.

Another finding on the relationship between household financial situation and SRH was that participants perceiving their financial situation as 'comfortable' or 'very comfortable' had even higher ORs (ranging from 1.33 to 1.59) of poor SRH than those with 'just getting by', although the results were not statistically significant. The reason why this association was found is unknown but some factors not included in this survey such as dietary habits, childhood economic difficulties, home ownership, neighborhood situation, social network, or physical exercise may partly explain the association or the results were simply by chance. However, further studies are warranted to draw a definite conclusion.

An unexpected finding was that higher educational attainment was related to poor SRH in this population. Most previous studies have observed that lower educational attainment relate to poorer SRH (Bobak, Pikhart, Hertzman, Rose, & Marmot, 1998; Honjo et al., 2006; Lahelma et al., 2004; von dem Knesebeck et al., 2003; White, Blane, Morris, & Mourouga, 1999), although there are some studies showing that educational attainment does not necessarily correlate with SRH (Osler, Heitmann, Hoidrup, Jorgensen, & Schroll, 2001; Wang, Iwasaki, Otani, Hayashi, Miyazaki, Xiao et al., 2005). It is not clear why workers with higher education attainment rated their health poor, but SME workers with higher education may work under higher job pressure and responsibility and multiple tasks with high workload, which may contribute to the development of poor SRH.

Behavioral Factors snd SRH

Among behavioral factors, current smoking was the only independent factor related to poor SRH. Women but not men who currently smoke had an independent association with poor SRH. As stated earlier, current smoking is a factor associated with poor SRH in both cross-sectional and prospective cohort studies. A population-based study specifically focused on the association between SRH and smoking reported that compared to never smoking women, current smoking women had OR of 1.95 (95% CI 1.2, 3.3) of poor SRH, whereas men had non-significant increase (OR=1.3, 95% CI 0.9, 1.9) by current smoking (Ho et al., 2003), consistent with our results. Several explanations are possible to this finding. First, women may experience more mental health problems than men by smoking. Previous studies have found that women rather than men having problems such as difficulty initiating and maintaining sleep (Franklin, Gislason, Omenaas, Jogi, Jensen, Lindberg et al., 2004; Nakata et al., *in press*), higher depressive symptoms (Benjet, Wagner, Borges, & Medina-Mora, 2004; Perez-Stable, Marin, Marin, & Katz, 1990; Son, Markovitz, Winders, & Smith, 1997), and poor mental health (Mino, Shigemi, Otsu, Ohta, Tsuda, Yasuda et al., 2001) by smoking. Second, women may experience higher social pressure than men not to smoke, especially in Asian countries (Mori, Sasaki, Iwanami, Araki, Mizuno, Kato et al., 2003). Women who persist in smoking despite such pressure may have more problems with psychosocial stress, quality of life, anxiety, depressed mood, social dysfunction, and impaired sleep, which may contribute to perceive their health poorer.

Health Related Factors and SRH

We found that mental health status as indicated by insomnia symptoms and depressive symptoms were independently associated with poor SRH. We also found that number of chronic disease under treatment and obesity (in men only) negatively correlated with SRH. Most studies including direct health outcomes or physical disability as independent variables observed a strong inverse association with SRH (Cott, Gignac, & Badley, 1999; Idler et al., 2000; Kivinen, Sulkava, Halonen, & Nissinen, 1998). For instance, Canadian household population interview survey found that illness related factors (any chronic condition or disability, pain severity, and any two week disability) as the strongest predictors of poor SRH including socioeconomic, demographic, lifestyle, and psychosocial resource variables (Cott et al., 1999). Kivinen et al. (1998) reported that strongest determinants of poor SRH were depression, coronary heart disease, and chronic lung disease among Finish men aged 70-89 years (Kivinen et al., 1998). A prospective study of IT and media workers observed that poor sleep quality at baseline was the strongest predictor of poor SRH at 1-year follow-up period (Hasson, Arnetz, Theorell, & Anderberg, 2006). A study by Okosun et al. (2001) reported that people with class II obesity (BMI>30) was consistently related to reduced self-rated health among white, black, and Hispanic population (Okosun et al., 2001). Thus it is plausible that poor health conditions as suffering from insomnia symptoms, depressive symptoms, obesity, and chronic disease are factors strongly associated with poor SRH in this sample.

Occupational/Organizational Factors and SRH

Among occupational factors, work hour and industry sector was associated with SRH in men while night/shift work schedule was associated with SRH in women. More than 8 hours of daily work in men had 1.6 times higher risk of poor SRH. We obtained similar results when cutoff point was at 9 hours of daily work or more (OR=1.7, 95% CI 1.2, 2.4), suggesting that overtime is a risk factor for poor SRH. Kopp et al. (2007) reported that weekend working hours are negatively correlated with SRH in both men and women while weekday working hours are positively correlated with SRH (Kopp et al., 2007). The authors concluded that healthier people work more and less healthy people work less during weekdays, but working in weekends may negatively influence SRH because of disturbance to non-working activities. Kaleta et al. (2006) also reported that long work hours (more than 42 hours/week) had negative impact on SRH (OR 2.0, 95% CI 1.1, 3.6) compared to 40-42 hours/week in male workers (Kaleta et al., 2006). In the same study, authors found that workers working less than 40 hours reported poor SRH with OR of 3.3 (95% CI 1.4, 7.7), suggesting workers who could not or do not work certain amount of time may already have had health-related difficulties or so. However, Kaleta et al. (2006) found no significant association in female workers in relation to work hours and SRH, consistent with current results. Although long hours of work seem detrimental to health, the relationship between work hours and health is rather complicated (Caruso, 2006; Iwasaki, Takahashi, & Nakata,

2006). Control over work time may be a key to reduce adverse effects of work hours on health.

Some industries (papermaking, printing, and chemical sectors) had higher prevalence of poor SRH than the textile industry (reference sector), especially in men. Industry sectors with poor working condition, i.e., exposure to toxic chemicals, poor work environment, and a high risk of occupational injuries or accidents may negatively contribute to SRH.

Night/shift work schedule was significantly associated with poor SRH in women. This finding is supported by the fact that night/shift workers experience various health problems than non-shift/daytime workers. Most prominent health issues in such population are poor sleep, chronic fatigue, and gastrointestinal complaints, i.e., the shift work disorders (Knutsson, 2003; Shen, Botly, Chung, Gibbs, Sabanadzovic, & Shapiro, 2006; Takahashi, Nakata, Haratani, Otsuka, Kaida, & Fukasawa, 2006; Takahashi, Tanigawa, Tachibana, Mutou, Kage, Smith et al., 2005). Thus it seems reasonable that night/shift workers to rate their health poorer than non-shift/daytime workers. In contrast, lack of association between night/shift work and poor SRH in men may be a result of healthy worker effect. We need to be aware of the fact that the relationship could be confounded by easiness to switch work schedules from night/shift work to daytime.

Strengths and Limitations of the Study

The strength of our study is that the survey included a wide range of variables to identify associated factors of SRH in workers of SMMEs. Multidimensional factors were included in the analysis to explain which factor could significantly contribute to poor SRH. Some variables considered to be unique to SMEs were also included.

Limitations are as follows. First, we did not ask physical and mental SRH separately. The results may change if we had asked them individually (Honjo et al., 2006; Mulvaney-Day, Alegria, & Sribney, 2007; Rohrer, Pierce, & Blackburn, 2005). Second, response bias may have occurred if the non-respondents differed from the respondents with respect to SRH. Of a total of 3,514 potential subjects, 923 (26.3%) refused to or could not participate in the survey at the initial recruitment. A major reason for non-participation was that the person responsible for the worksite did not have enough time to recruit workers or did not show any interest in the survey. Third, the data in this study derived from a single survey of workers in a geographically small area (Yashio city), which is not a representative sample of SMMEs in Japan. Fourth, data was obtained by self-reporting, which may introduce recall/reporting bias. Fifth, the cross-sectional design of this study limits the inferences of causality.

Conclusion

In conclusion, the present study demonstrated that poor SRH is prevalent in workers among SMMEs, and is associated with a number of risk factors that are modifiable. Such risk factors should be taken into account when attempting to improve health of workers in SMMEs.

ACKNOWLEDGEMENTS

This paper has been reviewed by Dr. Kenji Iwasaki, PhD, National Institute of Occupational Safety and Health, Japan, Dr. Yasumasa Otuka, PhD, Hiroshima University, and Mr. Rohit Verma, MSc, National Institute for Occupational Safety and Health, USA.

AUTHORS NOTES

All authors affirm the absence of any significant financial involvement in any organization with a direct commercial interest in the subjects of this manuscript.

The findings and conclusions in this report are those of the authors and do not necessarily represent the views of the National Institute for Occupational Safety and Health, USA.

REFERENCES

af Sillen, U., Nilsson, J.A., Mansson, N.O., & Nilsson, P. M. (2005). Self-rated health in relation to age and gender: influence on mortality risk in the Malmo Preventive Project. *Scandinavian Journal of Public Health,* 33(3), 183-189.

Amos, A., Currie, C., Hunt, S.M., & Martin, C. J.et al. (1990). Health-related behaviour in a small Scottish community. *Public Health,* 104(2), 131-140.

Andersen, F.K., Christensen, K. & Frederiksen, H. (2007). Self-rated health and age: a cross-sectional and longitudinal study of 11,000 Danes aged 45-102. *Scand J Public Health,* 35(2), 164-171.

Benjet, C., Wagner, F.A., Borges, G.G., & Medina-Mora, M. E. (2004). The relationship of tobacco smoking with depressive symptomatology in the Third Mexican National Addictions Survey. *Psychol Med,* 34(5), 881-888.

Benyamini, Y., Idler, E.L., Leventhal, H., et al. (2000). Positive affect and function as influences on self-assessments of health: expanding our view beyond illness and disability. *J Gerontol B Psychol Sci Soc Sci,* 55(2), P107-116.

Bobak, M., Pikhart, H., Hertzman, C., & Leventhal, E.A. (1998). Socioeconomic factors, perceived control and self-reported health in Russia. A cross-sectional survey. *Soc Sci Med,* 47(2), 269-279.

Caruso, C.C. (2006). Possible broad impacts of long work hours. *Ind Health,* 44(4), 531-536.

CDC (1996). Factors associated with self-perceived excellent and very good health among Blacks--Kansas, 1995. *Morbidity and Mortality Weekly Report,* 45(42), 906-911.

CDC. (1999). Identifying high-risk small business industries. The basis for preventing occupational injury, illness, and fatality. In DHHS (Ed.).

Cott, C.A., Gignac, M.A. & Badley, E.M. (1999). Determinants of self rated health for Canadians with chronic disease and disability. *J Epidemiol Community Health,* 53(11), 731-736.

Farmer, M.M., & Ferraro, K.F. (1997). Distress and perceived health: mechanisms of health decline. *Journal of Health and Social Behavior,* 38(3), 298-311.

Franklin, K.A., Gislason, T., Omenaas, E., Jogi, R., Jensen, E.J., Lindberg, E., et al. (2004). The influence of active and passive smoking on habitual snoring. *Am J Respir Crit Care Med,* 170(7), 799-803.

Froom, P., Melamed, S., Triber, I., et al. (2004). Predicting self-reported health: the CORDIS study. *Prev Med,* 39(2), 419-423.

Furuki, K., Hirata, M., & Kage, A. (2006). Nationwide survey of occupational health activities in small-scale enterprises in Japan. *Ind Health,* 44(1), 150-154.

Hasson, D., Arnetz, B.B., Theorell, T., & Anderberg, U.M. (2006). Predictors of self-rated health: a 12-month prospective study of IT and media workers. *Popul Health Metr,* 4, 8.

Heidrich, J., Liese, A.D., Lowel, H., & Keil, U. (2002). Self-rated health and its relation to all-cause and cardiovascular mortality in southern Germany. Results from the MONICA Augsburg cohort study 1984-1995. *Annals of Epidemiology,* 12(5), 338-345.

Hillen, T., Davies, S., Rudd, A.G., & Keil, U. (2003). Self ratings of health predict functional outcome and recurrence free survival after stroke. *J Epidemiol Community Health,* 57(12), 960-966.

Hirata, M., Kumagai, S., Tabuchi, T., Tainaka, H., Andoh, K., & Oda, H (1999). [Actual conditions of occupational health activities in small-scale enterprises in Japan: system for occupational health, health management and demands by small-scale enterprises]. *Sangyo Eiseigaku Zasshi,* 41(6), 190-201. (in Japanese)

Ho, S.Y., Lam, T.H., Fielding, R., & Janus, E. D. (2003). Smoking and perceived health in Hong Kong Chinese. *Social Science & Medicine,* 57(9), 1761-1770.

Honjo, K., Kawakami, N., Takeshima, T., Tachimori, H., Ono, Y., Uda, H., et al. (2006). Social class inequalities in self-rated health and their gender and age group differences in Japan. *J Epidemiol,* 16(6), 223-232.

Idler, E. L., & Benyamini, Y. (1997). Self-rated health and mortality: a review of twenty-seven community studies. *Journal of Health and Social Behavior,* 38(1), 21-37.

Idler, E. L., & Kasl, S. V. (1995). Self-ratings of health: do they also predict change in functional ability? *Journal of Gerontology: Psychological Sciences,* 50(6), S344-353.

Idler, E. L., Russell, L. B., & Davis, D. (2000). Survival, functional limitations, and self-rated health in the NHANES I Epidemiologic Follow-up Study, 1992. First National Health and Nutrition Examination Survey. *Am J Epidemiol,* 152(9), 874-883.

Ikeda, T., Nakata, A., Kobori, S., Hojo, M., & Sugishita, C. (2002). [Willingness to implement mental health measures among small-scale enterprise employers in Ohta ward, Tokyo, Japan]. *Sangyo Eiseigaku Zasshi,* 44(5), 200-207. (in Japanese)

Iwasaki, K., Takahashi, M. & Nakata, A. (2006). Health problems due to long working hours in Japan: working hours, workers' compensation (Karoshi), and preventive measures. *Ind Health,* 44(4), 537-540.

Kaleta, D., Makowiec-Dabrowska, T., Dziankowska-Zaborszczyk, E., & Jegier, A. (2006). Physical activity and self-perceived health status. *International Journal of Occupational Medicine and Environmental Health,* 19(1), 61-69.

Kaplan, G.A., Goldberg, D.E., Everson, S.A., Cohen, R.D., Salonen, R., Tuomilehto, J., et al. (1996). Perceived health status and morbidity and mortality: evidence from the Kuopio ischaemic heart disease risk factor study. *International Journal of Epidemiology,* 25(2), 259-265.

Karlson, B., Eek, F.C., Hansen, A.M., Garde, A. H., Osterberg, K., & Orbaek, P. (2006). Diurnal cortisol pattern of shift workers on a workday and a day off. *Scand J Work Environ Health,* Suppl 2, 27-34.

Kawachi, I., Kennedy, B. P., & Glass, R. (1999). Social capital and self-rated health: a contextual analysis. *Am J Public Health,* 89(8), 1187-1193.

Kennedy, B. P., Kawachi, I., & Prothrow-Stith, D. (1996). Income distribution and mortality: cross sectional ecological study of the Robin Hood index in the United States. *British Medical Journal,* 312(7037), 1004-1007.

Kivinen, P., Sulkava, R., Halonen, P., & Nissinen, A. (1998). Self-reported and performance-based functional status and associated factors among elderly men: the Finnish cohorts of the Seven Countries Study. *J Clin Epidemiol,* 51(12), 1243-1252.

Knutsson, A. (2003). Health disorders of shift workers. *Occup Med (Lond),* 53(2), 103-108.

Kopp, M. S., Stauder, A., Purebl, G., Janszky, I., & Skrabski, A. (2007). Work stress and mental health in a changing society. *Eur J Public Health.*

Kumagai, S., Hirata, M., Tabuchi, T., Tainaka, H., Andoh, K., & Oda, H. (2000). [Actual conditions of occupational health administration of small-scale enterprises in Japan: (II). Occupational health controls for hazardous and musculo-skeletally stressful working factors]. *Sangyo Eiseigaku Zasshi,* 42(5), 193-200. (in Japanese)

Laaksonen, M., Rahkonen, O., Martikainen, P., & Lahelma, E. (2005). Socioeconomic position and self-rated health: the contribution of childhood socioeconomic circumstances, adult socioeconomic status, and material resources. *Am J Public Health,* 95(8), 1403-1409.

Lahelma, E., Martikainen, P., Laaksonen, M., & Aittomaki, A. (2004). Pathways between socioeconomic determinants of health. *J Epidemiol Community Health,* 58(4), 327-332.

Lee, Y. & Shinkai, S. (2003). A comparison of correlates of self-rated health and functional disability of older persons in the Far East: Japan and Korea. *Arch Gerontol Geriatr,* 37(1), 63-76.

Leinonen, R., Heikkinen, E. & Jylha, M. (2001). Predictors of decline in self-assessments of health among older people--a 5-year longitudinal study. *Soc Sci Med,* 52(9), 1329-1341.

Lindstrom, M. (2005). Psychosocial work conditions, unemployment and self-reported psychological health: a population-based study. *Occup Med (Lond),* 55(7), 568-571.

Malmstrom, M., Sundquist, J. & Johansson, S.E. (1999). Neighborhood environment and self-reported health status: a multilevel analysis. *Am J Public Health,* 89(8), 1181-1186.

Martikainen, P., Lahelma, E., Marmot, M., Sekine, M., Nishi, N., & Kagamimori, S. (2004). A comparison of socioeconomic differences in physical functioning and perceived health among male and female employees in Britain, Finland and Japan. *Soc Sci Med,* 59(6), 1287-1295.

McCullough, M.E. & Laurenceau, J. P. (2004). Gender and the natural history of self-rated health: a 59-year longitudinal study. *Health Psychol,* 23(6), 651-655.

Miilunpalo, S., Vuori, I., Oja, P., Pasanen, M., & Urponen, H. (1997). Self-rated health status as a health measure: the predictive value of self-reported health status on the use of physician services and on mortality in the working-age population. *Journal of Clinical Epidemiology,* 50(5), 517-528.

Mino, Y., Shigemi, J., Otsu, T., Ohta, A., Tsuda, T., Yasuda, N., et al. (2001). Smoking and mental health: cross-sectional and cohort studies in an occupational setting in Japan. *Prev Med,* 32(4), 371-375.

Mori, T., Sasaki, T., Iwanami, A., Araki, T., Mizuno, K., Kato, T., et al. (2003). Smoking habits in Japanese patients with schizophrenia. *Psychiatry Res,* 120(2), 207-209.

Mossey, J. M., & Shapiro, E. (1982). Self-rated health: a predictor of mortality among the elderly. *Am J Public Health,* 72(8), 800-808.

Mulvaney-Day, N.E., Alegria, M. & Sribney, W. (2007). Social cohesion, social support, and health among Latinos in the United States. *Soc Sci Med,* 64(2), 477-495.

Mustard, C. A., Vermeulen, M. & Lavis, J.N. (2003). Is position in the occupational hierarchy a determinant of decline in perceived health status? *Social Science & Medicine,* 57(12), 2291-2303.

Nakata, A., Haratani, T., Kawakami, N., Miki, A., Kurabayashi, L., & Shimizu, H. (2000). Sleep problems in white-collar male workers in an electric equipment manufacturing company in Japan. *Ind Health,* 38(1), 62-68.

Nakata, A., Haratani, T., Takahashi, M., Kawakami, N., Arito, H., Kobayashi, F., et al. (2004a). Job stress, social support, and prevalence of insomnia in a population of Japanese daytime workers. *Soc Sci Med,* 59(8), 1719-1730.

Nakata, A., Haratani, T., Takahashi, M., Kawakami, N., Arito, H., Kobayashi, F., et al. (2004b). Association of sickness absence with poor sleep and depressive symptoms in shift workers. *Chronobiol Int,* 21(6), 899-912.

Nakata, A., Ikeda, T., Takahashi, M., Haratani, T., Fujioka, Y., Fukui, S., et al. (2005). Sleep-related risk of occupational injuries in Japanese small and medium-scale enterprises. *Ind Health,* 43(1), 89-97.

Nakata, A., Ikeda, T., Takahashi, M., Haratani, T., Hojou, M., Fujioka, Y., et al. (2006a). Non-fatal occupational injury among active and passive smokers in small- and medium-scale manufacturing enterprises in Japan. *Soc Sci Med,* 63(9), 2452-2463.

Nakata, A., Ikeda, T., Takahashi, M., Haratani, T., Hojou, M., Swanson, N.G., et al. (2006b). The prevalence and correlates of occupational injuries in small-scale manufacturing enterprises. *J Occup Health,* 48(5), 366-376.

Nakata, A., Takahashi, M., Haratani, T., Ikeda, T., Hojou, M., Fujioka, Y., et al. Association of active and passive smoking with sleep disturbances and short sleep duration among Japanese working population. *Int J Behav Med (in press).*

Nakata, A., Takahashi, M., Ikeda, T., Haratani, T., Hojou, M., & Araki, S. (2007). Perceived job stress and sleep-related breathing disturbance in Japanese male workers. *Soc Sci Med,* 64(12), 2520-2532.

Okosun, I.S., Choi, S., Matamoros, T., & Dever, G.E. (2001). Obesity is associated with reduced self-rated general health status: evidence from a representative sample of white, black, and Hispanic Americans. *Prev Med,* 32(5), 429-436.

Okosun, I.S., Seale, J.P., Daniel, J.B., & Eriksen, M.P. (2005). Poor health is associated with episodic heavy alcohol use: evidence from a National Survey. *Public Health,* 119(6), 509-517.

Osler, M., Heitmann, B.L., Hoidrup, S., Jorgensen, L.M., & Schroll, M. (2001). Food intake patterns, self rated health and mortality in Danish men and women. A prospective observational study. *J Epidemiol Community Health,* 55(6), 399-403.

Perez-Stable, E.J., Marin, G., Marin, B.V., & Katz, M.H. (1990). Depressive symptoms and cigarette smoking among Latinos in San Francisco. *Am J Public Health,* 80(12), 1500-1502.

Pijls, L.T., Feskens, E.J. & Kromhout, D. (1993). Self-rated health, mortality, and chronic diseases in elderly men. The Zutphen Study, 1985-1990. *Am J Epidemiol,* 138(10), 840-848.

Pikhart, H., Bobak, M., Siegrist, J., Pajak, A., Rywik, S., Kyshegyi, J., et al. (2001). Psychosocial work characteristics and self rated health in four post-communist countries. *J Epidemiol Community Health,* 55(9), 624-630.

Prager, E., Walter-Ginzburg, A., Blumstein, T., & Modan, B. (1999). Gender differences in positive and negative self-assessments of health status in a national epidemiological study of Israeli aged. *J Women Aging,* 11(4), 21-41.

Radloff, L. (1977). The CES-D Scale: a self-reported depression scale for research in general population. *Appl Psychol Meas,* 1, 385-401.

Rohrer, J.E., Pierce, J.R., Jr., & Blackburn, C. (2005). Lifestyle and mental health. *Prev Med,* 40(4), 438-443.

Seidell, J.C., Bakx, K.C., Deurenberg, P., Burema, J., Hautvast, J.G., & Huygen, F.J. (1986). The relation between overweight and subjective health according to age, social class, slimming behavior and smoking habits in Dutch adults. *Am J Public Health,* 76(12), 1410-1415.

Shen, J., Botly, L.C., Chung, S.A., Gibbs, A.L., Sabanadzovic, S., & Shapiro, C.M. (2006). Fatigue and shift work. *J Sleep Res,* 15(1), 1-5.

Shima, S., Shikano, T., Kitamura, T., & Asai, M. (1985). Reliability and validity of CES-D. *Jpn J Clin Psychiat,* 27, 717-723 (in japanese).

Son, B.K., Markovitz, J.H., Winders, S., & Smith, D. (1997). Smoking, nicotine dependence, and depressive symptoms in the CARDIA Study. Effects of educational status. *Am J Epidemiol,* 145(2), 110-116.

Stavem, K., Hofoss, D. & Aasland, O.G. (2003). Work characteristics and morbidity as predictors of self-perceived health status in Norwegian physicians. *Scand J Public Health,* 31(5), 375-381.

Svedberg, P., Lichtenstein, P. & Pedersen, N.L. (2001). Age and sex differences in genetic and environmental factors for self-rated health: a twin study. *Journal of Gerontology: Psychological Sciences,* 56(3), S171-178.

Takahashi, M., Nakata, A., Haratani, T., Otsuka, Y., Kaida, K., & Fukasawa, K. (2006). Psychosocial work characteristics predicting daytime sleepiness in day and shift workers. *Chronobiol Int,* 23(6), 1409-1422.

Takahashi, M., Tanigawa, T., Tachibana, N., Mutou, K., Kage, Y., Smith, L., et al. (2005). Modifying effects of perceived adaptation to shift work on health, wellbeing, and alertness on the job among nuclear power plant operators. *Ind Health,* 43(1), 171-178.

Unden, A.L. & Elofsson, S. (2006). Do different factors explain self-rated health in men and women? *Gend Med,* 3(4), 295-308.

von dem Knesebeck, O., Luschen, G., Cockerham, W.C., & Siegrist, J. (2003). Socioeconomic status and health among the aged in the United States and Germany: a comparative cross-sectional study. *Social Science & Medicine,* 57(9), 1643-1652.

Wang, N., Iwasaki, M., Otani, T., Hayashi, R., Miyazaki, H., Xiao, L., et al. (2005). Perceived health as related to income, socio-economic status, lifestyle, and social support factors in a middle-aged Japanese. *J Epidemiol,* 15(5), 155-162.

Weinberger, M., Darnell, J.C., Tierney, W.M., Martz, B. L., Hiner, S. L., Barker, J., et al. (1986). Self-rated health as a predictor of hospital admission and nursing home placement in elderly public housing tenants. *Am J Public Health,* 76(4), 457-459.

White, I.R., Blane, D., Morris, J.N., & Mourouga, P. (1999). Educational attainment, deprivation-affluence and self reported health in Britain: a cross sectional study. *J Epidemiol Community Health,* 53(9), 535-541.

Yen, I.H. & Kaplan, G.A. (1999). Poverty area residence and changes in depression and perceived health status: evidence from the Alameda County Study. *International Journal of Epidemiology,* 28(1), 90-94.

In: Social Sciences in Health Care and Medicine ISBN: 978-1-60456-286-6
Editors: J. B. Garner, T. C. Christiansen, pp. 167-180

Chapter 6

CHRONICALLY ILL PATIENTS' AND FAMILY CAREGIVERS' PERSPECTIVES ON THE USE OF COMPUTER TECHNOLOGIES IN FAMILY PRACTICE: IMPLICATIONS FOR THE DEVELOPMENT OF INFORMATIONAL CONTINUITY OF CARE

***Valorie A. Crooks*[1] *and Gina Agarwal*[2]**
[1]Department of Geography
8888 University Drive, Simon Fraser University
Burnaby, BC, CANADA, V5A 1S6
crooks@sfu.ca, Phone: (778)782-3507
[2]Department of Family Medicine
McMaster University, Hamilton, ON, L8P 4M3

ABSTRACT

Continuity of care is understood to be an enabling factor, leading to better health outcomes, and is positively correlated with having access to health services, increased patient satisfaction, and decreased emergency department use. More comprehensive care is viewed to be an outcome of having continuity of care. Further, continuity of care is also a core principle of health care planning. Central to establishing continuity of care is the development of a relationship between doctor and patient. The transfer of information between these parties facilitates the development of continuity in general and specifically informational continuity of care. Informational continuity of care refers to how well a patient's health information is able to 'travel' with him/her throughout the health service system including over time with the same practitioner and between practitioners in different settings including through primary, secondary, and tertiary care.

In this chapter we draw on the findings of a study conducted in Ontario, Canada to support our contention that patients and family caregivers play a significant role in establishing informational continuity of care within family practice. We draw on findings from two primary datasets: (1) in-depth interviews (n=24) with both chronically ill patients and family caregivers who frequently speak on behalf of a chronically ill relative during medical appointments, and (2) a systematic review of the role that patients, doctors, and information technology play in establishing informational continuity of care. We combine the findings of these datasets in a methodologically innovative way in order to consider the use of computer technologies in information transfer and management in the interaction between doctor and patient/caregiver in the family practice setting. The findings reveal that chronically ill patients and family caregivers do indeed care about *how* information is recorded by doctors and that this shapes the doctor-patient interaction. The findings also show that they have strong opinions of the role(s) that computer technologies should play during the interaction specifically. We conclude this chapter by considering the implications of the findings for family doctors and the practice of family medicine.

INTRODUCTION

Continuity of care is a hallmark of quality health service delivery (Xu, 2002) and one of four principles of Canada's family medicine system (Moore & Busing, 1993). There are numerous definitions of continuity which include the following commonly cited characteristics: the availability of information in a medical record; the availability and/or constancy of a clinician; having a usual source or place of care; keeping follow-up appointments; providing seamless and coordinated care during transitions; and having an ongoing commitment to the patient (Donaldson, 2001). Continuity is understood to be an enabling factor, leading to better health outcomes, and is positively correlated with having access to health services, patient satisfaction, and decreased emergency department use (Xu, 2002). More comprehensive care is viewed to be an outcome of having continuity of care (Xu, 2002). Continuity of care is also a core principle of health care planning, although access tends to be seen as a more pressing planning concern (Grey et al., 2003). Central to establishing continuity of care is the development of a relationship between doctor and patient (Grey et al., 2003). The transfer of information between these parties facilitates the development of continuity in general and specifically informational continuity of care (Grey et al., 2003; Manious, Goodwin & Stange, 2004).

There is no single definition of continuity of care (Donaldson, 2001). Rather, three interrelated dimensions of continuity are recognized: (1) informational (availability of recorded information); (2) longitudinal (having a regular site of care); and (3) relational/interpersonal (development of a trusting relationship between doctor and patient over time) (Saultz & Albedaiwi, 2004). Informational continuity refers specifically to how well a patient's health information is able to 'travel' with him/her throughout the health service system including over time with the same practitioner and between practitioners in different settings including through primary, secondary, and tertiary care (Haggerty et al., 2003). Most research regarding informational continuity sets as its goal to facilitate information transfer between health professionals and especially from family doctors to specialists and surgeons. Thus, a particular area of inquiry pertains to the use of health informatics and information technology to assist with establishing informational continuity (Kibbie, Phillips & Green, 2004). This is because, as Hamilton et al. (2003, p.929) suggest: "Most general practices now use computers for their record keeping. This has many advantages, principally because computerised records are easier for retrieval of information.

High quality record keeping is useful for continuity of care, and may be essential for medicolegal purposes."

The purpose of this chapter is to investigate patients' perspectives on the use of technology, and specifically computers and EMRs (as tools of health informatics), in establishing informational continuity of care *within* family medicine; in doing so we break with the tendency to focus on the transfer of information between practitioners or different types of care. Our focus is on the transfer of information within family medicine in two specific types of interpersonal interactions: (1) between chronically ill patient and family doctor; and (2) between someone who is an unpaid family caregiver for a chronically ill individual and family doctor. We consider these interactions because it is our contention that the patient's and family caregiver's role(s) in establishing informational continuity of care have been underconceptualized and are mostly missing from this area of health services research. Further, because chronic illnesses are those for which there is no cure, the establishment of two-way information transfer is particularly important in order to control symptoms, prevent progression (where possible), and promote self-care and management (each of which is an important element of managing chronic illness [Thorne et al., 2004]) which is why they are our focus.

In this chapter we draw on the findings of 24 in-depth interviews with patients and family caregivers and the results of a systematic review in addressing our overall purpose in an innovative integrated analysis of these two datasets. Such a multi-method approach addresses calls made within both the social science and health science literatures to recognize the importance of integrating methodologies and research techniques in order to advance our state-of-knowledge regarding pressing issues (e.g. Morse 2003; Tashakkori & Teddlie, 2003). In the present study, the interviews are used to illustrate the 'place' that computers should occupy in the doctor-patient interaction and in the practice space while the findings of the systematic review are used to consider the role(s) of information technologies in the establishment and maintenance of informational continuity of care.

In the section that follows we provide an overview of both study methods. Following this is a discussion of the main findings of the integrated analysis. Specifically, three issues related to informational continuity of care are the focus: (1) confidentiality of recorded information; (2) recording and storing of contextual patient information; and (3) how and when information is recorded in the practice space. In the final section of this chapter we offer a concluding discussion that draws together a summary of the findings with consideration of the implications for both the establishment and maintenance of informational continuity of care and for family doctors and the practice of family medicine.

METHODS

The study we report on here was conducted in the summer of 2006. We discuss the methods for collecting our two datasets separately in this section.

Systematic Review

A comprehensive literature scan was performed for the systematic review. The electronic databases MEDLINE (OVID) (1966 – week 1, May, 2006), CINAHL (OVID) (1982 – week 1, May, 2006), EMBASE (1980 – week 1, May, 2006), PSYCHINFO (1806 – week 1, May, 2006), and Web of Science (1900 – week 1, May, 2006) were thoroughly searched. Three sets of questions were used to guide the systematic review:

- Set 1: Is there informational continuity of care in family practice? How is informational continuity established, developed, and/or maintained in family practice? What are the different dimensions of informational continuity of care in family practice?
- Set 2: What is the role of patients in establishing/maintaining informational continuity of care in family practice? What is the role of family caregivers in establishing/maintaining informational continuity of care in family practice? What is the role of technology in establishing/maintaining informational continuity of care in family practice? What is the role of the doctor in establishing/maintaining informational continuity of care in family practice?
- Set 3: Are patient contributions to informational continuity of care welcomed/accepted by family doctors? How do family doctors use patient/caregiver historical information?

Articles in English pertaining to humans which were deemed relevant to the search questions were retrieved. All reference lists for the included articles were hand searched for additional citations. We devised the search strategy using existing articles and keywords obtained from broad literature searches on the electronic databases identified above. Search terms were refined through an iterative and collaborative process of reviewing outcomes of preliminary keyword searches in the databases. As shown in Table 1, the search strategy included two intersecting areas of inquiry: (1) family medicine; and (2) informational continuity of care. Extra terms were added to focus the articles identified on the questions to be answered by the review.

Titles obtained from the initial searches were independently reviewed by both investigators. Articles of all study types were included so as to be sure to obtain a comprehensive body of relevant literature to review. Articles focusing on issues outside of family medicine or primary care were excluded, as were those which reviewed continuity of care in general or other types of continuity that did not explicitly mention informational continuity. After independently selecting titles, meetings were held to discuss the inclusion and exclusion of articles that the investigators disagreed about. Following this, abstract review and then full article review took place.

A structured data extraction form was developed to ensure that articles accepted for review were appraised in a consistent way. On the form, information was recorded regarding the nature of the study design, the analytic technique employed, and the quality of interpretation. We also extracted material from the articles pertaining to the three sets of questions guiding the review. Also recorded on the form was a listing of any references from the article to be followed up on and an indication of whether to accept or reject the article for the systematic review.

Table 1. Systematic review search terms

Subject terms	MeSH (Medical Subject Headings) terms
Family practice	Family Practice/ or family medicine.mp. or general practice.mp. or primary care.mp. or Primary Health Care/ or general practitioner.mp. or Physicians, Family/ or Primary Health Care/ or Family Practice/ or family practitioner.mp. or primary care physician.mp. or family physician.mp. or family doctor.mp. or Primary Health Care/ or primary care clinician.mp. or Community Health Centers/ or health care clinic.mp. or primary health care clinic.mp. or primary health care*.mp. or family clinic.mp.
Informational continuity of care	"Continuity of Patient Care"/ or informational continuity of care.mp. or Physician-Patient Relations/ or medical records.mp. or Medical Records/ or Medical Records Systems, Computerized/ or written medical records.mp. or electronic medical records.mp. or Mental Recall/ or Memory/ or remembered information.mp. or knowledge.mp. or Knowledge/ or Knowledge Bases/ or notes.mp. or casenotes.mp. or Medical History Taking/ or medical history.mp. or patient history.mp. or past medical history.mp. or Physician-Patient Relations/ or Communication/ or communication of information.mp. or patient charts.mp. or Medical Records Systems, Computerized/ or patient records.mp. or patient medical history.mp. or doctor-patient communication.mp. or doctor-patient interaction.mp. or professional knowledge.mp. or physician-patient relations.mp. or Physician-Patient Relations/ or Health Knowledge, Attitudes, Practice/ or lay knowledge.mp.
Establishment & maintenance	Establish*; Maint*; Develop*
Dimensions	Dimension*; Aspect*; Level*

A total of 193 articles were obtained from all five bibliographic databases, 151 of which were original articles (after removal of duplicates). The kappa agreement scores for the 151 articles reviewed at the title/abstract stage was 0.673 (std. error of 0.17 and sig. of 0.004) which is reflective of a high level of agreement between the investigators regarding which articles to include in or exclude from the review. Fifty six articles were retained following the title and abstract reviews and identification of additional references from the bibliographies of reviewed articles. Of these, 33 articles were included in the final review. We excluded 23 reviewed articles because they did not contain the correct elements required for inclusion once the full paper was read and data were extracted, and three articles were unobtainable. Contained in Figure 1 is a visual overview of the steps noted here.

IDENTIFICATION
193 articles source from 5 databases
151 remain after removal of duplicates
↓
TITLE & ABSTRACT REVIEW
112 excluded
39 selected for review (3 unobtainable)
↓
ARTICLE REVIEW 1
25 included
11 excluded
↓
20 new articles identified from references of reviewed papers
↓
ARTICLE REVIEW 2
8 included
12 excluded
↓
OUTCOME
33 articles accepted for review

Figure 1. Overview of systematic review process

In-Depth Interviews

The purpose of conducting the in-depth interviews was to learn more about how chronically ill patients and family caregivers prepare to share information with family doctors during doctor-patient interactions. Semi-structured guides were used for interviews with both groups. In-depth interviews are known to generate rich data (Johnson, 2002) and semi-structured formats allow for the probing of topics not included in the guide but that are raised by the participants (Holstein & Gubrium, 1995), both of which were viewed as being important for this type of exploratory study. The guides were divided into four main sections of questions: (1) health status and history; (2) relationship with family doctor; (3) doctor-patient interactions; and (4) demographics. In the guide for caregivers, the questions posed made reference to their role in preparing for the care recipient's appointments and interacting with the recipient's doctor. Questions in the doctor-patient interactions section inquired about how appointments were prepared for, how one determines what should be discussed during appointments, how frequently one's illness history is discussed during appointments, how information is recorded by the doctor during appointments, and perceived differences between hand written and computer managed charts. Answers from these questions are drawn upon in the analytic discussion that follows.

Prior to being interviewed all respondents were informed of their rights as a participant in a research study and signed consent forms. All participants were also asked to select a pseudonym which are the names used in the remainder of this chapter. Before any interviews took place approval for the study was given by the research ethics board at McMaster University.

A total of 24 people participated in the in-depth interviews, 14 of whom had chronic illnesses (11 women, 3 men) and ten of whom were caregivers for someone who had a chronic illness (7 women, 3 men). Interviews were conducted between May and September of 2006. All participants lived in the 'Golden Horseshoe' area of the province of Ontario, Canada, and most were located in the city of Hamilton. Interviews were conducted at a location of the participant's choosing; 17 took place in the home of the individual or care recipient, five were held in a public setting, and the remaining two were conducted in the participant's place of work. With few exceptions, the interviews lasted for between 30 minutes and one hour. In order to enhance consistency, all interviews were conducted by the same research assistant.

Many strategies were simultaneously employed in order to recruit potential participants for the study. Posters were placed in numerous hospitals, grocery stores, and health care clinics in and around the Hamilton area. Several local caregiver and chronic illness support groups and agencies were sent information about the study. Personal and professional networks of the investigators and the research assistant who conducted the interviews were also drawn upon. Finally, participants from previous studies who met the recruitment criteria of the current study (namely that they lived in the area and belonged to one of the two respondent groups) were mailed information letters. A total of 32 potential participants contacted us about participating in an interview, 24 of whom eventually did. Those who did not participate either did not meet our recruitment criteria or were not available for an interview during the temporal period of data collection.

All interviews were digitally recorded and transcribed verbatim. Once all transcribing was completed the files were uploaded into a qualitative data management software program, NVivo©. Following this the investigators worked collaboratively to develop a coding scheme. The steps involved in coding scheme development were to: (1) independently review two transcripts from each participant group and identify major themes; (2) hold a meeting to discuss the emerging themes and lay out the coding framework; and (3) finalize the scheme and enter it into the data management program. Though the foci of the interviews for both participant groups were the same, because different questions were asked and different issues emerged it was decided to develop two separate schemes, one for each group, that contained some overlapping codes. The findings we present here, however, do not rely on the use of our coded data. Specifically, we performed keyword searches within the dataset for terms that related to technology (e.g. computer, electronic, technology) and extracted this information into a separate file. Extracted data were reviewed in order to identify both confirmation with the systematic review findings and also dissenting viewpoints. Both investigators reviewed the extracted data independently in order to confirm their interpretation. We thus triangulated the data emergent from the interviews with findings from the systematic review while also employing investigator triangulation for the purpose of confirmation.

RESULTS

The findings we present in this section combine the results of both the systematic review and in-depth interviews in an integrated analysis. Our unique integration of these two datasets provides a methodologically innovative way to examine informational continuity of care, one which has not been used before.

Confidentiality of Recorded Information

The systematic review revealed that *how* information is stored, managed, and transferred is an important part of establishing informational continuity of care within family practice. Medical records reflect the quality of care provided (Starfield et al., 1979) and family doctors are the gatekeepers to this information in that they can restrict others from having access to these files and as such a patient's medical history (Hjortdahl, 1992; Mandl, Szolovits & Kohane, 2001). However, concerns were raised regarding the level of confidentiality afforded by electronic medical records (EMRs) specifically (Schers et al., 2003; Mandl, Szolovits & Kohane, 2001; Wardman et al., 2000). An outcome of this is that patients may be reluctant to share information with family doctors over concern that others may be able to access their computerized records (Schers et al., 2003). This concern was articulated by two interview participants who said:

> Julie: ...it feels a little scary from the confidentiality point of view to have everything on the computer. And I know logically that doesn't make sense because the same people and...rules apply no matter what, but somehow it's like, oh, with a touch of button all your information could go somewhere.

> Agnes: I don't have any objections or worries about it [computerized or written records] either way. Um, the issue is to have good record keeping and if entering that into a computer directly that is regularly backed up and the files are backed up. I'm okay with that, but I wouldn't be real happy if it went onto somebody's Blackberry or all went onto you know, into a file and you know, the lights went out and it was all gone. And so...I don't care where it [stored] is but I want to make sure that it's accessible and there is some level of confidentiality around it as well.

These comments illustrate the specific types of concerns participants shared with regard to confidentiality.

Despite confidentiality concerns, most participants viewed the use of EMRs to be an appropriate way for a family doctor to store medical information and also saw them as reflective of a modern practice. In fact, doctors who did not use computers in the practice room or did not show evidence of keeping electronic records of some sort were frequently described as "old school" or "old fashioned" by interview participants. One study reviewed further suggested that older doctors may find it difficult to use EMRs due to a lack of familiarity with such a recording system (Rowan et al., 2002). Yet the (multi-site) search capabilities, coordination of records, and timeliness afforded by the EMR makes it an attractive way to record and share health information (Kibbie, Phillips & Green, 2004; Litaker et al., 2005; Rigby et al., 1988; Rowan et al., 2002; Schers et al., 2003) and it can thus become a tool central to the establishment of informational continuity of care.

Recording and Storing of Contextual Patient Information

The type(s) and quality of information recoded by the family doctor during and after the doctor-patient interaction was another concern raised by the systematic review and supported by both groups of participants. Recording certain types of information has the ability to enhance the effectiveness of care provided (Starfield et al., 1979). More specifically, recording contextual or anecdotal information regarding an individual's lifestyle, social situation, and family is viewed as not just appropriate but also needed in order to develop informational continuity of care (Freer, 1980; Hjortdahl, 1992; Manious et al., 1988). Participants expressed concern regarding whether and how this contextual information is recorded (and not just remembered). Specifically, several suggested that this type of information is more likely to be recorded in a hand written record as opposed to an EMR:

> George: Depends on how the computer record is set up. If it's set up as a simple check list, I don't think it's as accurate, but if it's set up where you can put in some anecdotal remarks then it's just as appropriate [as a written record].
>
> Margaret: But to me it's just better that she [the family doctor] does it by hand and writes everything down that you say.
>
> Di'Ianni: My personal opinion is the computer tends to formulate answers and it's useful for formulating information but not useful for anecdotal information unless the doctor recognizes that limitation and strives to overcome it in using a computer... Oh, I definitely think that the anecdotal information from a, from written notes is the most accurate [form of record keeping].

Regardless of how such contextual or anecdotal information about the patient gets recorded (by hand or EMR) it is viewed as being important by the participants.

Having patients or family caregivers share contextual information, thus, is an element of establishing informational continuity in family practice if we understand that such continuity begins with the interaction between doctor and patient. However, such personal/social/anecdotal information is regularly not recorded in medical records (Starfield et al., 1979). This can be a deliberate strategy on the doctor's behalf so that s/he becomes the sole keeper of such knowledge (Freeman, Olesen & Hjortdahl, 2003), or can be an outcome of not having to regularly share patient files with others and thus transmit this information (Freeman, 1984). It also reflects the fact that this information is difficult to record (Freeman, 1984). However, it is important to remember that while the patient record contains points of information, it is the family doctor who has accumulated knowledge based on what has been shared during past interactions that can bring those information points together for medical purposes (e.g. diagnosis, preventative care) (Hjortdahl, 2001).

How and When Information is Recorded in the Practice Space

Most participants were ambivalent about how information was recorded by their family doctor, whether by hand notes or on computer, as long as it was accurate, accessible, and safe. When asked about whether or not it was appropriate for computers to be used in the practice space, all but one participant agreed this was acceptable. The participant who disagreed stated that "they're harder to clean germs off of."

While the presence of a computer within the practice space was not viewed as problematic, how it was used during the appointment was of concern to participants. Many agreed that it is okay for a doctor to search for information in an EMR or from a database during the appointment or to fill out an electronic prescription script to print off. What was more contentious is the practice of recording information in the patient record on the computer during the appointment itself. As these participants' comments reveal, such an act is seen to lead to more impersonal interactions:

> Beth: ...yeah, they [the doctor] may miss some little thing that you told them because they're looking down [at the keyboard] or you don't feel that it's an interaction, it feels too scientific then.

> Tim: I mean it's probably easier with most people to take the [written] notes and interact during the examination rather than, you know, than turning and typing on a keyboard or whatever they do.

> Huck: I know technology is a good thing, and I know it's better as far as the doctor is concerned, but it seems funny to be sitting there typing away on the computer [during an appointment]. It just seems like okay, like those minutes I could use talking or you could be doing something.

> Di'Ianni: I can't see a doctor talking to me working on a keyboard with their focus on a screen you know. So I don't know...it might be advantage if information we're later transferred to computers.

Though the use of EMRs, and thus the practice of recording health information via computer, can facilitate the establishment of, and even enhance, informational continuity of care (Litaker et al., 2005), the participants' responses indicate that one must be sensitive as to how and when this information is recorded in the practice space. Interestingly, there was no discussion of this issue in any of the reviewed articles.

Conclusion

Continuity of care is a dynamic concept. This study has shown that there are many factors that need to be considered when attempting to establish and maintain informational continuity of care including the type of information that gets stored and the confidentiality of the recording system. The in-depth interviews revealed that the participants shared many of the concerns regarding information transfer and sharing identified in the existing literature through the systematic review. For example, concerns over the ability of EMRs to remain confidential were raised in both review articles and by the interview participants. Such concerns could potentially lead individuals to not share personal details during appointments for fear that they will somehow be leaked to others, thereby negatively affecting the establishment of informational continuity of care. These concerns are reflective of a larger finding from the interviews; that patients and family caregivers do care how their medical information is stored and managed both during the doctor-patient interaction and thereafter.

Conducting the systematic review confirmed our contention that the views of patients and caregivers are mostly missing from the existing body of literature regarding informational continuity of care. Though not explicitly discussed in this chapter, the interviews revealed that members of both groups spent time determining what to discuss during appointments with family doctors, confirming that informational continuity truly begins with them as it is some or all of the information they *decide* to share that ultimately gets recorded in the medical record. Because time was invested in such preparation it is not surprising to learn that the participants we interviewed, both chronically ill individuals and family caregivers alike, cared how this information was recorded by their family doctor.

Locating a place for recording social, familial, and other anecdotal or contextual information (e.g. job type, personal stressors, interpersonal relationships) in the medical record, whether hand written or computer managed, was raised as a priority both in the systematic review and interview findings. This is particularly important for people managing chronic illnesses and their caregivers as the development of an accurate personal *and* medical history is necessary for many reasons. For example, such information is important to the regular family doctor because these factors of individuals' social and personal environments are crucial to developing personalized chronic illness management programs. The family doctor will also use the recorded and remembered information from repeated contacts with their patients to build a 'social map' of a patient and his/her family that can be drawn upon as needed (Holden, 1994). Visits to patients' homes allow family doctors to further build on this information and their understanding of a patient's 'social map' (McWhinney, 1997). However, in order for one's non-regular family doctor or specialist to be able to gain a working knowledge of the factors that may be shaping cycles of symptom exacerbation and/or remission these details must be recorded, particularly as the regular family doctor's accumulated remembered information cannot be accessed in such an instance. They must also be recorded in the chance that a doctor's remembered information is, or becomes, inaccurate or incomplete.

The findings of this work have multiple implications for how family doctors organise information sharing and recording in their practices. Information should be recorded and stored in a secure fashion, in such a way that patients and family caregivers feel confident that their personal details will not be inadvertently divulged to anyone else. Policies regarding the use of computers, passwords, and computer screen hibernation when leaving a patient in the room must also be set and enforced by each practice. Data should be kept in an encrypted way, including laboratory results and consult notes. Furthermore, medical records should be better organised for recording contextual and anecdotal information, and perhaps patients/family caregivers could be given access to a certain portion of their file in which they could add pertinent parts of their social, familial, and even medical histories on their own. Attention to the validation of the EMR can also assist in the maintenance of informational continuity in that we must be assured that the most up-to-date information is entered in the correct fashion in all instances. Finally, patients' (including family caregivers) views and opinions need to be incorporated into any future computerised medical record policies and perhaps these policies should be made transparent and known to patients.

ACKNOWLEDGEMENTS

We are grateful to the participants who shared their time and stories with us. We would also like to acknowledge the assistance of our research assistant, Mirjana Vuksan, in undertaking this study. Development of this research was supported by 'Health Care, Technology and Place: An Interdisciplinary Capacity Enhancement Team Grant' from the Institute of Health Services and Policy Research (IHSPR), Canadian Institutes of Health Research (CIHR).

Valorie Crooks received stipendiary funding through a CIHR Strategic Training Postdoctoral Fellowship in HCTP and a Canadian Health Services Research Foundation/CIHR Postdoctoral Fellowship in Health Services Research during the study period. Gina Agarwal is funded by a Post Doctoral Fellowship award from the Canadian Diabetes Association and also received stipendiary funding through a CIHR Strategic Training Postdoctoral Fellowship in HCTP during the study period.

REFERENCES

Donaldson, M.S. (2001). Continuity of Care: A Reconceptualization. *Medical Care Research and Review*, *58*(3), 255-290.

Freeman, G. (1984). Continuity of Care in General Practice: a Review and Critique. *Family Practice*, *1*(4), 245-252.

Freeman, G.K., Olesen, F. & Hjortdahl, P. (2003). Continuity of care: an essential element of modern general practice? *Family Practice*, *20*(6), 623-627.

Freer, C.B. (1980). Health diaries: a method of collecting health information. *Journal of the Royal College of General Practitioners*, *30*, 279-282.

Grey, D.P., Evans, P., Sweeney, K., Lings, P., Seamakr, D., Seamakr, C., Dixon, M., & Bradley, N. (2003). Towards a theory of continuity of care. *Journal of the Royal Society of Medicine, 96*, 160-166.

Haggerty, J.L., Reid, R.J., Freeman, G.K., Starfield, B.H., Adair, C.E., & McKendry, R. (2003). Continuity of care: a multidisciplinary review. *BMJ*, *327*, 1219-1221.

Hamilton, W.T., Round, A.P., Sharp, D., & Peters, T.J. (2003). The quality of record keeping in primary care: a comparison of computerized, paper and hybrid systems. *British Journal of General Practice, 53*, 929-933.

Hjortdahl, P. (1992). The Influence of General Practitioners' Knowledge about their Patients on the Clinical Decision-Making Process. *Scand Journal of Primary Health Care, 10*, 290-294.

Hjortdahl, P. (2001). Continuity of care – going out of style? *British Journal of General Practice*, *51*, 699-670.

Holden H. (2004). The social geography of general practice. *British Journal of General Practice, 54*, 72-75.

Holstein, J.A. & Gubrium, J.F. (1995). *The Active Interview*. Thousand Oaks, California: Sage Publications.

Johnson, J. (2002). In-depth Interviewing. In J.F. Gubrium & J.A. Holstein (Eds.), *Handbook of Interview Research: Context & Method* (pp. 103-119). Thousand Oaks, California: Sage Publications.

Kibbie, D.C., Phillips, R.L. & Green, L.A. (2004). The Continuity of Care Record. *American Family Physician, 70*(7), 1220-1222.

Litaker, D., Ritter, C., Ober, S., & Aron, D. (2005). Continuity of care and cardiovascular risk factor management: Does care by a single clinician add to informational continuity provided by electronic medical records? *The American Journal of Managed Care, 11*(11), 689-696.

Mandl, K.D., Szolovits, P. & Kohane, I.S. (2001). Public standards and patients' control: how to keep electronic medical records accessible but private. *BMJ, 322*, 283-286.

Manious, A.G., Baker, R., Love, M.M., Gray, D.P., & Gill, J.M. (2001). Continuity of Care and Trust in One's Physician: Evidence from Primary Care in the United States and the United Kingdom. *Family Medicine, 33*(1), 22-27.

Manious, A.G., Goodwin, M.A. & Stange, K.C. (2004). Patient-Physician Shared Experiences and Value Patients Place on Continuity of Care. *Annals of Family Medicine, 2*(5), 452-454.

McWhinney, I. (1997). A Textbook of Family Medicine 2nd Edition. New York, NY: Oxford University Press.

Moore, L. & Busing, N. (1993). Continuity of Care in the Family Medicine Residency. *Canadian Family Physician, 39*, 531-534.

Morse, J.M. (2003). Principles of mixed methods and multimethod research design. In A. Tashakkori & C. Teddlie (Eds.), *Handbook of mixed methods in social and behavioural research* (pp. 189-208). Thousand Oaks, California: Sage Publications.

Rigby, M., Roberts, R., Williams, J., Clark, J, Savill, A., Levy, B., & Mooney, G. (1998). Integrated record keeping as an essential aspect of a primary care led health service. *BMJ, 317*, 579-582.

Rowan, M.S., Lawson, B., MacLean, C., & Burge, F. (2002). Upholding the Principles of Primary Care in Preceptors' Practices. *Family Medicine, 34*, 744-749.

Saultz, J.W., & Albedaiwi, W. (2004). Interpersonal continuity of care and patient satisfaction: a critical review. *Annals of Family Medicine, 2*(5), 445-451.

Schers, H., Van Den Hoogen, H., Grol, R., & van den Bosch, W. (2003). Continuity of information in general practice – patient views on confidentiality. *Scandinavian Journal of Primary Health Care, 21*, 21-26.

Starfield, B., Steinwachs, D., Morris, I., Bause, G., Siebert, S., & Westin, C. (1979). Concordance Between Medical Records and Observations Regarding Information on Coordination of Care. *Medical Care, XVII*(7), 758-766.

Tashakkori, A. & Teddlie, C. (2003). *Handbook of Mixed Methods in Social and Behavioural Research*. Thousand Oaks, California: Sage Publications.

Thorne, S.E., Harris, S.R., Mahoney, K., et al. (2004). The context of health care communication in chronic illness. *Patient Education and Counselling, 54*, 299-306.

Wardman, L., Rout, J., Ormiston, P., Nagle, J., Munshi, S., Kirby, A. et al. (2000). Patients' knowledge and expectations of confidentiality in primary health care: a quantitative study. *British Journal of General Practice, 50*, 910-902.

Xu, K.T. (2002). Usual Source of Care in Preventative Service Use: A Regular Doctor versus a Regular Site. *HSR: Health Services Research, 37*(6), 1509-1529.

In: Social Sciences in Health Care and Medicine ISBN: 978-1-60456-286-6
Editors: J. B. Garner, T. C. Christiansen, pp. 181-198

Chapter 7

THE MODERATING EFFECT OF CONCERN FOR FACE ON HELP-SEEKING INTENTION AMONG INTIMATE PARTNER ABUSED PREGNANT WOMEN

***Ying Lau*[1*] *and Kin Sun Chan*[2]**

[1]RN, RM, IBCLC, B. Health Science, B. Nursing (Hon), MN, PhD
School of Health Sciences, Macao Polytechnic Insititute, Macau SAR, China
[2]B. Social Science (Hon), M. Phil, PhD
Faculty of Social Sciences and Humanities, The University of Macau, Macau SAR, China

ABSTRACT

Objective(s): (1) To examine concern for face and different forms of Intimate Partner Violence (IPV) on formal or informal help-seeking intention; and (2) To examine the moderating effect of concern for face on formal or informal help-seeking intention among different groups of pregnant women who suffer from IPV.

Design: A retrospective cross-sectional comparative quantitative study at a university-affiliated regional hospital among 1,200 Hong Kong Chinese pregnant women.

Measurements: The Protective and Acquisitive Face Orientation (PAFO) scale (Short Form) and the modified Cohen's Willingness to Seek Help scale were used to measure concern for face and help-seeking intention. The different forms of IPV were investigated by using the Revised Conflict Tactics Scale (CTS-2).

Results: The results of hierarchical regression models found that women with "Psychological Aggression" significantly negatively associate with formal help intention after adjusting for socio-demographic variables. Women with one subscale of Protective Face Concern: "Keep a low profile to avoid attention (KLP)" was found to negatively associate

* Corresponding author: Alameda Dr. Carlos D'Assumpcao No.335-341, "Centro Hotline" 5 Ander, Macau.Telephone: (853) 66144064 (MOBILE), (853) 83998615 (OFFICE). E-mail: ylau@ipm.edu.mo.

with formal and informal help-seeking intention after adjustment ($p < 0.05$). The moderating effects of "Physical Assault" and KLP on informal help-seeking intention were found.

Conclusion: IPV and concern for face have an inhibitive effect on the intention to seek help. Implications and limitations are also discussed.

Keywords: Help-Seeking Intention; Concern for Face; Intimate Partner Violence.

Introduction

Intimate Partner Violence (IPV) is a serious and pervasive public health concern (Tjaden & Thoennes, 1998). Legal and legislative reforms have broadened the options for battered women, while researchers have shed light on IPV's prevalence, causes, consequences, and potential solutions. As the knowledge base has expanded, conceptualizations of the problem have also shifted. Until recently, the most common research approach to IPV was to investigate the personal characteristics of the perpetrator or the victim (Koss et al., 1994). Although this kind of individual level approach had validity, it rendered invisible the larger sociocultural context in which IPV occurs, and implicitly conceptualized violence as stemming from individual pathology or deviance, ignoring the important ways in which violence is embedded within social contexts and cultures.

The literature has found that IPV victims are more likely to seek help compared to non-victims (Lipsky, Caetano, Field, & Larkin, 2006) but that Asian women would be less likely to report incidents of IPV than women from other racial/ethnic groups (Bauer, Rodriguez, Quiroga, & Flores-Ortiz, 2000; Lee & Au, 1998; Tjaden & Thoennes, 1998). Indeed, in several studies regarding Asian women, participants tended to report IPV incidents and seek help only when the violence reached a severe or crisis level (Abraham, 2000; Huisman, 1996). IPV within the Asian family context, especially among Chinese families, has a long documented history (Mayer & Coulter, 2002). Studies have also shown that many women among the Chinese population are still routinely abused (Meng, 1999; Wang, 1999), and that Chinese women do not normally report IPV experiences; instead, evidence surfaces only in the most serious cases. IPV scholars suggest that culturally different women may cope with IPV differently (Abraham, 2000). Delay in seeking or reluctance to seek help is sometimes a result of the unavailability of relevant support, but in other cases is explained by some underlying causes (Bui, 2003). However, the empirical evidence is too sparse to clarify the development of such behavior. Thus, the need for further research is clear and imperative.

Help-Seeking Intention

Help-seeking is conceptualized as a coping strategy used by people to reduce stress (Karabenick, 1998). It is a process that comprises several components: (1) An individual becomes aware of a problem or a need. (2) Resources may be needed to alleviate the problem. (3) These resources need to be obtained from other people. (4) The individual has to communicate in some way with these other people. Therefore, help-seeking intention is a complex behavioral process. However, not all requests for help are motivated by deficits, problems, or needs (Wang, 2002). A cognitive theory from general literature on help-seeking in "stigmatizing" situations suggests three relevant processes or stages of seeking help in the IPV context: defining the problem, deciding to seek help, and selecting a source of support, and that the individual, interpersonal, and sociocultural factors that influence decision making at each of these stages are relevant factors in the face of violence (Liang, Goodman, Tummala-Narra, & Weintraub, 2005).

Help-seeking intention involves some deliberation (Nadler, 1990) and the way that individuals appraise the potential costs and benefits of soliciting help is important in the deliberation process; personality disposition and cultural beliefs influence cognitive appraisal and coping choices (Lazarus & Folkman, 1984). The decision to seek assistance from others is influenced by various factors that include socio-demographic variables such as age, educational level (Coker, Derrick, Lumpkin, & Aldrich, 2000), total monthly income (Coker, Derrick, Lumpkin, & Aldrich, 2000), supportive networks (Chatzifotiou & Dobash, 2001), and interpersonal relationships (Kaukinen, 2004). While many of these studies have examined the demo-socio-economic variables, very few studies have explored the cultural aspects linked to the help-seeking tendency (Raj & Silverman, 2002). This study attempted to understand one of the important cultural factors – concern for face – and to investigate how the face issue influences help-seeking intention.

Concern for Face and Help-Seeking Intention

The term "face" is defined as the positive social value a person effectively claims for himself by the line others assume he has taken during a particular contact (Goffman, 1967). From the symbolic interaction perspective, Goffman proposed that face was what he called "public performance". According to Goffman's work, face is fundamental to a sense of self in terms of socially approved attributes. Brown and Levinson (1987) defined "face" as the public self-image that every member wants to claim for himself (Brown & Levinson, 1987). Chou (1996) defines "face" as the public representation of self (Chou, 1996). In other words, face is the public image that one wants to project for others. Hence, concern for face can be interpreted as concern for the protection and enhancement of one's public image.

While face is recognized by all societies (Goffman, 1955), it assumes a particular importance in Chinese culture (Hu, 1944). According to Gao, et al. (1996), in Chinese culture, concern for one's reputation is conceptualized in two ways: as face (*lian*) and image (*mianzi*) (Gao, 1996; King & Myers, 1977). While face may be defined as something that "...represents the confidence of society in the integrity of an individual's moral character, the loss of which makes it impossible for him/her to function properly in the community, image stands for the kind of prestige or reputation achieved through getting on in life, through success and ostentation" (Hu, 1944, p. 45). In other words, face is related to the protection of one's public image and the need to avoid losing face in public, while image is concerned with the projection and the claiming of one's public image. To the Chinese, concern for face makes a person vulnerable not only to what others have said, but also in anticipation of potential gossip. This anticipation usually creates tremendous pressure for the Chinese, so much so that it has a controlling effect on behavior. Concern for face has a familial dimension for the Chinese as well. While losing face in public is considered to bring shame on the family, gaining face can bring glory to the family (Schneiderman, 1995). Family members are expected to know how to keep secrets and hide their shame from the public. To conclude, concern for face serves to regulate the perceived appropriate social behavior of the Chinese, thus maintaining social harmony.

Chou (1996) defined concern for face as the public representation of self (Chou, 1996). There are two types of face orientation: protective face orientation (PFO) and acquisitive face orientation (AFO). Conceptually, people who are high in PFO are more concerned about behavior and situations that involve a possibility of losing face, and will therefore attempt to avoid inappropriate behavior and entering into potential face-threatening situations. They also tend to adopt self-effacing attributions more readily, perceive a greater loss of face, and exhibit cautious and withdrawal behavior more readily (Chou, 1996). On the other hand, people with high AFO are eager to enter into possible face-gaining situations and, like those with high PFO, tend to adopt self-serving attributions of outcomes more readily (Chou, 1996). However, when people with high AFO are confronted with potential face-threatening situations, they may conceal that specific situation from others and avoid admitting any weakness. To conclude, people who are high in PFO and AFO negatively associate their intention to seek help through either formal or informal channels.

The Relationship between Concern for Face and IPV on Help-Seeking Intention

Unique forms of help-seeking behavior have been significantly associated with different races and ethnicities among IPV victims (Lipsky, Caetano, Field, & Larkin, 2006). The literature on help-seeking in Chinese communities has focused on the investigation of various determinants of help-seeking, including both situational mediators and personal differences (Wang, 2002). Some studies have found that "the nature of problems" is an important factor in determining the willingness of people to seek help and their choice of helper among the Chinese population (Boey, 1999; Ho, 1994).

In general, the Chinese population regards the problem of IPV as a family problem rather than a social problem (Tang, Lee, & Cheung, 1999). Chinese people with traditional beliefs tend to believe that a family problem is private family affair (*jia shi*) that should not be handled by people outside the family (*wai ren*), and that letting "outside" people know about a family problem is embarrassing (Leong & Lau, 2001; Shek, 1998). When the problem of IPV does occur, outside intervention is strongly discouraged for fear this will bring shame and dishonor to the family (Ho, 1990) and seeking help from an "outsider" means confronting cultural prohibitions against causing a loss of face for oneself as well as one's family (Xu, 1998). Suffering and perseverance are valued virtues and divorce is not common in Chinese culture (Lee, 1996). Women are recognized for enduring hardship and are discouraged from discussing IPV when it occurs (Catolico, 1997). Chinese women who experience IPV often live within the cultural milieu (Lee & Au, 1998). They also face tremendous cultural pressure when they try to break away from the abusive cycle because the maintenance of harmonious relationships is stressed (Hu & Chen, 1999). Therefore, by disclosing IPV to an outsider, a woman may put herself into a face-threatening situation that involves the possibility of losing face.

In addition, because the acquisition of face is very important to the Chinese, there is constant pressure to avoid having the family name regarded in a bad light by others by concealing IPV (Leong & Lau, 2001). Even when a woman recognizes the problem of IPV by herself, her desire to gain face at all costs can also prevent her from seeking help from others (Dasgupta & Warrier, 1996). There is a primary way of conceptualizing the interrelationships among IVP, concern for face and help-seeking intention using a moderator hypothesis. According to this hypothesis, concern for face may act as an accelerator that may exacerbate the negative effects of IPV on help-seeking intention. Thus, it is hypothesized that for women with high PFO and AFO, interactions with various forms of IPV are negatively associated with help-seeking intention from either formal or informal resources. However, no study has directly explored the relationship between concern for face and willingness to seek help among Chinese women who suffer from IPV.

The Purpose of the Study

The present study attempts to examine the relationship between concern for face and different forms of IPV, and the moderating effect of these two variables on the intention to seek help. This is a crucial study area that must be addressed if culturally relevant interventions are to be designed to facilitate IPV disclosure and support services in this population.

Method

For the present study, which is a retrospective cross-sectional comparative study, the following three hypotheses were established: (1) Women who experience different forms of IPV (physical, psychological, sexual or injury-causing) have a negative association with help-seeking intention (either formal or informal); (2) Women who have concern for face (either high PFO or high AFO) have a negative association with help-seeking intention; and (3) There are moderating effects between various forms of IPV and concern for face on the help-seeking intentions of Chinese women.

Sample

Assuming a true prevalence of 16%, as estimated by the previous Hong Kong study (Leung, Leung, Lam, & Ho, 1999), then at the 95% confidence interval for the estimates from this study to have a margin of error of +/-2% would require around 1200 participants. Therefore, 1,200 post-natal mothers participated in the study, a number which is considered to be adequate for the detection of IPV. The sample was recruited from a university-affiliated regional public hospital on the south-western side of Hong Kong Island which serves a population of over 1.2 million people.

Measures

The instruments used were all self-administered questionnaires. In addition to exploring socio-demographic variables (e.g., age, educational level, length of marriage, monthly family income, place of birth, and support network), one item from Cohen's *willingness to seek help scale* was selected and modified to measure an individual's willingness to seek help (Cohen, 1999) in dealing with a hypothetical situation of intimate partner abuse during pregnancy, because a majority of women are not aware of, hide or deny IPV, even where IPV is experienced (Edin & Hogberg, 2002). ("If I experienced psychological aggression, physical assault, sexual coercion or injury by my partner during pregnancy, I would seek help from others"). The underlying principle for the questions asked was borrowed from the concept of the contingent valuation method (Olsen & Smith, 2001). The advantage of the contingent valuation method elicits a hypothetical answer that is highly sensitive to the real preferences of individuals (Klose, 1999). Respondents were given dichotomous answers (Yes/ No). Another item was used to explore the various help-seeking behaviour of respondents, i.e., "If I sought help from others, whom would I approach for help?" Respondents were given only one choice for their "primary" (first choice) helper from both informal and formal channels. Informal resources included partner's family members, own family members, and friends; formal resources included physicians, nurses, medical social workers and police. A linguistic validation process (included translation into Cantonese, review, and back-translation by two experts) was carried out for these two items.

The short form of the Protective and Acquisitive Face Orientation (PAFO) scale was used to measure the general trend of peoples' protective and acquisitive motives in face-relevant situations (Wang, 2002), which is a modified version of a 50-item version (Chou, 1996). It consists of 20 items and contains two major subscales: the Protective Face Orientation subscale (P-subscale) and the Acquisitive Face Orientation subscale (A-subscale). The P-subscale consists of four factors: keeping a low profile to avoid attention (P1); avoiding making mistakes (P2); downplaying public acclaim (P3); and protecting face through modesty (P4). The A-subscale includes two factors: attracting attention through ostentation (A1) and getting ahead through social achievement (A2) (Wang, 2002). Respondents were asked to select one of 4 levels of agreement. Higher scores indicated that respondents have a high degree of concern for face. The psychometric properties of the Chinese version have been analyzed in two previous unpublished theses carried out among Chinese working adults and university student samples (Chou, 1996; Wang, 2002) which suggest that the items were found to be satisfactory in terms of the validity and reliability of the PAFO scale (Chou, 1996; Wang, 2002).

However, the validity and reliability of the scale used were tested because no published evidence is available. First, we tested the validity of the scale used in our sample by examining the structural similarity of this scale to the PAFO scale. The factor analysis (VARIMAX) of 20 items produces four components in this study that explain 45.98 % of the variance (Table 1). These results demonstrate that the construct of the scale is similar to the PAFO scale used in previous studies. The four components with new categories of items were used to measure concern for face in this study. The PAFO scale was found to be reliable as the Cronbach's α coefficients of the four components used in this study were .70 to .82.

Table 1. Factor analysis of Protective and Acquisitive Face Orientation Scale (PAFO) (short form) in this study

		Components			
		1	2	3	4
1	Cautious/ conscious of making mistakes				0.563
2	Not talk much to call for attention		0.668		
3	Keep strength in low profile		0.737		
4	Talk conservatively / not show off		0.679		
5	Wait for people to discover my strength		0.446		
6	To be a celebrity	0.661			
7	Being supported and respected	0.667			
8	Honor family and ancestors	0.654			
9	Admire prestigious / powerful / high status people	0.724			
10	Strengths be presented to others	0.405			
11	Happy with people's attention / admiration	0.583			
12	Like grand houses / offices / cars	0.672			
13	Achieve success slowly and safety				0.598
14	Concern basic dignity's intake			0.467	
15	Success known to people	0.409			
16	Seized opportunity to be leader	0.604			
17	Be modest about one's talent /learning			0.622	
18	Peaceful unless face being derogated			0.678	
19	Leave room for retreat when asking favors			0.509	
20	Be the person who is admired by others	0.653			
Total Variance Explained (%): 45.98 %		19.78	13.88	6.76	5.56

Component 1: A-subscale 1 and A-subscale 2 (A1 & A2) [A-subscale1: Attracting attention through ostentation and A-subscale 2: Getting ahead through social achievement]

Component 2: P-subscale 1 (P1) [P-subscale: Keep low profile to avoid attention]

Component 3: P-subscale 3 and 4 (P3 & P4) [P-subscale 3: Downplaying public acclaim and P-subscale 4: Protecting face through modesty]

Component 4: P-subscale 2 (P2) [P-subscale 2: Avoidance of making mistake]

The Revised Conflict Tactics Scale (CTS-2) was used to measure different forms of IPV (Straus et al 1996). Responses to particular items were summed to create the following subscales: psychological aggression; physical assault; sexual coercion and injury. The reliability and validity of the CTS2 was satisfactory (Straus et al., 1996). The Chinese version has been used, based on a previous study (Chan, 2001). The Cronbach's αcoefficient of the CTS-2 was 0.85 in this study, suggesting good internal consistency.

Data Analysis

The SPSS/PC 13.0 software package was used for statistical analysis. Factor analysis (VARIMAX) was used to test the validity of the PAFO scale used and Cronbach's α coefficients were used to test the reliability of three instruments. Analyses of variance (ANOVAs) and Chi-square (X^2) tests were used to compare socio-demographic characteristics, various form of IPV, and the concern for face among groups with various degrees of help-seeking intention (formal or informal).

To test the moderating effect of the concern for face in the relationship between different forms of IPV and help-seeking intention, a series of hierarchical regression models were constructed and the predictive variables, including socio-demographic variables, four forms of IPV and four subscales of the PAFO scale, were added in the first block (model 1), where the dependent variable was help-seeking intention (formal or informal). In the second block (model 2), an interaction term between four forms of IPV and four subscales of the PAFO scale was added in different models (Baron & Kenny, 1986). Centered variables (i.e., dividing the variables by their deviation score forms so that their means are zero) were used for the IPV and concern for face variables to lessen multicollinearity due to the interaction terms used. The intercorrelations among all variables examined ranged from 0.11 to 0.48, revealing that multicollinearity was not a problem in this study. Hostmer and Lemshow's goodness-of-fit (HL-GOF) test was used to fit the models (Hosmer Jr. & Lemershow, 2000).

RESULTS

The study was approved in June 2002 by the Hospital Institutional Review Board. The consent of the women to participate was obtained after explaining the nature, purpose, and potential risks of the study. A total of 1,265 Chinese Hong Kong women in three postnatal wards were invited to participate in the study from July 2002 to February 2003. Among the participants, 65 (5.1%) declined to participate and the primary reasons given were wound pain, tiredness, being too busy taking care of their babies, and reluctance to disclose information. The remaining 1,200 women (the respondent rate = 94.9%) completed the questionnaires.

Table 2. Characteristics of Participants with various Seeking Help Intentions

Characteristics of participants		Entire Sample (n=1200)	Non seeking Help (n=222)	Informal seeking help (n=708)	Formal seeking help (n=270)
Socio-demographic characteristics		*N (%)*	N (%)	N (%)	N (%)
Age*	≦25	235 (19.6)	60 (27.0)	126 (17.8)	49 (18.1)
	> 26	965 (80.4)	162 (73.0)	582 (82.2)	221 (81.9)
Educational level	≦Primary	79 (6.6)	19 (8.6)	48 (6.8)	12 (4.4)
	≥ Secondary	1121 (93.4)	203 (91.4)	660 (93.2)	258 (95.6)

Characteristics of participants		Entire Sample (n=1200)	Non seeking Help (n=222)	Informal seeking help (n=708)	Formal seeking help (n=270)
Years in Hong Kong**	< 1 year	254 (21.2)	67 (26.4)	135 (19.1)	52 (19.3)
	≥ 1 year	946 (78.8)	155 (69.8)	573 (80.9)	218 (80.7)
Length of marriage*	< 1 year	269 (22.4)	65 (29.3)	149 (21.0)	55 (20.4)
	≥ 1 year	931 (77.6)	157 (70.7)	559 (79.0)	215 (79.6)
Total family income* (Hong Kong Dollar)	< $10,000	453 (37.8)	115 (51.8)	226 (31.9)	112 (41.5)
	≥ $10,000	747 (62.3)	107 (48.2)	482 (68.1)	158 (58.5)
Supportive Network:					
Instrumental support provided	Yes	1086 (90.5)	190 (85.6)	651 (91.9)	245 (90.7)
	No	114 (9.5)	32 (14.4)	57 (8.1)	25 (9.3)
Psychological support Provided	Yes	1091 (90.9)	192 (86.5)	657 (92.8)	242 (89.6)
	No	109 (9.1)	30 (13.5)	51 (7.2)	28 (10.4)
Communication with participant's family	≥ 1 year	1150 (95.8)	212 (95.5)	687 (97.0)	251 (93.0)
	< 1 year	50 (4.2)	10 (4.5)	21 (3.0)	19 (7.0)
Supportive partner	Yes	1081 (90.1)	191 (86.0)	649 (91.7)	241 (89.3)
	No	119 (9.9)	31 (14.0)	59 (8.3)	29 (10.7)
Supportive extended family	Yes	924 (77.0)	164 (73.9)	550 (77.7)	210 (77.8)
	No	276 (23.0)	58 (26.1)	158 (22.3)	60 (22.02)
Intimate partner violence during pregnancy					
Psychological aggression		106 (79.1)	27 (20.1)	59 (44.0)	20 (14.9)
Physical assault		49 (36.6)	10 (7.5)	26 (19.4)	13 (9.7)
Sexual coercion		66 (49.3)	14 (10.4)	33 (24.6)	19 (14.2)
Injury		24 (17.9)	7 (5.2)	11 (8.2)	6 (4.5)
Concern for face		M(SD)	M(SD)	M(SD)	M(SD)
Protective and Acquisitive Face Orientation Scale (PAFO)		52.61 (4.81)	52.77 (4.12)	52.62 (4.99)	52.47 (4.86)
Protective Face Subscale (PFO)					
Keeping a low profile to avoid attention (P1)**		11.63 (1.57)	**11.87 (1.55)**	**11.64 (1.59)**	**11.44 (1.51)**
Avoiding making mistakes (P2)		6.06 (0.75)	6.04 (0.68)	6.05 (0.75)	6.11 (0.79)
Down playing public acclaim & Protecting face through modesty (P3 & P4)		11.23 (1.38)	11.14 (1.24)	11.30 (1.44)	11.11 (1.34)
Acquisitive Face Subscale (AFO)					
Attracting attention through ostentation and Getting ahead through social achievement (A1 & A2)		23.69 (3.78)	23.71 (3.28)	23.65 (3.87)	23.80 (3.92)

Table 2. Continued

Characteristics of participants	Entire Sample (n=1200)	Non seeking Help (n=222)	Informal seeking help (n=708)	Formal seeking help (n=270)
Informal resources (First Choice):				
Participant's own family		--	368 (51.97)	--
Partner's family		--	33 (4.66)	--
Friends		--	307 (43.36)	--
Formal resources (First Choice):				
Doctors		--	--	12 (4.44)
Nurses		--	--	0 (0.00)
Social workers		--	--	188 (69.63)
Police		--	--	70 (25.93)

*$p < 0.05$; **$p < 0.01$. M(SD) = Median (Standard Deviation)
Chi-square *(X^2)* test and ANOVA test

More than half of the respondents (59.0%) adopted an intention to seek informal help in dealing with a hypothetical situation of IPV during pregnancy, as shown in Table 2. The participants' own family members (52.0%) and their friends (43.4%) were the main sources of informal help. Only 22.5% adopted formal help-seeking behavior and none sought the help of nurses in this study. Socio-demographic characteristics were found to result in no significant differences among the non seeking help, formal seeking help and informal seeking groups, other than in the cases of age, years lived in Hong Kong, length of marriage and total family income (Table 2). 106 (8.8 %), 66 (5.5%), 49 (4.1%), and 24 (2.0%) of the respondents had experienced psychological aggression, physical assault, sexual coercion and injury respectively as confirmed by the CTS-2. The mean score of the P-subscale of protective concern for face (P1) was significantly higher among non-help-seeking groups ($p < 0.05$), as shown in Table 2.

Table 3. Hierarchical Regression models of Concern for face and Intimate Partner Violence on Formal Help Seeking Intention

	Formal help seeking intention (N = 270) ‡				
	Model 1	Model 2	Model 3	Model 4	Model 5
Intimate partner violence during pregnancy	OR (95% CI)	OR (95% CI)	OR (95% CI)	OR (95% CI)	OR (95% CI)
Psychological aggression (PsA)	**0.33 (0.13, 0.83)****	**0.30 (0.11, 0.80)***	**0.35 (0.14, 0.89)***	**0.36 (0.14, 0.93)***	**0.30 (0.12, 0.80)**
Physical assault (PA)	2.29 (0.66, 7.99)	2.25 (0.61, 8.33)	2.56 (0.55, 11.93)	2.15 (0.58, 8.01)	3.48 (0.81, 14.97)

Intimate partner violence during pregnancy	Formal help seeking intention (N = 270) ‡ Model 1	Model 2	Model 3	Model 4	Model 5
Sexual coercion (SC)	1.67 (0.60, 4.62)	1.85 (0.62, 5.52)	1.65 (0.58, 4.73)	1.63 (0.56, 4.74)	1.89 (0.62, 5.74)
Injury (IN)	0.56 (0.13, 2.35)	0.57 (0.13, 2.46)	0.43 (0.09, 2.17)	0.55 (0.12, 2.18)	0.00 (0.00, --)
Concern for Face: *Protective Face Subscale*					
Keeping a low profile to avoid attention (P1)	**0.77 (0.67, 0.89)*****	**0.77 (0.67, 0.89)*****	**0.76 (0.66, 0.88)*****	**0.77 (0.66. 0.88)*****	0.09 (0.00, 0.14)
Avoiding making mistakes (P2)	1.20 (0.91, 1.59)	1.20 (0.91, 1.60)	1.21 (0.91, 1.60)	1.22 (0.92, 1.62)	1.58 (0.00, 0.03)
Down playing public acclaim & Protecting face through modesty (P3&4)	1.08(0.92, 1.26)	1.07 (0.91, 1.26)	1.07 (0.92, 1.26)	1.08 (0.92, 1.26)	0.00 (0.00, --)
Concern for Face: *Acquisitive Face Subscale*					
Attracting attention through ostentation and Getting ahead through social achievement (A1&2)	1.01 (0.95, 1.06)	1.01 (0.95, 1.06)	1.01 (0.95, 1.06)	1.01 (0.95, 1.06)	6.07 (0.00. 115)
Moderating Effect (Interaction Effect): Intimate partner violence interact with concern for face					
PsA X Concern for face					
PsA X P1		1.01 (0.81, 1.25)			
PsA X P2		0.99 (0.83, 1.17)			
PsA X P3&4		0.98 (0.75, 1.28)			
PsA X A1&2		1.08 (0.88, 1.33)			
PA X Concern for face					
PA X P1			0.84 (0.62, 1.14)		
PA X P2			0.97 (0.81, 1.17)		
PA X P3&4			1.05 (0.79, 1.39)		
PA X A1&2			1.00 (0.81, 1.24)		
SC X Concern for face					
SC X P1				0.99 (0.79, 1.25)	
SC X P2				0.92 (0.78, 1.09)	
SC X P3&4				0.97 (0.77, 1.23)	
SC X A1&2				1.09 (0.86, 1.38)	

Table 3. Continued

	Formal help seeking intention (N = 270) ‡				
	Model 1	Model 2	Model 3	Model 4	Model 5
IN X Concern for face					
IN X P1					0.00 (0.00, --)
IN X P2					4.73 (0.00, 143)
IN X P3&4					0.00 (0.00, --)
IN X A1&2					0.00 (0.00, --)

‡Non-seeking help group (reference)

p-value of Goodness of fit test (Hosmer & Lemeshow test) * p-value < 0.05; ** p-value < 0.01

Results from a multiple logistic regression model after adjusting for socio-demographic variables (age, educational level, place of birth, length of marriage, total family income, and supportive network).

Table 4. Hierarchical Regression models of Concern for Face and Intimate Partner Violence on Informal Help Seeking Intention

	Informal help seeking intention (N=708) ‡				
	Model 1	Model 2	Model 3	Model 4	Model 5
Intimate partner violence during pregnancy	OR (95% CI)	OR (95% CI)	OR (95% CI)	OR (95% CI)	OR (95% CI)
Psychological aggression (PsA)	0.71 (0.38, 1.35)	0.65 (0.34, 1.25)	0.76 (0.40, 1.45)	0.71 (0.37, 1.33)	0.71 (0.37, 1.35)
Physical assault (PA)	1.52 (0.54, 4.25)	1.57 (0.52, 4.72)	1.28 (0.37, 4.41)	1.41 (0.50, 3.98)	1.52 (0.52, 4.45)
Sexual coercion (SC)	0.99 (0.43, 2.27)	1.03 (0.44, 2.44)	0.94 (0.40, 2.22)	1.01 (0.42, 2.39)	1.01 (0.44, 2.33)
Injury (IN)	0.57 (0.16, 1.97)	0.59 (0.16, 2.21)	0.59 (0.15, 2.33)	0.63 (0.18, 2.27)	0.55 (0.16, 1.95)
Concern for Face: *Protective Face Subscale*					
Keeping a low profile to avoid attention (P1)	**0.86 (0.77, 0.97)***	**0.87 (0.77, 0.97)***	**0.85 (0.76, 0.95)***	**0.86 (0.77, 0.97)***	**0.87 (0.77, 0.97)***
Avoiding making mistakes (P2)	0.92 (0.72, 1.16)	0.91 (0.72, 1.16)	0.92 (0.73, 1.17)	0.92 (0.73, 1.17)	0.92 (0.73, 1.16)
Down playing public acclaim & Protecting face through modesty (P3&4)	1.13 (1.00, 1.28)	1.13 (0.99, 1.28)	1.12 (0.99, 1.27)	1.13 (1.00, 1.28)	1.13 (1.00, 1.28)
Concern for Face: *Acquisitive Face Subscale*					
Attracting attention through ostentation and Getting ahead through social achievement (A1&2)	1.01 (0.97, 1.06)	1.01 (0.97, 1.06)	1.02 (0.97, 1.06)	1.02 (0.97, 1.06)	1.01 (0.97, 1.06)

	Informal help seeking intention (N=708) ‡				
	Model 1	Model 2	Model 3	Model 4	Model 5
Moderating Effect (Interaction Effect): Intimate partner violence interact with concern for face					
PsA X Concern for face					
PsA X P1		0.98 (0.78, 1.22)			
PsA X P2		1.00 (0.86, 1.16)			
PsA X P3&4		1.09 (0.93, 1.29)			
PsA X A1&2		1.07 (0.91, 1.25)			
PA X Concern for face					
PA X P1			**0.83 (0.63, 1.08)***		
PA X P2			0.95 (0.80, 1.13)		
PA X P3&4			1.00 (0.86, 1.16)		
PA X A1&2			1.09 (0.87, 1.34)		
SC X Concern for face					
SC X P1				1.02 (0.80, 1.31)	
SC X P2				0.91 (0.78, 1.05)	
SC X P3&4				0.98 (0.85, 1.12)	
SC X A1&2				1.10 (0.92, 1.31)	
IN X Concern for face					
IN X P1					1.09 (0.78, 1.52)
IN X P2					1.00 (0.86, 1.16)
IN X P3&4					1.02 (0.79, 1.32)
IN X A1&2					0.99 (0.83, 1.18)

‡Non-seeking help group (reference)

p-value of Goodness of fit test (Hosmer & Lemeshow test) * p-value < 0.05; ** p-value < 0.01

Results from multiple logistic regression models after adjusting for socio-demographic variables (age, educational level, place of birth, length of marriage, total family income, and supportive network).

Table 3 and Table 4 show the results of the hierarchical logistic regression models for the four forms of IPV, concern for face and the interaction terms of these two variables in different combinations on their intention to seek help via formal and informal channels after controlling for socio-demographic variables. The Odds Ratio (OR) of Psychological Aggression (PsA) (OR = 0.30 to 0.36) was significantly associated with formal help-seeking intention ($p < 0.05$) from Model 1 to Model 5, suggesting that women who experience PsA are less likely to seek formal help. Therefore, this finding partially supported the first hypothesis. The OR of P1 (OR = 0.76 to 0.89) was consistently significantly associated with informal and formal help-seeking intention after adjustment from Model 1 to Model 5 (Tables 4 and 5). This finding indicated that women who keep a lower profile to avoid attention are less likely to seek formal or informal help. Thus, the second hypothesis was partially confirmed. As indicated in Model 3 in Table 4, the interaction term between Physical Assault (PA) and P1 was significant. The result showed that the women who have a higher level of protective face orientation in terms of P1 might escalate the negative linkage between the PA and informal help-seeking intention. The result partially supported our third hypothesis.

DISCUSSION

Psychological Aggression and Concern for Face

In this study, the results showed that the majority of IVP took the form of PsA that was negatively related to formal help-seeking intention. The possible explanations might be related to the perception that psychological abuse is less likely to be punished, for example, by way of legal sanctions, when compared to physical or sexual abuse (Jacobson, 1994). Recent studies have also found that psychological aggression is more acceptable among Chinese people than among Western ethnic groups (Iavicoli, Grivres, Wilets, Kriesman, & Amir, 2001). Therefore, women might not seek formal help in the event of psychological abuse. However, one should not underestimate the psychological trauma that women suffer from psychological aggression (Tang, Wong, Cheung, & Lee, 2000).

Concern for Face and Help-Seeking Intention

This study also reveals that women who have concern for face in terms of "keeping a low profile to avoid attention (P1)" are less likely to adopt an intention to seek either formal or informal help. According to Chou (1996), individuals who adhere to this aspect of concern for face are sensitive to face-losing situations, and, to the extent possible, avoid entering into situations where they might experience embarrassment and shame. Clear boundaries of self-disclosure exist in the Chinese culture, as demonstrated by the expression that "family disgrace should not be revealed to an outsider" (*jia chou bu ke wai yang*) (Ng & Ingram, 1989). Therefore, concern for face may play a powerful role in abused women's decisions about whether or not to seek help from friends, family, or outside agencies. The possible explanation may be related to Asian cultural traditions that emphasize family privacy and fear of divorce and gender roles that give men superior social status, which may prevent many women from seeking help outside the family, even when they define the IPV as a problem (Liang, Goodman, Tummala-Narra, & Weintraub, 2005).

Moderating Effect of Physical Assault and Concern for Face on Informal Help-Seeking Intention

Our findings indicated that for women who experience Physical Assault (PA). the maintenance of a low profile to avoid attention (KLP) might have a negative impact on the intention to seek informal help. Therefore, KLP may accelerate the negative linkage of PA and informal help-seeking intention. One possible explanation could be associated with the fact that physically assaulted women are most likely to isolate themselves (Moraes & Reichenheim, 2002) and tend not to communicate with relatives or friends (Campbell, Oliver, & Bullock, 1998). If women concerned with protective face conceal incidents of PA, the perpetrators are likely use this vulnerability to control and assert their authority and to continue the cycle of violence (Campbell, 2002). Furthermore, because women's experiences of PA have left them frightened and ashamed, it is difficult for them to be assertive and positive in planning their lives (Peckover, 2003) and it is often difficult for them to remember the family members or friends who have helped them out in the past (Caeser, 1998). Since IPV rarely ceases without outside intervention, the consequences of delay in seeking help can be serious and the adverse impacts of IPV may be cumulative.

CONCLUSION

The findings of this study provide some initial evidence of the influence of concern for face on the pathway to the intention to seek help associated with various forms of IPV in Hong Kong. The study has several implications. Firstly, women with protective face concern are reluctant to seek help from both informal and formal channels and none would seek help from nurses. It is important for nurses to reach out to this target group in the form of health education and in the planning of a culture-specific intervention with a special focus on concern for face. Secondly, it is essential for nurses to identify face issues which are often subtly expressed through the everyday language and behavior of women with IPV. Supportive, sensitive, and non-judgmental communication skills can greatly facilitate such disclosures (Bacchus, Mezey, & Bewley, 2002). Thirdly, traditional Chinese notions have a strong influence on people who believe that IPV is a private matter and do not see its serious social consequences. It is therefore necessary to cultivate a new public opinion about IPV.

In spite of the contributions it makes to the literature, this study has several limitations. Firstly, while it examined the cultural variable of the concern for face, it overlooked a number of other important factors such as interpersonal relationships, social networks and personality attributes. Secondly, the use of a cross-sectional survey design in this study could not capture the causal relationships among IPV, concern for face, and help-seeking behavior. Such relationships could be examined much more clearly through a longitudinal design. Finally, the inclusion of only Chinese groups in this study is unlikely to have contributed significantly to the understanding of the continuum of culturally unique differences about concern for face and help-seeking intention in a multicultural city such as Hong Kong. Future research in these areas is warranted.

REFERENCES

Abraham, M. (2000). Speaking the unspeakable: Marital violence among South Asian immigrants in the United States. New Brunswick: Rutgers University Press.

Bacchus, L., Mezey, G. & Bewley, S. (2002). Women's perceptions and experiences of routine enquiry for domestic violence in a maternity service. British Journal of Obstetric and Gynecology, 109, 9 -16.

Baron, R.M., & Kenny, D.A. (1986). The moderator-mediator variable distinction in social psychological research: conceptual, strategic, and statistical considerations. Journal of Personality and Social Psychology, 51, 1173 - 1182.

Bauer, H., Rodriguez, M., Quiroga, S., & Flores-Ortiz, Y. (2000). Barriers to health care for abused Latina and Asian immigrant women. Journal of Health Care for the Poor and Underserved, 11, 33 - 44.

Boey, K.W. (1999). Help-seeking preference of college students in urban China after the implementation of the 'open-door' policy. International Journal of Social Psychiatry, 45(2), 104 - 117.

Brown, P. & Levinson, S.C. (1987). Politeness: some universals in language usage London: Cambridge University Press.

Bui, H.N. (2003). Help-seeking behavior among abused immigrant women: A case of Vietnamese American women. Violence Against Women, 9(2), 207 - 239.

Caeser, P. (1998). Exposure to violence in the families of origin among wife abusers and martially nonviolent men. *Violence and Victims, 3*, 49-63.

Campbell, J.C., Oliver, C.E. & Bullock, L.F.C. (1998). Dynamics of battering during pregnancy. In J. C. Campbell (Ed.), *Empowering survivors of abuse* (pp. 81 - 89). Thousand Oaks, CA: SAGE.

Catolico, O. (1997). Psychological well-being of Cambodian women in resettlement/. *Advanced in Nursing Science, 19*, 75 - 84.

Chan, K.L. (2001). *An evaluation study of group therapy for male batters and intervention strategies*. Hong Kong: Hong Kong Family Welfare Society and Department of Social Work and Social Administration, University of Hong Kong.

Chatzifotiou, S. & Dobash, R. (2001). Seeking informal support: Marital violence against women in Greece. *Violence Against Women, 7*(9), 1024 - 1050.

Chou, M.L. (1996). *Protective and acquisitive face orientation: a person by situation approach to face dynamic in social interaction.* Unpublished doctoral dissertation, University of Hong Kong, Hong Kong.

Cohen, B.Z. (1999). Measuring the willingness to seek help. *Journal of Social Service Research, 26*(1), 67 - 82.

Coker, A.L., Derrick, C.D., Lumpkin, J.K., & Aldrich, T.E. (2000). Help seeking for intimate partner violence and forced sex in South Carolina. *American Journal of Preventive Medicine, 19*(4), 316 - 320.

Dasgupta, S., & Warrier, S. (1996). In the floor steps of "Arundhati": Asian India women's experience of domestic violence in the U. S. *Violence Against Women, 2*, 238 - 259.

Edin, K. E., & Hogberg, U. (2002). Violence against pregnant women will remain hidden as long as no direct questions are asked. *Midwifery 18*, 268 - 278.

Gao, G. (1996). Self and others: a Chinese perspective on interpersonal relationship. In W. B. Gudykunst, S. Ting-Toomey & T. Nishida (Eds.), *Communication in personal relationships across culture*. Thousand Oaks: SAGE Publications.

Goffman, E. (1955). On face-work: an analysis of ritual elements in social interaction. *Psychiatry, 18*, 213 - 231.

Goffman, E. (1967). *Interaction ritual: essays on face-to-face behavior*. New York: Basic Books.

Ho, C. (1990). An analysis of domestic violence in Asian American communities: a multicultural approach to counseling. *Women and Therapy, 9*(1 - 2), 129 - 150.

Ho, K.M.J. (1994). *A study on help-seeking pattern among young people in Hong Kong*. Hong Kong.: University of Hong Kong.

Hosmer Jr, D.W., & Lemershow, S. (2000). *Applied logistic regression*. Wiley: New York.

Hu, H.C. (1944). The Chinese concept of face. *American Anthropologist, 46*, 45 - 64.

Hu, X. & Chen, G. (1999). Understanding cultural values in counseling Asian families. In K. S. Ng (Ed.), *The family psychology and counselling series: Counseling Asian families from a system perspective* (pp. 27 - 37). Alexandria, VA: American Counselling Association.

Huisman, K. (1996). Wife battering in Asian American communities: Identifying the service needs of an overlooked segment of the U.S. population. *Violence Against Women, 2*, 260 - 283.

Iavicoli, L., Grivres, S., Wilets, I.F., Kriesman, E., & Amir, T. (2001). Cultural attitudes towards domestic violence. *Academic Emergency Medicine, 8*, 462.

Jacobson, N.S. (1994). Rewards and dangers in researching domestic violence. *Family Process, 33*, 81 - 85.

Karabenick, S.A. (1998). Help seeking as strategic resources. In S. A. Karabenick (Ed.), *Strategic help seeking*. Mahwah: NJ Lawrence Erlbaum Associates, Inc., Publishers.

Kaukinen, C. (2004). The help-seeking strategies of female violent-crime victims: the direct and conditional effects of race and the victim-offender relationship. *Journal of Interpersonal Violence, 19*(9), 967 - 990.

King, A. Y.C. & Myers, J.T. (1977). *Shame as an incomplete conception of Chinese culture: A study of face*. Hong Kong: The Chinese University of Hong Kong Social Research Centre.

Klose, T. (1999). The contingent valuation method in health care. *Health Policy, 47*(2), 97 - 123.

Koss, M.P., Goodman, L.A., Browne, A., Fitzgerald, L.F., Keita, G.P., & Russo, N.F. (1994). *No safe haven: Male violence against women at home, at work, and in the community*. Washington, DC: American Psychological Association.

Lazarus, R. & Folkman, S. (1984). *Stress, appraisal, coping*. New York: Singer.

Lee, E. (1996). Asian American families: an overview. In G. McGoldrick, G. Giordao & J.K. Pierce (Eds.), *Ethnicity and family therapy* (pp. 227 - 247). New York: Guilford.

Lee, M. & Au, P. (1998). Chinese battered women in North America: their experiences and treatment. In A. Roberts (Ed.), *Battered women and their families: intervention and treatment programs* (pp. 448 - 482). New York: Springer.

Leong, F.T.L. & Lau, A.S.L. (2001). Barriers to providing effective mental health services to Asian Americans. *Mental Health Services Research, 3*, 201 - 214.

Leung, W.C., Leung, T.W., Lam, Y.Y., & Ho, P.C. (1999). The prevalence of domestic violence against pregnant women in a Chinese community. *International Journal of Gynecology and Obstetrics, 66*(1), 23-30.

Liang, B., Goodman, L.A., Tummala-Narra, P., & Weintraub, S. (2005). A theoretical framework for understanding help-seeking processes among survivors of intimate partner violence. *American Journal of Community Psychology, 36*(1/2), 71 - 84.

Lipsky, S., Caetano, R., Field, C.A., & Larkin, G.L. (2006). The role of intimate partner violence, race, and ethnicity in help-seeking behaviors. *Ethnicity and Health, 11*(1), 81 - 100.

Mayer, B.W. & Coulter, M. (2002). Psychological aspects of partner abuse: Part two of a two-part series. *American Journal of Nursing, 102*(6), 24AA-24CC.

Meng, L. (1999). Enduring violence and staying in marriage: Stories of battered women in rural China. *Violence Against Women, 5*(1469 - 1493).

Moraes, C.L. & Reichenheim, M.E. (2002). Domestic violence during pregnancy in Rio de Janeiro, Brazil. *International Journal of Gynecology and Obstetrics, 79*, 269 - 277.

Nadler, A. (1990). Help-seeking behaviors as a coping resource. In M. Rosenbaum (Ed.), *Learned resourcefulness: on coping skills, self-control, and adaptive behaviors* (pp. 127 - 162). New York: Springer.

Ng, R. S.Y. & Ingram, S.C. (1989). *Chinese culture in Hong Kong*. Hong Kong: Asia 2000.

Olsen, J.A. & Smith, R.D. (2001). Theory versus practice: a review of 'willingness-to -pay' in health and health care. *Health Economics, 10*(1), 39 - 52.

Peckover, S. (2003). 'I could have just done with little more help': an analysis of women's help-seeking from health visitors in the context of domestic violence. *Health and Social Care in the Community, 11*(3), 275 - 282.

Raj, A. & Silverman, J. (2002). Violence against women immigrant women: The roles of culture, context, and legal immigrant status on intimate partner violence. *Violence Against Women, 8*(3), 367 -398.

Schneiderman, S. (1995). *Saving face: America and the politics of shame* (1st ed.). New York: Alfred A. Knopf.

Shek, D.T L. (1998). Help-seeking patterns of Chinese parents in Hong Kong. *Asia Pacific Journal of Social Work, 8*(1), 106 - 119.

Tang, C., Lee, A. & Cheung, F.M. (1999). Violence against women in Hong Kong. In F. M. Cheung (Ed.), *Breaking the silence: Violence against women against women in Asia.* Hong Kong: Equal Opportunities Commission.

Tang, C.S.K., Wong, T., Cheung, F.M.C., & Lee, A. (2000). Exploring how Chinese define violence against women: a focus group study in Hong Kong. *Women's Studies International Forum, 23*, 197-209.

Tjaden, P. & Thoennes, N. (1998). *Prevalence, incidence, and consequences of violence against women: Finding from the National Violence against Women Survey.* Washington, DC: U. S. Department of Justice.

Wang, H. (2002). *Help seeking tendency on situation of threat to self-esteem and face-losing.* Unpublished doctoral dissertation, The University of Hong Kong, Hong Kong.

Wang, X. (1999). Why are Beijing women beaten by their husbands? A case analysis of family violence in Beijing. *Violence Against Women, 5*, 1493 - 1505.

Xu, X. (1998). *Chinese understanding of domestic violence.* Unpublished manuscript, The John Hopkins University.

In: Social Sciences in Health Care and Medicine ISBN: 978-1-60456-286-6
Editors: J. B. Garner, T. C. Christiansen, pp. 199-211

Chapter 8

SELF-MANAGEMENT OF CHRONIC DISEASE IN HEALTHCARE: THE ROLE OF PHARMACY

Lorraine Smith, Ines Krass and Carol Armour
Faculty of Pharmacy
The University of Sydney, 2006, AUSTRALIA
lsmith@pharm.usyd.edu.au
Tel: 61 2 9036 7079
Fax: 61 2 9351 4391

ABSTRACT

Improvements in the quality of biomedical care have resulted in a change in disease trends. In the twenty-first century, in developed countries, it is estimated that 80% of healthcare funds are now being directed towards the care and support of those with chronic diseases. The last decade has seen a rapid change in the role of the community pharmacist. There is a pressing need for increasing healthcare professionals' theoretical and practical knowledge of patient self-management, as well as their skills in helping their patients who have a chronic disease to manage effectively their illness on a daily basis. Pharmacists have high levels of therapeutic knowledge and skills, and are very often the first, and most common, point of contact for people with chronic illness. Community pharmacies offer accessible and convenient venues for patients with chronic disease to gain support for improving their self-management skills. Thus, pharmacists are in an ideal position to contribute to the improved quality of care of patients with a chronic disease. This chapter will discuss the theoretical issues surrounding self-regulation of illness behavior, the concept of illness self-management, and how these constructs can be applied to deliver effective self-management programs. The methods we adopted for a number of our research projects trialing community pharmacy disease programs, along with the results, will be used to illustrate these ideas. Importantly, the generic application of these programs to a range of disease states, and healthcare settings, will also be discussed.

Introduction

The rise of the biomedical model of healthcare has transformed the diagnosis, treatment and health outcomes of ill and injured people. Longevity has increased through the effective treatment of infection and the development of vaccines, and advances in technology have resulted in dramatic improvements in surgical techniques. With these improvements in the quality of biomedical care, disease trends have altered. Although people in developed countries now live longer, chronic disease is on the rise, and, as we enter the twenty-first century, it is estimated that the global burden of chronic disease will account for almost three quarters of all deaths (WHO, 2005). In countries such as Australia up to 80% of healthcare funds are now being directed towards the care and support of those with chronic diseases (AIHW, 2006). The reasons for an increase in chronic disease are complex, but are due to a combination of lifestyle and ageing factors: as the body ages, so does its organs; as standards of living have increased so have sedentary habits and over-eating; cigarette smoking and over-consumption of alcohol are resulting in diseases with long-term and devastating effects. In addition, genes are now recognized as playing a much larger role than previously thought in the development of chronic and life threatening diseases. These factors increase the risk of people developing a chronic disease during their lifetime.

By its very nature, chronic disease involves long-term illness accompanied by the presence of symptoms, often on a daily basis, which can be resistant to treatment. The biomedical model of healthcare is inadequate in its capacity to effectively treat chronic illness. Alternative models of healthcare, which recognize that the responsibility for management of the illness cannot remain with the healthcare professional but must be shared with the patient, are necessary to maximize health outcomes and quality of life for those living with a chronic disease. Effective healthcare for those living with chronic illness also requires the participation of community-based rather than hospital-based healthcare professionals (HCP). However, the healthcare sector has been tardy in recognizing the concomitant need for increasing healthcare professionals' theoretical and practical knowledge of patient self-management, and the necessary skills for working with their patients who have a chronic disease to maximize effective chronic care.

This chapter will outline the theoretical underpinnings of chronic disease self-management, and discuss the roles that community pharmacists can adopt in promoting patient self-management of chronic illness. These issues will be illustrated with examples from our research programs which have developed and implemented a range of self-management interventions through community pharmacies in Australia.

The Process of Self-Regulation of Illness Behaviour

Mastery of self-regulatory processes has been recognized for many years as a powerful determinant of behaviour change across a variety of domains, such as education (Pintrich, 2000; Zimmerman, 1990) and health (Horne & Weinman, 2002; Leventhal et al., 2003). This is supported by a significant body of theoretical literature (for example, Bandura 1997, 1993, 1986; Carver & Scheier, 1998; Leventhal & Mora, 2005; Maes & Karoly, 2005). Self-regulation is concerned with modifying one's behaviour through a combination of cognitive, emotional and behavioural processes, in response to environmental demands (Carver and Scheier, 1998). Johnson (1999) suggests that individuals will regulate their behaviour in an effort to align desired personal goals with actual reality.

Leventhal et al (2003) propose that these are conscious processes, and this involves monitoring symptoms, adjusting behaviour accordingly and appraising the effects of the modified behaviour. We would argue that for many people, self-regulation of illness is not necessarily a conscious behaviour, but that HCPs can provide an important service by assisting their patients to make explicit the cognitive and behavioural processes that they need to undertake in order to effectively manage their chronic condition. In chronic health care settings, the effectiveness of the care provided by HCPs is determined by the extent to which the patient actively monitors and self-regulates his or her health-related behaviours.

In addition to these self-regulatory processes, a range of specific personal beliefs and behaviours are necessary for optimal self-management of chronic illness (Battersby et al., 2004; Horne & Weinman, 2002). Patients are more likely to be effective in the day to day management of their condition if they:

- have a sound understanding of their illness as well as its treatment,
- are willing to participate in treatment decisions,
- have a capacity to establish and maintain good working relationships with healthcare professionals (HCPs) involved in the treatment of the illness,
- are able to take medications as directed,
- are aware of symptom severity and symptom control, and
- are confident in their ability to undertake and execute these tasks.

However, making changes to lifestyle and adapting to living with a chronic illness can, for many patients, appear to be in some respects overwhelming or unachievable. This may be for a variety of reasons: some patients have unrealistic expectations about what they should be able to do and enter a cycle of failing to make positive changes, loss of personal control and declining confidence. For other patients simply knowing *what* to do about making changes to lifestyle and *how* to start can be difficult.

Interventions Applying Principles of Self-Regulation of Illness Behaviour

Applying the theory of self-regulation of illness behaviour to the clinical management of chronic illness has resulted in a model of self-management that HCPs can implement to help improve their patients' management of chronic illness (Bandura 2005; Horne & Weinman, 2002; Leventhal et al., 2003; Maes et al., 2005; Wright et al., 2003). This model comprises a series of steps involving the development of explicit goals and strategies, in consultation with the HCP, which will address problem areas of health and illness of personal relevance to the patient. In order for the nominated goals and strategies to be effective, the patient also needs to know how to monitor their progress towards the achievement of their set goals. The model stipulates that these patient-driven processes require timely and supportive feedback by the HCP. Most importantly, this model of intervention is delivered through a written medium, so that the steps in the process (goals, strategies, monitoring, feedback) are reinforced, provide guidance to the patient and are addressed at follow-up appointments between patient and HCP. In keeping with the model of self-regulation of illness behaviour further written information would be provided for the patient. This would include relevant medical information regarding the illness, written in lay terms.

Goal setting can help patients adopt a more planned and explicit approach to managing their chronic illness. Effective goal setting helps the patient to make changes in lifestyle, and it plays a key role in problem solving. A strength of this approach is that it facilitates the acquisition of skills and confidence by the patient. It also helps to maximize personal investment, thereby increasing the likelihood of successful behaviour change. Mastery of these important behaviours is guided by the step-by-step nature of the intervention and the opportunity for regular support and feedback from the HCP. This mastery will contribute positively to patients' confidence in their ability to undertake the necessary tasks for effective self-management of their illness.

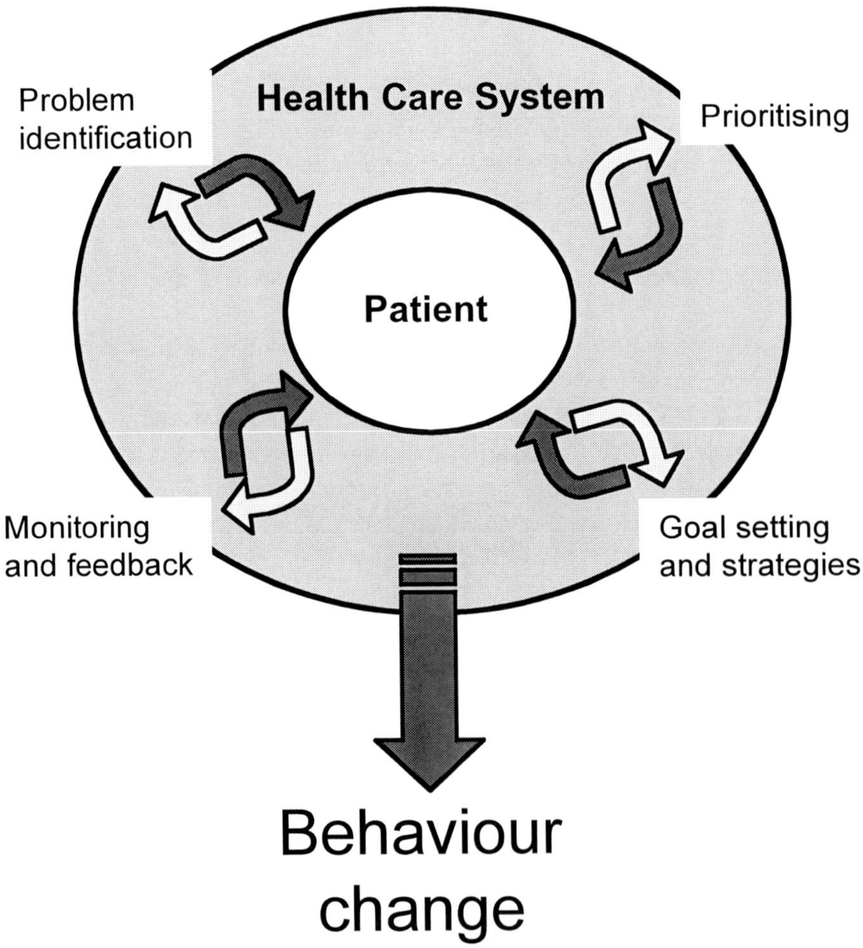

Figure 1. The process of supporting self-regulation of illness behaviour in patients.

COMMUNITY PHARMACY-BASED CHRONIC DISEASE INTERVENTIONS

Over the last decade the role of the community pharmacist has extended beyond the traditional boundaries of the expert dispensing of medications, to include a range of health-related services, such as cholesterol checks and blood pressure monitoring. More recently, community pharmacy-based chronic disease state service models have been developed, implemented and evaluated in Australia (Armour et al., 2004; Armour et al., 2007; Gordois et al., 2007; Krass et al., 2007a, 2007b; Saini et al., 2004; Smith et al., 2007; Taylor et al., 2005). Community pharmacists are ideally placed to provide specialist support to patients for optimizing their chronic disease self-management practices. This is because pharmacists are highly accessible by the general public, often being the first point of HCP contact for the patient, and their therapeutic knowledge is extensive.

Research conducted by the Pharmacy Practice Research Team at the Faculty of Pharmacy, University of Sydney, has shown that these types of services can have positive effects on patient self-management of chronic conditions such as asthma, allergic rhinitis and type 2 diabetes, and, that community pharmacies can be an appropriate setting for the delivery of such a model (Smith et al., 2007; Smith et al., 2005).

Asthma Intervention Models

Asthma

Asthma is a chronic inflammatory disorder, characterized by bronchoconstriction, inflammation and hyper-responsiveness of the airways. People with asthma experience symptoms of wheezing, chest tightness, breathlessness and coughing, particularly during the night or early morning. Asthma attacks tend to be episodic, however inflammation of the airways is chronically present (GINA, 2006). The disease is one of the most common chronic diseases in western countries (AIHW, 2005; Castro et al., 2003; Warschburger et al., 2004).

As asthma is a chronic condition it requires patients to actively self-manage their condition on a day to day basis. Patients need to constantly review their symptoms, medications, and lifestyle and make adjustments in their behaviour. These are cognitive and behavioural processes, the success of which are mediated by the patient's ability and motivation to recognize the presence of symptoms, assess the severity of these symptoms and their relationship to daily activities, and subsequent modification of medications and behaviour.

However, research has indicated that with respect to the management of asthma these self-management attributes are not widespread (Clark & Partridge, 2002). Despite campaigns, promotional activities and professional schemes aimed at improving asthma management practices (Coughlin et al., 2000; Reid et al., 2000; Ruffin et al., 1999) achieving effective patient management of the disease remains problematic.

In our work over the last seven years we have trained community pharmacists to work with asthma patients using a variety of self-management intervention models. In one of our first studies, pharmacists were trained to help their patients set goals, but the intervention did not include the subsequent steps of strategy development or monitoring (Saini, Krass &

Armour, 2004). In this study the goals patients set focused on medication usage, attaining a written action plan and trigger avoidance. The results of this study indicated significant improvements in asthma severity, perceived asthma control, adherence to medications and asthma knowledge. Evaluation of this model suggested that the extent to which the goal setting component of the intervention contributed to these outcomes could not be determined as it was part of a larger asthma care model of intervention. Feedback from this study also indicated that pharmacists found the collaborative goal-setting process difficult to operationalise with their patients.

A subsequent intervention study sought to redress these issues by adopting a more patient- rather than clinical-focus. This was achieved by incorporating more detailed pharmacist education in self-regulation theory and intervention, material aids such as workbooks, communications skills and the inclusion of regular visits between patient and HCP to enable feedback to take place. Furthermore, this project (Smith et al., 2007) was designed to focus almost entirely on patient self-regulation of asthma management behaviour. The key components of the self-regulatory model – goals, strategies, monitoring, rewards and feedback – were included in the intervention. Our pharmacists were trained to facilitate rather than direct their patient's self-management behaviours. This was achieved by encouraging the patient to select those problem areas of asthma control that were of personal rather than clinical relevance, to set achievable goals directly relating to those problem areas, and to devise appropriate strategies for achieving those goals.

CASE STUDY – 'Roberto', aged 18

Roberto sets as his primary goal that of remaining on court for an entire basketball game without having to come off early due to an exacerbation of asthma symptoms. As the pharmacist and Roberto review his typical basketball preparation activities it emerges that inadequate symptom control and no physical warmup are occurring prior to the game. Addressing these shortcomings become strategies for achieving the goal. In Roberto's workbook the Goal is written down: "Last whole game without coming off early". The Strategies to achieve this goal are also written down: "(1) Use reliever medication 20 minutes before game. (2) Wear warm clothes before going on court. (3)Do stretching exercises 10 minutes before game." The goal and strategies are noted in the Roberto's workbook, along with space to record monitoring of the effectiveness of the strategies to achieve the goal. This allows for targeted feedback to take place between Roberto and his pharmacist at his regular follow up visits.

Implementation of this self-regulatory model to guide patient behaviour enables the identification of problem areas of asthma control, and a structured step-wise process for Roberto to improve his asthma control. This process builds a means for him to acquire the cognitive and behavioural attributes necessary for optimal daily management of his chronic illness. It also provides guidance for the pharmacist, and can ultimately contribute to improvements in clinical as well as psychosocial outcomes, as Figure 2 below illustrates.

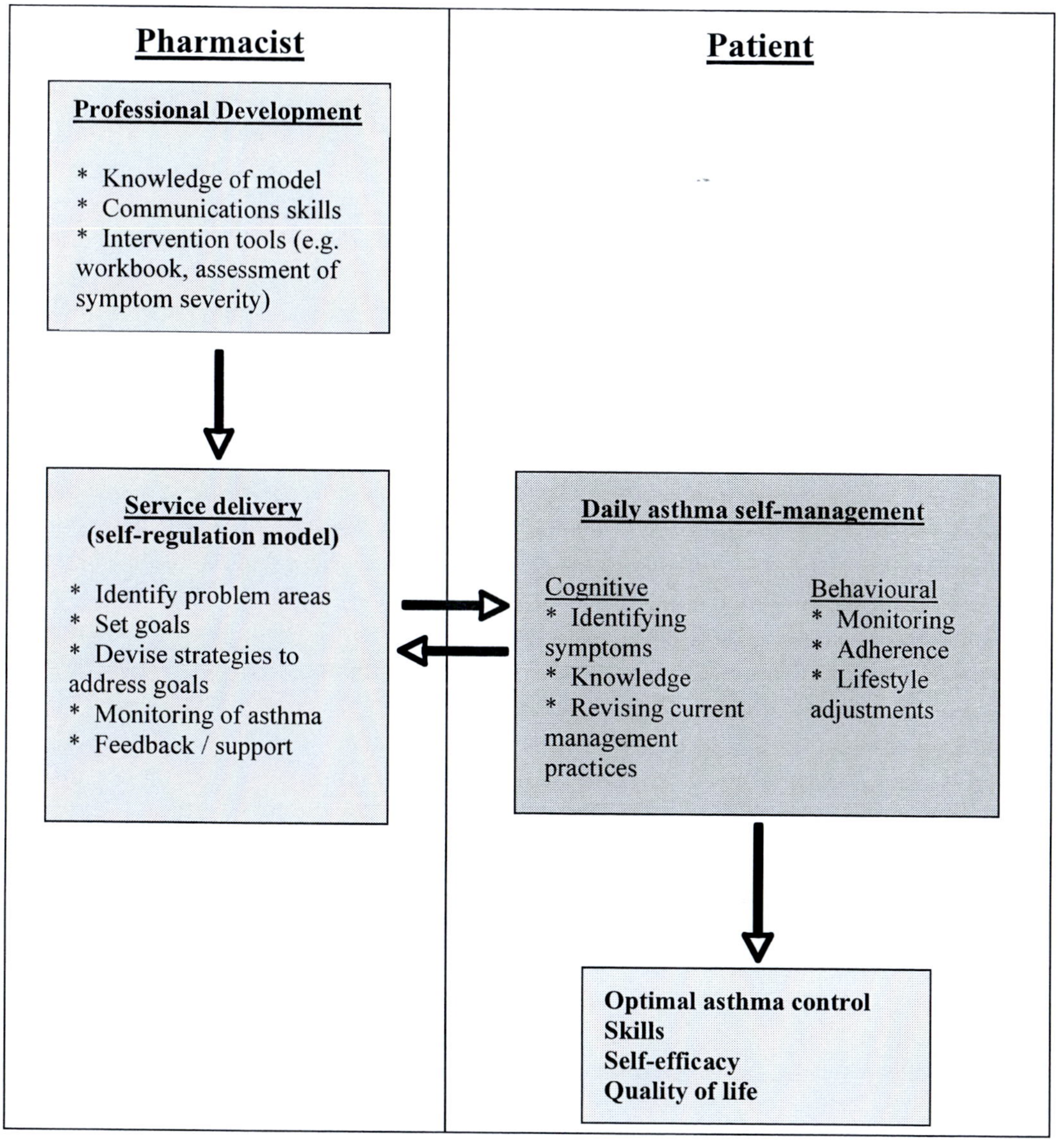

Figure 2. Pharmacist-Patient Model of Asthma Self-Regulation.

Subsequent analysis of the data from this parallel, controlled study has indicated improvements in asthma self-efficacy and asthma quality of life ($ps < 0.05$) when compared to the control group (Smith et al., 2007). Patient satisfaction with this intervention was very high (Smith et al., 2005), with patients reporting that the goals- and strategies- setting process they engaged in with their pharmacist as an extremely useful process. Patients also reported the medical information and goal setting sections of the workbook as either very- or extremely- helpful aids.

A further study conducted by the Sydney University Pharmacy Practice team sought to incorporate these patient-focused components of a disease state management service within a clinically focused model. The Pharmacy Asthma Care Program (PACP) was a multi-site project conducted across three states of Australia involving 57 community pharmacies. The project was designed to identify people who may be at risk of poorly controlled asthma and offer them a specialized service comprising an on-going cycle of assessment, goal setting, monitoring and review. Patients' asthma severity was assessed, spirometry (lung function) was conducted, asthma inhaler device use and adherence to medications were reviewed, and personal goals regarding asthma control were set. When this was done not only was patient retention and satisfaction extremely high but also clinical outcomes such as asthma severity, use of asthma reliever and preventer medications showed significant improvement (Armour et al., 2007).

The results of these two asthma intervention models showed that providing structured, *process-oriented* support is associated with improvements in patient skills in day to day management of asthma. These interventions contributed to improvements in patients' asthma related quality of life and self-efficacy, and increased their personal investment and autonomy in the management of their illness.

However, these positive outcomes raised more questions regarding self-regulatory processes, and we sought to further investigate the nature of patient self-management practices. Specifically, we were interested in understanding the extent to which personal autonomy influences self-management and health outcomes, and how clinical treatment guidelines might be more closely aligned with patients' personal goals for treatment. To these ends, we devised an intervention model to explore patient autonomy in treatment goals for intermittent allergic rhinitis. We hypothesized that the greater the patient autonomy in nominating goals and devising strategies the better the health outcome.

Allergic Rhinitis Intervention Model

Allergic Rhinitis

Allergic Rhinitis (AR) is an inflammatory disorder of the nasal mucosa, in response to allergen exposure. The most common allergens include pollens, moulds, dust mites, animal dander, tobacco smoke and pollution-related materials (Bousquet et al., 2001). Symptoms include a watery, runny nose; sneezing, nasal pruritus and congestion (Walls et al., 2005). However, patients also report ocular, respiratory and sleep disturbances as related symptoms (Bousquet et al., 2005). AR has a significant impact on patient morbidity and quality of life.

Our model tested the impact of patient-set goals versus pharmacist-set goals on symptom severity and quality of life in a pre-post test intervention study (O'Connor et al., 2007). Community pharmacists were trained to either (i) encourage their patients to nominate goals relating to managing their AR symptoms, along with strategies to achieve those goals, or to (ii) provide the patient with two pre-determined goals which were based on clinical treatment guidelines - 'eliminate hay fever symptoms' and 'avoid triggers'. In the latter intervention group the pharmacist asked the patient what their particular symptoms and AR triggers were and devised strategies relevant to the symptoms and triggers. For both groups the goals and strategies were written on a goals card for the patient to keep and bring with them to their visits to the pharmacist for the duration of the study.

Significant improvements were achieved in both symptom severity and quality of life for both groups. However, contrary to expectations, the pharmacist-set goals intervention group had significantly greater improvements in symptom severity. Close inspection of the goals and strategies data for the two groups showed important differences: the goals and strategies in the pharmacist-set goals group were more explicit, better structured and more achievable. For example, typical strategies of the pharmacist-set goals group were *Stay indoors when windy, Get carpets cleaned.* In contrast, in the patient-set goals group typical strategies were *Avoid Triggers; Live in a fairly dust free home.* Clearly, the pharmacist-set group goals are more achievable than the patient-set group goals. In the patient-set goals group the goals are unrealistic because they are of too general a nature and too difficult to achieve.

We concluded that healthcare practitioner input which encouraged patient participation but which at the same time provided structure was necessary in order for the patient to achieve a process for optimal self-management behaviour. Thus, tailoring clinical guidelines to individual patient needs and making explicit the implicit supports the cognitive process of goal attainment.

Type 2 Diabetes Care Model

Another example of effective pharmacy based chronic disease state management which actively engages the patient is a community pharmacy diabetes care model implemented and tested in several trials in the Australian community pharmacy setting (Armour et al, 2004, Krass et al, 2007, Krass et al, 2007).

Type 2 Diabetes

Type 2 diabetes mellitus is a complex metabolic disorder primarily characterized by insulin resistance. Insulin resistance is assumed to be present when the biological effects of insulin, the key hormone in blood glucose regulation, are severely impaired in the liver, muscles and adipose tissues (Kahn, 2003). In response to the onset of insulin resistance, the body reacts by increasing the secretion of insulin by the pancreatic β-cells. In the early stages of type 2 diabetes, this enhanced secretion can compensate for the reduced insulin sensitivity. However, pancreatic β-cell function decreases progressively, causing hyperglycemia and finally leading to clinically evident type 2 diabetes (Strumvoll et al 2005).

The most recent and robust trial was the Pharmacy Diabetes Care Program, a randomized controlled trial conducted in 56 pharmacies from a representative sample of urban and rural areas in four Australian states. Intervention patients received a service which comprised an on-going cycle of assessment, management and review which focused on support of diabetes self-management. This was provided at regular intervals over 6 months in the pharmacy. Control patients were assessed at 0 and 6 months and received no intervention. For those who received the service there were significant improvements in glycaemic control as shown by average falls of 1mmol/L in blood glucose levels and 1% in HbA_{1C}. Collectively, these studies demonstrated that regular visits to the pharmacy by patients with type 2 diabetes to receive self-management support, education and monitoring translated into better control of diabetes and thus better health outcomes (Krass et al 2007).

Are Principles of Self-Management Generalisable?

From our experience we would argue, yes, principles of disease state self-management are generalisable. We have found positive effects in two different disease states and in different models ranging from a heavy clinical focus to a primarily self-management focus where these principles were integrated. Regardless of the primary focus of the intervention model, patients were provided the opportunity to learn life long problem solving skills relating to their disease. Furthermore, these skills are 'transferable', that is, they can be adopted for use in a variety of situations. This is because the *process* has been taught, as opposed to simply providing solutions or courses of action to address the problem. So too, these process skills are generalisable by pharmacists in their care of patients with a wide range of disease states. Again, the process of problem identification, and steps required for effective problem solving can be adapted according to the needs of the patient and the requirements of their disease.

A strength of this model of self-management is that a fundamental underlying principle involves tailoring heathcare interventions to the particular needs of the patient. In our current community pharmacy healthcare models this approach is novel. In the future the challenge will be to re-orient HCPs thinking from the position of 'what must I do to change this patient's behaviour?', to 'what can I do to work with this particular patient so that their personal engagement in their healthcare is activated?' The difference in orientation is important: the former takes a healthcare system perspective whilst the latter takes a patient perspective.

Conclusion

There is wide scope for further research into patient self-management of chronic conditions and Australian studies are indicating promising results from community pharmacy-led interventions. The Australian Government has recognized the role of patient self-management in its Chronic Disease Strategy and is devoting considerable sums of money to research in this area. From our recently conducted studies we know that pharmacists are well-placed to deliver healthcare services focusing on teaching and supporting patients specific and life-long skills in self-management – at the same time as improving clinical outcomes - and that their patients report high levels of satisfaction with such services.

References

Armour C, Bosnic-Anticevich S, Brillant M, Burton, D., Emmerton, L., Krass, I., Saini, B., Smith, L., & Stewart, K. (2007) Pharmacy asthma care program (PACP) improves outcomes for patients in the community. Thorax 62:496-502.

Armour, C., Taylor, S, Hourihan, F, Smith, C., & Krass, I. (2004). Pharmacists leading the way in diabetes care – disease state management *JAPhA,* 44:455-466.

Australian Institute of Health & Welfare. (2005). Asthma in Australia.

Australian Institute of Health and Welfare (2006). *Australia's Health 2006.* AIHW cat. no. AUS 73. Canberra: AIHW.

Bandura, A. (1986). *Social Foundations of Thought and Action: A Social Cognitive Theory.* Englewood Cliffs, NJ: Prentice-Hall, Inc.

Bandura, A. (1993). Perceived self-efficacy in cognitive development and functioning. *Educational Psychologist, 28,* 17-148.

Bandura, A. (1997). *Self-Efficacy: The Exercise of Control.* New York: Freeman.

Bandura, A. (2005). The primacy of self-regulation in health promotion. *Applied Psychology and International Review, 54* (2), 245-254.

Battersby, M.W., Ask, A., Reece, M.M., et al. (2004). The Partners in Health scale: The development and psychometric properties of a generic assessment scale for chronic condition self-management. *Australian Journal of Primary Health, 9,* 41-52.

Bousquet, J., van Cauwenberge, P., Khaltaev, N.; WHO Panel (2001). Allergic rhinitis and its impact on asthma. ARIA, in collaboration with the World Health Organisation. J Allergy Clin Immunol, 108 Suppl: S1-S315.

Bousquet, J., Neukirch, F., Bousquet, P.J., Gehano, P., Klossek, J.M., Le Gal, M., & Allaf, B. (2005). Severity and impairment of allergic rhinitis in patients consulting in primary care. J Allergy Clin Immunol, 117:158-162.

Carver, C.S. & Scheier, M.F. (1998). *On the Self-Regulation of Behavior.* Cambridge: Cambridge University Press.

Castro, M., Zimmermann, N.A., Crocker, S., Bradley, J., Leven, C., Schechtman, K.B. (2003). Asthma intervention program prevents readmissions in high healthcare users. *Am J Respir Crit Care Med,* 168(9):1095.

Clark, N.M. & Partridge, M.R. (2002). Strengthening asthma education to enhance disease control. *Chest, 121*(5), 1661-1669.

Global Strategy for Asthma Management and Prevention, Global Initiative for Asthma (GINA) 2006. Available from: http://www.ginasthma.org.

Coughlin, J., Wilson, A. & Gibson, P. (2000). *Summary Report of the 1999 Evidence-based Review of the Australian Six Step Asthma Management Plan.* NSW Health.

Goeman, D., Aroni, R., Stewart, K., Sawyer, S., Thien, F., Abramson, M., & Douglass, J. (2002). Patients' views of the burden of asthma: a qualitative study. *Medical Journal of Australia, 177,* 295-299.

Gordois, A., Armour, C., Bosnic-Anticevich, S., Brillant, M., Burton, D., Emmerton, L., Krass, I., Saini, B., Smith, L., & Stewart, K. (2007). Cost effectiveness analysis of a pharmacy asthma care program in Australia. *Disease Management and Health Outcomes, 15,* 387-396.

Hicks, R. & Harris, G. (2001). Identifying patients with asthma whose beliefs and attitudes may place them 'at risk': The development and initial validation of the Asthma Navigator. *Journal of Applied Health Behaviour, 3,* 1-7.

Horne, R. & Weinman, J. (2002). Self-regulation and self-management in asthma: exploring the role of illness perceptions and treatment beliefs in explaining non-adherence to preventer medication. *Psychology and Health, 17*(1), 17-32.

Johnson J.E. (1999). Self-regulation theory and coping with physical illness. Res Nurs Health, *22*(6):435-48.

Kahn S.E. (2003). The relative contributions of insulin resistance and beta-cell dysfunction to the pathophysiology of Type 2 diabetes. Diabetologia, 46:3-19.

Krass, I., Taylor, S.J., Smith. C., & Armour, C.L. (2006). The pharmacist's role in continuity of care in type 2 diabetes: an evaluation of a model. *J Pharm Technol,* 22: 3-8.

Krass, I, Armour, C., Mitchell, B., Brillant, M., Dienaar, R., Hughes, J., Lau, P., Peterson, G., Stewart, K., Taylor, S., & Wilkinson, J. (2007). Pharmacy Diabetes Care Program: Analysis of two screening methods for undiagnosed type 2 diabetes in Australian community pharmacy. *Diabetes Research and Clinical Practice, 75*, 339-347.

Krass, I., Armour, C., Mitchell, B., Brillant, M., Dienaar, R., Hughes, J., Lau, P., Peterson, G., Stewart, K., Taylor, S., & Wilkinson, J. (2007). The Pharmacy Diabetes Care Program: Evaluating the impact of a diabetes service model delivered by community pharmacists in Australia. *Diabetic Medicine, 24*, 677-683.

Leventhal, H., Brissette, I. & Leventhal, E.A. (2003). The common-sense model of self-regulation of health and illness. In, L.D. Cameron & H. Leventhal (eds.) *The self-regulation of health and illness behaviour.* Routledge, London.

Leventhal, H. & Mora, P.A. (2005). Is there a science of the processes underlying health and illness behaviours? *Applied Psychology An International Review, 54*(2), 255-566.

Maes, S., & Karoly, P. (2005). Self-regulation assessment and intervention in physical health and illness. *Applied Psychology An International Review, 54*(2), 267-299.

Marks, G., Dunn, S. & Woolcock, A. (1992). A scale for the measurement of quality of life in adults with asthma. *Journal of Clinical Epidemiology, 45,* 461-472.

Narhi, U., Airaksinen, M. & Enlund, H. (2001). Pharmacists solving problems in asthma management – experiences from a one-year intervention programme in Finland. *The International Journal of Pharmacy Practice, March,* 55-59.

O'Connor, J., Seeto, C., Saini, B., Bosnic-Anticevich, S., Krass, I., Armour, C., & Smith, L. (2007). Healthcare professional versus patient goal setting in intermittent allergic rhinitis. *Patient Education and Counseling, 70*(1), 111-117.

Pintrich, P.R. (2000). The role of goal orientation in self-regulated learning. In M. Boekaerts, P.R. Pintrich, & M. Zeidner (Ed.), *Handbook of Self-Regulation* (pp. 451-502). Academic Press: San Diego, CA.

Put, C., van den Bergh, O., Lemaigre, V., Demedts, M., & Verleden, G. (2003). Evaluation of an individualized asthma programme directed at behavioural change. *European Respiratory Journal, 21,* 109-115.

Reid, D., Abramson, M., Raven, J., & Walters, H. (et al. (2000). Management and treatment perceptions among young adults with asthma in Melbourne: The Australian experience from the European Community Respiratory Health Survey. *Respirology, 5,* 281-287.

Ruffin, R.E., Wilson, D., Southcott, A.M., Smith, B., & Adams, R.J. (1999). A South Australian population survey of the ownership of asthma action plans. *Med J Aust, 171,* 348-351.

Saini, B., Krass, I. & Armour, C. (2004). Development, implementation, and evaluation of a community pharmacy-based asthma care model. *The Annals of Pharmacotherapy, 38,* 1954-60.

Smith, L., Bosnic-Anticevich, S., Mitchell, B., Krass, I., Saini, B., & Armour, C. A (2007). Treating Asthma with a Self-Management Model of Illness Behaviour in an Australian Community Pharmacy Setting. *Social Science & Medicine, 64,* 1501-1511.

Smith, L., Bosnic-Anticevich, S., Saini, B., Mitchell, B., Quah, S., Krass, I., & Armour, C. (2005). Collaborative goal setting in community pharmacy #2: towards the effective self-management of asthma. Australian Psychological Society Annual Conference, Melbourne, September.

Stumvoll M, Goldstein B.J. & van Haeften T.W. (2005). Type 2 diabetes: principles of pathogenesis and therapy. *Lancet,* 365:1333-46.

Taylor, S.J., Milanova, T., Hourihan, F., Krass, I., Coleman, C., & Armour, C.L. (2005). A cost effectiveness analysis of a community pharmacist initiated disease state management service for type 2 diabetes mellitus. *Int. J. Pharm. Prac. 13,* 33-40.

Thoonen, B., Schermer, T., Jansen, M., Smeele, I., Jacobs, A., Grol, R., van Schayck, O. (2002). Asthma education tailored to individual patient needs can optimise partnerships in asthma self-management. *Patient Education and Counselling, 47,* 355-360.

Tobin, D., Wigal, J., Winder, J.., Holroyd, K., & Creer, T. (1987). The "Asthma Self-Efficacy Scale". *Annals of Allergy, 59,* 273-277.

Walls R.S., Heddle R.J., Tang M.L.K., Basger, B.J., Solley, G.O., & Yeo, G.T. (2005). Optimising the management of allergic rhinitis: an Australian perspective. *Med J Aust,* 182:28-33.

Warschburger, P., Busch, S., Bauer, C.P., Kiosz, D., Stachow, R., & Petermann, F. (2004). Health-related quality of life in children and adolescents with asthma: results from the ESTAR Study. *J Asthma,* Jun; 41(4):463-70.

Wright, C.C., Barlow, J.H., Turner, A.P., & Bancroft, G.V. (2003). Self-management training for people with chronic disease: An exploratory study. *Brit. J. Hlth Psych, 8,* 465-476.

World Health Organisation (WHO) (2005). *Preparing a health care workforce for the 21st century: The challenges of chronic conditions.* Geneva:WHO.

Zimmerman, B.J. (1990). Self-regulating academic learning and achievement: The emergence of a social cognitive perspective. *Educational Psychology Review, 2,* 173-201.

In: Social Sciences in Health Care and Medicine ISBN: 978-1-60456-286-6
Editors: J. B. Garner, T. C. Christiansen, pp. 213-221

Chapter 9

LOOKING BEYOND THE INDIVIDUAL: THE IMPACT OF AN INTIMATE PARTNER ON HEALTH AND HEALTH BEHAVIORS

Gregory G. Homish
Department of Health Behavior
School of Public Health and Health Professions
The State University of New York at Buffalo
and
Research Institute on Addictions
The State University of New York at Buffalo

Much of the research on risk factors for substance use, mental health, and physical health in adults has largely focused on individual risk factors. Although of great importance, individual risk factors are only one component of understanding individuals' risk. Understanding other factors, such as relational influence processes (i.e., influence from family, peers, and the community) are also important for public health efforts. Among adult couples, an intimate partner can be a powerful influence of change, motivating an individual to make positive changes or seek treatment for problems; however, intimate partners can also be a source of negative influence causing the escalation or relapse of problematic or negative behaviors or blocking treatment and intervention efforts. The goal of this commentary is to provide background on why relational processes are important and to describe how these processes can be used to improve health. On the basis of empirical findings regarding relational processes, we make a number of recommendations for individuals and health care practitioners to begin to consider the larger domain of risk and protective factors.

WHY CONSIDER BROADER SOCIAL NETWORK FACTORS?

Individuals do not exist within a vacuum; therefore, it is possible that ideas, attitudes and behaviors can be shaped by other influences. These influences can be from a variety of individuals within the larger social network—work colleagues, acquaintances, friends, immediate family, extended family, etc. As we have argued elsewhere (Homish & Leonard, 2006), and in accord with other researchers (e.g., Rempel & Rempel, 2004; Westmaas, Wild, & Ferrence, 2002), one of the most powerful sources of social influence among adults is likely an intimate partner. Influence from an intimate partner can function via indirect or direct pathways to cause changes in behaviors (Umberson, 1987). Lewis and Rook (1999) describe the indirect process as "when a person internalizes a sense of obligation to one or more significant others" (page 63). Direct social control processes involve prompting, regulation, or persuasion by a significant other (Lewis & Rook, 1999; Umberson, 1987). Social control processes can lead to either health enhancing behaviors or health compromising behaviors (Lewis & Rook, 1999). Among intimate partners, it is possible that a variety of direct and indirect processes are involved in increasing risk or decreasing risk for changes in partners' health behaviors over time.

In What Areas Do Partners' Directly or Indirectly Influence Change?

There is a substantial body of research that documents that behaviors of intimate partners can influence each other's behavior across a variety of domains. For instance, in a study of married couples and retirement decisions, almost half of retired husbands and wives reported that their spouse influenced their decision to retire (Smith & Moen, 1998). In another study of partner influence, a male partner's beliefs about breastfeeding predicted his partner's breastfeeding duration even after considering the woman's own beliefs about breastfeeding (Rempel & Rempel, 2004). Partner influence has also been found in other domains, such as contraception (e.g., Kerns, Westhoff, Morroni, & Murphy, 2003), food choices (e.g., Bove, Sobal, & Rauschenbach, 2003; Homish & Leonard, in press), and political beliefs (e.g., Jennings & Stoker, 2000).

Evidence of how partners influence each other has also been observed with respect to mental and physical health outcomes, although the processes underlying the influence may be quite different. Beach and colleagues (2006) suggest that some issues that may not initially be of clinical interest, can increase risk for a partner's onset or relapse of a disorder. For example, the association between a wife's depression and husband's depression and wife's depression and husband's anger were assessed in a sample of women with osteoarthritis (Druley, Stephens, Martire, Ennis, & Wojno, 2003). The depression construct, however, was depressive symptoms, not necessarily a clinical diagnosis. Results revealed that wives' initial depression and anger were related to increases in husbands' anger over time. Thus, although the depressive symptoms may not have initially appeared clinically significant, they nonetheless related to changes in husbands' behavior over time. Tower and Kasl (1996) tested the longitudinal influence of one spouse's depressive symptoms and changes in his/her partner's depressive symptoms over time. After controlling for a variety of covariates (age, education, race, financial strain, and chronic illness), changes in depressive symptoms were related to changes in partner's depressive symptoms over time. Similarly, Homish, Leonard, and Kearns-Bodkin (2006) found that both husbands' and wives' alcohol problems related to marriage were significantly associated with increased depressive symptomatology among wives. Thus, relational processes appear important in not only intimate couples' decision making processes, but also in the mental health of both members of the relationship.

Extending beyond mental health issues, evidence suggests that social network influences, in particular that of an intimate partner, are also important when considering changes in substance use. With respect to smoking, Daly and colleagues (1993) examined late onset smoking initiation (women who started smoking at 17 years old or older) and found that women whose significant others also smoked were significantly more likely to start smoking compared to women whose partners did not smoke. Similarly, relapse to smoking may be related to a partner's behaviors. Severson et al. (1995) found that among women who stopped smoking during pregnancy, the strongest predictor of relapse was a smoking partner. Others have also found that relapse was related to living with smokers (Homish & Leonard, 2005). Collins and colleagues (1990) found that social influence processes were the most important predictor of long term smoking outcome. Relational processes are also involved in cessation of smoking. Individuals are more likely to stop smoking when their partners are nonsmokers (McBride et al., 1998) and they have more confidence in their ability to remain a nonsmoker when their partner does not smoke (Severson et al., 1995).

There is also evidence of partner influence with respect to alcohol use behaviors. In a general population survey conducted in Quebec, Canada, wives' frequency of drinking was found to be positively related to their husbands' drinking (Demers, Bisson, & Palluy, 1999). Although not as robust, there was also a significant association between husbands' drinking and wives' frequency of heavy drinking (5 or more drinks). In another cross-sectional study of substance use and married couples, Graham and Braun (1999) found that having a partner who drinks was associated with higher levels of drinking. In two separate longitudinal studies of alcohol use and marriage, one spouse's drinking was related to his/her partner's alcohol use one year later (Leonard & Eiden, 1999; Leonard & Mudar, 2003, 2004). Evidence of partner influence has also been found in treatment samples. In a longitudinal study of alcoholism treatment outcome, patients whose spouses consumed more alcohol had worse outcomes (Moos, Finney, & Cronkite, 1990).

Research with respect to partner influence on marijuana or other illicit substances is present, but more limited. Social influence factors involved in drug use have tended to focus on parents, peers, and siblings but have excluded influence of an intimate partners drug attitudes and behaviors (for a discussion of this, see Yamaguchi, 1990). Kandel (1984) used a large sample of young adults to assess social influence processes involved in marijuana use. After controlling for demographic variables and other substance use, having a spouse or partner who used marijuana was a correlate of current marijuana use for both men and women. However, these findings are based on cross-sectional data. In a more recent investigation, Yamaguchi and Kandel (1997) hypothesized that over time, spouses would influence each other's marijuana use; however, their findings did not support this hypothesis. In their report, the two assessments were, on average, 5 ½ years apart, so it is possible that any potential partner influence was missed due to such a long assessment interval. In contrast to the findings reported by Yamaguchi and Kandel, Homish, Leonard, & Cornelius (2007) found one partner's marijuana use was longitudinally predictive of increased risk for marijuana use in the other partner over the first four years of marriage. This persisted after considering the effect of well known, individual level risk factors such as cigarette smoking, heavy drinking, and negative affect.

Falba and Sindelar (2008) examined the longitudinal relation between one partner's physical health factors (exercise, cholesterol screening and obtaining a flu shot) and his or her partner's health behaviors. After controlling for relevant covariates, it was consistently found that when one spouse improves his or her behavior, the other spouse is also likely to improve their health behavior. Similarly, Homish and Leonard (in press) examined how premarital health behaviors of one spouse (frequency of healthy eating, frequency of unhealthy eating, following a regular exercise routine, and attending routine medical screening) longitudinally impacted the health behaviors of their partners over the first four years of marriage. Importantly, the health behaviors of one partner prior to marriage were longitudinally predictive of the partners' health behaviors over the first four years of marriage. For example, individuals with higher levels of exercise prior to marriage had partners who engaged in higher levels of exercise throughout the next four years. These findings were true for each outcome and remained significant after controlling for sociodemographic factors.

In sum, a considerable body of evidence has been developing to suggest that among adult, intimate partners, there is a significant influence processes involved between the partners. This influence process may be direct or indirect, and appears to exist for a variety of attitudes, behaviors, and health conditions. That is, the process extends from general relationship issues into a variety of mental health, substance use, and physical health domains. The mechanisms of the influence, however, are not clear. Nonetheless, intimate partners appear to be a powerful source of influence. This influence can promote positive health behavior changes.

Other Factors to Consider

Evidence suggests that intimate partners can influence changes in each others physical and mental health conditions. In addition to the process of change that can occur directly or indirectly, there is also an inherent similarity between adult, intimate that cannot be ignored. This similarity between partners exists across a wide range of behaviors and condtions. For example, Houts and colleagues (1996) found that among newlywed couples, there was a greater similarity among leisure activities and division of household task that would be expected by chance. More directly relevant to the current report, however, the similarity between partners' health-related behaviors is an important factor to consider when designing, implementing, or assessing health interventions. In a longitudinal study of newly married couples, Homish and Leonard (in press) found a similarity in dietary habits. This similarity existed for both healthy eating habits as well as unhealthy eating habits. High levels of concordance also occur among other behaviors such as smoking (Homish & Leonard, 2005; Sutton, 1993), alcohol use (Leonard & Eiden, 1999; Leonard & Mudar, 2003), and illicit drug use (e.g., Homish, Leonard, & Cornelius, 2007; Leonard & Homish, 2005; Yamaguchi & Kandel, 1993).

In addition to concordance among health-related behaviors, empirical evidence also suggests a concordance among disorders. Galbaud Du Fort and colleagues (1998) examined concordance for psychiatric disorders in a sample of 519 couples. Significant associations between male and female partners were found for major depression, mania, alcohol abuse or dependence, and drug abuse or dependence. Others have also found concordance for mental health diagnoses between intimate partners (Lindeman et al., 2002; McLeod, 1993). This high level of concordance between intimate partners is not limited to mental health conditions. Stimpson and Peek (2005) found that there was a high concordance for hypertension, diabetes, arthritis and cancer among intimate partners even after controlling for age, education, body mass index, smoking, and drinking. This is consistent with other research. For example, in a recent review of 103 studies, Meyer and colleagues commented that "The research overwhelmingly suggests evidence of concordant mental and physical health" (p. 2297, Meyler, Stimpson, & Peek, 2007).

In sum, the very nature of intimate partnerships is such that members of the relationship have a high degree of interdependence. This interdependence allows for influence processes to potentially occur. Additionally, intimate partners have a high degree of concordance for certain behaviors. This is in accord with compatibility theories that suggest that couples with greater levels of similarity are more likely to have greater marital functioning (Levinger and Rands, 1985). Whether this similarity exists as a result of an assortative mating process or rather some type of contagion, convergence or influence is outside the scope of this commentary. The fact that concordance is often present, however, is one of the key elements to understanding how relational processes can relate to health behaviors.

Recommendations/Considerations for Researchers and Health Care Providers

On the basis of concordance and direct and indirect social influence processes, a number of important considerations emerge. These considerations are in three general areas: health promotion activities, disease/disorder screening, and treatment and intervention. The first domain, health promotion, involves the conscious awareness that individuals' behaviors and attitudes can be modified by the social network. It is important to note that although concordance was found for disorders, it was also found for behaviors—behaviors that either are factors that increase risk or factors that decrease risk for disease development. Therefore, in terms of promoting positive health change, it is important to consider the social network. Stimpson and Peek (2005) suggest that health promotion activities should begin to target family systems. By targeting family systems, it possible that "collateral health effects" can be realized (p. 185, Christakis, 2004); that is, the health behaviors of one partner causing changes in the partner's behaviors. In fact, Chow and colleagues consider the failure to consider the families of patients with premature coronary artery disease "an obvious but neglected target for primary intervention" (p. 481, Chow, Dominiczak, Pell, Pell, Walker, & O'Dowd).

Understanding relational processes is also important when considering the detection of disease or disorders. Currently, most health care providers assess an individuals' risk for a disease or disorder on the basis of two major factors: individual level risk factors and family history. For example, when considering risk for cancer, clinicians will ask if the individual smokes and if they have any first degree relatives who had cancer or died from cancer. These two broad domains are vitally important. However, social network factors, such as the health and health behaviors of intimate partner can also be important. For example, Hippisley-Cox and Pringle (1998) found that the risk for hypertension doubles when a spouse has hypertension. These findings persisted after considering the impact of age, diabetes, and BMI. Thus, knowledge of partner risk factors, coupled with knowledge of individual level risk and family history, can be a powerful, more complete screening approach. Additionally, partners can be influential in engaging one another in routine health screening. For example, Van Jaarsveld and colleagues (2006) examined factors that related to increasing motivation to attend colorectal screening and found that inviting both husbands and wives to attend colorectal screening increase the motivation to attend the screening among wives. Further, invitation of both members increasing the likelihood that both men and women would actually attend the screening.

Finally, relational risk factors can be a critical factor in the success or failure of intervention efforts. Falba and Sindelar discuss the possibility of spillover effects. The example they provide relates to smoking cessation; that is, although only one member is involved in an intervention to stop smoking, they may learn coping skills and other tools that can also help their partner quit smoking. This may be a direct process (e.g., a new ban on smoking in the house) or indirect (e.g., one individual visualizing the success of his/her partners smoking cessation efforts). In terms of an empirically based example of a spillover effect, or alternatively, a reciprocal influence process (e.g., Stimpson and Peek, 2005) is provided from the work of White and colleagues (1991). They examined changes in dietary habits in a sample of women enrolled in a program to reduce their dietary fat compared to a group of comparison women. Husbands were not enrolled in the program. Husbands with wives in the intervention, compared to husbands whose wives were in the control group, also reduced their dietary fat consumption.

Conclusion

The goal of this commentary was two-fold. First, we were interested in providing empirical evidence of the importance of relational processes. That is, understating how the broader social network, in particular intimate partners, relates to health and health behavior changes. The second goal was to provide a series of recommendations for researchers as well as health care providers. These recommendations include considering how much information can be provided by the health behaviors and condition of on an intimate partner and to communicate how vital an intimate partner can be in both positive and negative changes in health. Future work will need to explore the mechanism of action for the influence processes, determine when and under what conditions the influence process is most effective (e.g., health promotion, health intervention, etc), and to determine when the influence process is detrimental (e.g., direct influence causing increased stress to the individual and the relationship).

References

Beach, S.R.H., Wamboldt, M.Z., Kaslow, N.J., Heyman, R.E., & Reiss, D. (2006). Describing Relationship Problems in DSM-V: Toward Better Guidance for Research and Clinical Practice. *Journal of Family Psychology, 20*(3), 359-368.

Bove, C.F., Sobal, J. & Rauschenbach, B.S. (2003). Food choices among newly married couples: convergence, conflict, individualism, and projects. *Appetite, 40*(1), 25-41.

Chow, C.K., Dominiczak, A.F., Pell, J.P., Pell, A.C.H., Walker, A., & O'Dowd, C. (2007). Families of patients with premature coronary heart disease: an obvious but neglected target for primary prevention. *BMJ, 335*(7618), 481-485.

Christakis, N.A. (2004). Social networks and collateral health effects (Vol. 329, pp. 184-185): Br Med Assoc.

Collins, R.L., Emont, S.L. & Zywiak, W.H. (1990). Social influence processes in smoking cessation: postquitting predictors of long-term outcome. *J Subst Abuse, 2*(4), 389-403.

Daly, K.A., Lund, E.M., Harty, K.C., & Ersted, S.A. (1993). Factors associated with late smoking initiation in Minnesota women. *American Journal of Public Health, 83*(9), 1333.

Demers, A., Bisson, J. & Palluy, J. (1999). Wives' convergence with their husbands' alcohol use: social conditions as mediators. *J Stud Alcohol, 60*(3), 368-377.

Druley, J.A., Stephens, M.A. P., Martire, L.M., et al. (2003). Emotional congruence in older couples coping with wives' osteoarthritis: Exacerbating effects of pain behavior. *Psychology & Aging, 18*(3), 406-414.

Falba TA, Sindelar JL. (2008). Spousal Concordance in Health Behavior Change. *Health Services Research.* (43)96-116.

Galbaud du Fort, G., Bland, R.C., Newman, S.C., & Boothroyd, L.J. (1998). Spouse similarity for lifetime psychiatric history in the general population. *Psychol Med, 28*(4), 789-802.

Graham, K. & Braun, K. (1999). Concordance of use of alcohol and other substances among older adult couples. *Addictive Behaviors, 24*(6), 839-856.

Hippisley-Cox, J. & Pringle, M. (1998). Are spouses of patients with hypertension at increased risk of having hypertension? A population-based case-control study. *Br J Gen Pract, 48*(434), 1580-1583.

Homish, G.G. & Leonard, K.E. (in press). Spousal Influence on General Health Behaviors in a Community Sample. *American Journal of Health Behavior.*

Homish, G. G. & Leonard, K.E. (2005). Spousal Influence on Smoking Behaviors in a US Community Sample of Newly Married Couples. *Social Science & Medicine, 61*, 2557-2567.

Homish, G.G. & Leonard, K.E. (2006). Relational Processes and Alcohol Use: The Role of One's Spouse. In E. Y. Brozner (Ed.), *New Research on Alcohol Abuse and Alcoholism* (pp. 19-33). Hauppauge: Nova Science.

Homish, G.G., Leonard, K.E. & Cornelius, J.R. (2007). Predictors of marijuana use among married couples: the influence of one's spouse. *Drug and Alcohol Dependence.* 33(2), 279-291.

Homish, G.G., Leonard, K.E. & Kearns-Bodkin, J.N. (2006). Alcohol use, alcohol problems, and depressive symptomatology among newly married couples. *Drug Alcohol Depend, 83*(3), 185-192.

Houts, R.M., Robins, E. & Huston, T.L. (1996). Compatibility and the development of premarital relationships. *Journal of Marriage & the Family, 58*(1), 7-20.

Jennings, M.K. & Stoker, L. (2000). *Political Similarity and Influence between Husbands and Wives* (No. 2001-14). Berkeley, CA: Institute of Governmental Studies, University of California, Berkeley.

Kandel, D.B. (1984). Marijuana users in young adulthood. *Arch Gen Psychiatry, 41*(2), 200-209.

Kerns, J., Westhoff, C., Morroni, C., & Murphy, P.A. (2003). Partner Influence on Early Discontinuation of the Pill in a Predominantly Hispanic Population. *Perspectives on Sexual and Reproductive Health, 35*(6), 256-260.

Leonard, K. E. & Eiden, R.D. (1999). Husband's and wife's drinking: unilateral or bilateral influences among newlyweds in a general population sample. *J Stud Alcohol Suppl, 13*, 130-138.

Leonard, K. E. & Homish, G.G. (2005). Changes in Marijuana use Over the Transition into Marriage. *Journal of Drug Issues, 35*(2), 409-430.

Leonard, K.E. & Mudar, P. (2003). Peer and partner drinking and the transition to marriage: a longitudinal examination of selection and influence processes. *Psychol Addict Behav, 17*(2), 115-125.

Leonard, K.E. & Mudar, P. (2004). Husbands' influence on wives' drinking: testing a relationship motivation model in the early years of marriage. *Psychology of Addictive Behaviors, 18*(4), 340-349.

Lewis, M.A. & Rook, K.S. (1999). Social Control in Personal Relationships: Impact on Health Behaviors and Psychological Distress. *Health Psychology, 18*(1), 63-71.

Levinger, G. & Rands, M. (1985). Compatibility in marriage and other close relationships. In W. J. Ickes (Ed.), *Compatible and incompatible relationships* (pp. 309-331). New York: Springer-Verlag.

Lindeman, S., Kaprio, J., Isometsa, E., Poikolainen, K., Heikkinen, M., Hamalainen, J., et al. (2002). Spousal resemblance for history of major depressive episode in the previous year. *Psychol Med, 32*(2), 363-367.

McBride, C.M., Curry, S.J., Grothaus, L.C., Nelson, J.C., Lando, H., & Pirie, P.L. (1998). Partner smoking status and pregnant smoker's perceptions of support for and likelihood of smoking cessation. *Health Psychology, 17*(1), 63-69.

McLeod, J.D. (1993). Spouse concordance for depressive disorders in a community sample. *J Affect Disord, 27*(1), 43-52.

Meyler, D., Stimpson, J.P. & Peek, M.K. (2007). Health concordance within couples: A systematic review. *Social Science & Medicine, 64*(11), 2297-2310.

Moos, R.H., Finney, J.W. & Cronkite, R.C. (1990). *Alcoholism treatment: context, process, and outcome*. New York: Oxford University Press.

Rempel, L.A. & Rempel, J.K. (2004). Partner influence on health behavior decision-making: Increasing breastfeeding duration. *Journal of Social and Personal Relationships, 21*(1), 92-111.

Severson, H.H., Andrews, J.A., Lichtenstein, E., Wall, M., & Zoref, L. (1995). Predictors of smoking during and after pregnancy: a survey of mothers of newborns. *Preventive Medicine, 24*(1), 23-28.

Smith, D.B. & Moen, P. (1998). Spousal Influence on Retirement: His, Her, and Their Perceptions. *Journal of Marriage and the Family, 60*(3), 734-744.

Stimpson, J.P. & Peek, M.K. (2005). Concordance of chronic conditions in older Mexican American couples. *Prev Chronic Dis, 2*(3), 1-7.

Sutton, G.C. (1993). Do men grow to resemble their wives, or vice versa? *Journal of Biosocial Science., 25*(1), 25-29.

Tower, R.B. & Kasl, S.V. (1996). Depressive Symptoms Across Older Spouses: Longitudinal Influences. *Psychology and Aging, 11*(4), 683-697.

Umberson, D. (1987). Family status and health behaviors: social control as a dimension of social integration. *J Health Soc Behav, 28*(3), 306-319.

van Jaarsveld, C.H., Miles, A., Edwards, R., & Wardle, J. (2006). Marriage and cancer prevention: does marital status and inviting both spouses together influence colorectal cancer screening participation? *J Med Screen, 13*(4), 172-176.

Westmaas, J.L., Wild, T.C. & Ferrence, R. (2002). Effects of Gender in Social Control of Smoking Cessation. *Health Psychology, 21*(4), 368-376.

White, E., Hurlich, M., Thompson, R.S., et al. (1991). Dietary changes among husbands of participants in a low-fat dietary intervention. *Am J Prev Med, 7*(5), 319-325.

Yamaguchi, K. (1990). Drug use and its social covariates from the period of adolescence to young adulthood. Some implications from longitudinal studies. [Review] [34 refs]. *Recent Developments in Alcoholism, 8*, 125-143.

Yamaguchi, K. & Kandel, D.B. (1993). Marital Homophily on Illicit Drug Use among Young Adults: Assortative Mating or Marital Influence? *Social Forces, 72*, 505-528.

Yamaguchi, K. & Kandel, D.B. (1997). The influence of spouses' behavior and marital dissolution on marijuana use: Causation or selection. *Journal of Marriage and the Family, 59*(1), 22-36.

In: Social Sciences in Health Care and Medicine ISBN: 978-1-60456-286-6
Editors: J. B. Garner, T. C. Christiansen, pp. 223-233

Chapter 10

INFORMAL CAREGIVING TO CHILDREN WITH HIV/AIDS IN TOGO: MEASURES AND CONCEPTS

Ami R. Moore
University of North Texas

In Africa, it was very common that older family members make important health decisions when young members are sick (Seeley, Kajura, Bachengama, Okongo, Wagner, & Mulder, 1993; Foster 2000). Traditionally, the extended family and clan had been the backbone of the African family system as they had provided help and support to its members whenever needed, especially in times of crises (Foster, 2000). However, because of the unprecedented demands and needs of people living with HIV/AIDS, these institutions may not be able to meet these challenges.

Additionally, because of modernization and individualism prevalent in urban areas, the roles of the extended family in times of need may be weakened (Foster & Williamson, 2000). In fact, AIDS is an exorbitant disease, and currently, most Africans cannot afford effective antiviral therapies. Some families have spent their life savings on loved ones with AIDS but have not seen any improvement in the health of the sick (Moore & Henry, 2005; Family Health International, 2001; UNICEF, 2002). Also, stigma associated with HIV/AIDS has made it difficult for family members to cope with the disease and openly talk about their loved ones who are either HIV positive or have AIDS. Consequently, extended family members or clans may be reluctant to help because of fear of being stigmatized or the inability to care for a sick family or provide assistance because of poverty.

In general, caregiving has a negative impact on the health and well-being of caregivers. Caregiving to people living with AIDS is a stressful activity (Turner & Pearlin, 1989; Pearlin, Aneshensel, & LeBlanc, 1997) that can lead to anxiety and depression (Folkman et al., 199; LeBlanc et al., 1997; Land & Hudson, 2002). Furthermore, caregiving to children with HIV/AIDS is believed to be extraordinarily challenging because when a child is affected usually one parent or both are affected as well (Bettoli-Vaughan et al, 1998). Thus, caring for a child with AIDS can threaten the family unit (Lesar & Maldonato, 1997) by creating additional medical, psychosomatic, and financial strains on the family (Lesar et al, 1995).

Living with AIDS affects the family unit as a whole. It changes behaviors of infected children and challenges their physical and mental abilities (Lesar & Maldonato, 1997).

Caregivers of children living with AIDS face many demands on their families' limited resources, both from the children as well as from other infected family members. This only adds to the burden of stress that the caregivers may already be experiencing. However, studies have indicated that effective coping strategies may reduce the level of stress and anxiety among caregivers (McCubbin & Thompson, 1987; Graffi & Minnes, 1989). Furthermore, a few studies report that caregiving has some positive influences on caregivers. For instance, Atkins & Amenta (1991) and Carlisle (2000) found that caregivers obtained benefits and rewards in the process of caring for a person with HIV/AIDS.

The study proposes to examine informal caregiving to children with HIV or AIDS in Togo in order to generate empirical indicators that will be used to develop caregiving measures. Informal caregiving has become an important outlet for people living with AIDS since AIDS is a chronic disease that eventually incapacitates its victims. Moreover, the health care system is poorly developed in Africa (Merson & Rosenfield, 2000), with scarce resources for people with AIDS. Thus, the plight of family members and friends who are caretakers of a loved one with AIDS is compounded.

Researchers have developed instruments to measure the level of stress and anxiety among people giving care to loved ones or close relatives afflicted with chronic and debilitating illnesses; for example the Hopkins Symptom Checklist (Derogatis, Lipman, Rickles, Uhlenhuth, & Covi, 1974); the CES-D measure (Radloff, 1977) and measures of stress by Pearlin, et al. (1990; 1997). Unfortunately, these measures of caregiving experiences have all been developed in the western societies which are economically and culturally different from African societies. Because these measures tend to be culture specific (Aranda & Knight, 1997; Horowitz & Reinhard, 1995), they cannot adequately assess the experiences of informal caregivers in Africa where the effects of HIV/AIDS has been the most severe. Transporting measures from non-African settings may not translate the concepts and experiences of the caregivers in ways that are intelligible and meaningful to African caregivers. Thus, developing instruments to measure caregivers to children with HIV/AIDS is necessary to make intervention programs efficacious. This study attempts to develop an instrument that will measure caregiving experiences of people caring for children with HIV or AIDS in Togo.

SETTING

Togo is located in the western coast of Africa. With an estimated population of 6.1 million inhabitants, Togo's primary economic activity is subsistence agriculture (Wikipedia, 2007). A significant percent of the Togolese population was living below the national poverty line: 32.3% in 2002 (UNDP, 2006). An estimated prevalence rate of HIV among adults aged 15 to 49 is 3.2 % with 88,000 AIDS orphans in the beginning of 2007 (UNESCO, 2007). It is noteworthy to report that this prevalence rate has declined from a high of 6% in 2000 (UNAIDS/WHO, 2000). However, the impact of HIV/AIDS in Togo is enormous and especially deleterious among the poor who seem to be the most affected by this epidemic (Moore & Williamson, 2003; Moore & Henry, 2005).

METHODS

Participants, Procedure and Analysis

Subjects were convenience-sampled from HIV/AIDS centers in Lomé, Togo. Because of the sensitive nature of the study, we asked the directors at three centers that provide services to people with HIV/AIDS and their families to recruit for the study primary caregivers of children aged 0 to 15 who was HIV positive or had AIDS. We had established working relations with these centers since 2001. It is important to note that 'Unite de Recherche Demographique[1]' in Lomé, Togo--a demographic institute--helped with the study. They provided a demographer statistician, an expert in social and demographic research, who assisted the author with the study.

We explained the study protocol to the directors who selected five of their employees who had at least a Bachelor's degree in Social Sciences to help with the study. The five employees were trained by the author for two days. As part of their training, they also watched the author conduct the first 10 qualitative interviews and later the first 10 surveys. In order to maintain conformity, regular meetings were held to discuss the interviews. To be included, a participant had to be a current primary caregiver and had used the centers' services in the past.

First, through in-depth interviews, the caregiving experiences of 30 caregivers were assessed in July, 2006. Caregivers were asked to give a detailed description of all the things they did from dawn to dusk to the seropositive child. They were also asked to describe ways they managed caregiving demands; for example, what they did specifically when they had ups and downs. They were asked to list all the people they disclosed the serostatus of the child to and the reason(s) for disclosure. They were also asked to list all the family members and others that provided any kind of support and specify what the person did.

Interviews were in French or Ewe (one of the native languages in Togo). They were tape-recorded. They lasted on average about 60 minutes. Tapes were transcribed verbatim. Second, the author and the statistician demographer analyzed the transcripts independently. Quality assurance in the form of inter-coder reliability was enhanced by meetings in which interview content was discussed and conceptual themes debated. Recurrent themes and phrases were classified and grouped into categories. The data were reduced by consensus to key conceptual themes and phrases such as disclosure, coping, impact of antiretroviral drugs (ARVs), etc.

The following section briefly describes the main findings of the qualitative study from which the measures were derived. Caregivers carefully selected people to whom they disclosed the serostatus of the child they were caring for because they feared discrimination and stigma upon disclosure. Most of them did not have any support from family and friends. Family and friends were even at times unaware of the serostatus of the child. Caregivers relied heavily on their faith to overcome the daily challenges of caring for a child with HIV/AIDS. They had substantial financial difficulties meeting the needs of the child they were caring for. For instance, they were for the most part unable to provide nutritious foods to the child. Caring for a child with HIV/AIDS is a taxing activity that affects other activities of

[1] Unité de Recherche Démographique is one of the respected research institutes in Togo. It collects data for national and international institutions such as Demographic and Health Surveys (DHS) data for Macro International Inc.

the caregivers. For example, most of the caregivers had either stopped their income generating activities or changed them in order to have time to care for the child.

Also, because of the advanced age and the health status of some caregivers, they felt that they should not be caring for a child. Yet, all of the caregivers reported gratitude for having antiretroviral drugs available at a very nominal price, although at times they were financially unable to buy them. Caregivers took extra care for the child because they did not want either to expose the child to other infections or expose others to HIV. Caregivers used different means to cope with the challenges of caring for a child with HIV/AIDS. Some prayed more, others listened more to music.

From the conceptual themes and phrases, we created questions that reflected the caregiving experiences. Whenever possible, we tried to retain verbatim phrases for the questions. It is important to note that, originally, there were 66 items created. However, during the several meetings that we had, the items were reduced to 50 because some did not fit the concepts. These questions were structured following the principal topics gathered from the qualitative study. For instance, from the theme 'disclosure', two categories of questions were created. One depicted caregivers' disclosure of the child's serostatus to family members and the other depicted caregivers' disclosure of the child's serostatus to people they felt can provide them some help. These questions went through a series of pretests and revisions. A set of Likert-style frequency descriptors was used for all response options (4—completely agree; 3—agree; 2—somewhat agree; 1—disagree). The questions were subsequently administered to 207 caregivers from September to December, 2006 in Lomé, the capital city of Togo and the surrounding towns. Because of missing cases, only 201 surveys were analyzed.

FINDINGS

Table 1 presents the descriptive statistics of the caregivers and the children. It can be noted that caregivers were mainly females (about 73%). They were on average 41.66 years and had on average 8.62 years of education. The majority of the caregivers were caring for their nephews or nieces. Most of the caregivers were seronegative (44%). They mostly identified themselves as catholic (about 47%). Over half of the children had lost their biological parents. Most of the children were on ARVs (80%). The ones who were not on therapy were either too young or had a high CD4 count.

The 11 dimensions that describe informal caregiving experiences of children with HIV/AIDS in Togo are: disclosure, expression of faith, financial difficulties, family support, impact of caregiving demands on other activities, personal and social norms, impact of antiretroviral drugs, supplemental efforts made for the child, coping with stress of caregiving, positive comparision, and profound meaning of child's serostatus. Table 2 describes the measures and the reliability (alpha) values. Internal consistency—Cronbach's α for the scales vary from 0.43 (disclosure to families) to 0.91 (supplemental effort). Overall, the scales are relatively quite reliable. Two thirds of the Chronbach's α values are greater than 0.60.

Table 1. Descriptive statistics of caregivers and children caring for

Gender	Female	72.60
	Male	27.40
Marital Status	Married	43.30
	Cohabiting	4.50
	Single	11.90
	Divorce/separated	14.40
	Widowed	25.90
Religion	Catholicism	47.30
	Protestantism	13.40
	Other Christian religion	29.40
	Islam	4.50
	Traditional religion	2.50
	Other	2.10
	None	1.00
Serostatus of caregivers	Positive	32.80
	Negative	43.80
	Don't know	23.40
Caregiver's relation to child	Parent	23.40
	Aunt/uncle	39.30
	Grandparent	25.90
	Brother/sister	4.00
	Other	7.40
Status of biological parents of the child		
Father	Deceased	51.70
	Ill	7.00
	Abandoned child	14.40
	Living with child	14.90
	Other	12.40
Mother	Deceased	53.20
	Ill	20.90
	Abandoned child	3.00
	Living with child	17.40
	Other	5.50
Gender of child	Female	54.70
	Male	45.30
Child attending school	Yes	70.10
	No	29.90
Average age caregivers (years)	41.66	
Average years of education	8.62	
Average age children	7.00	
Average monthly expenses	27,601.27 CFA ($1=500)	

Table 2: Constructs and reliability (alpha) of each scale.

A. Disclosure

These are some propositions about people with whom you shared the child's positive serostatus. Which of the propositions best describes your situation? Please answer any one of the statements.

I. Family member **(alpha = 0.43)**

a. Disclose serostatus of child to my family members (2.34).
b. Disclose serostatus of child to members of other family (1.73).
c. Disclose serostatus of child to child's siblings (1.43).

II. Provider of help **(alpha = 0.63)**

a. Disclose child's serostatus to people who can financially help me (2.01).
b. Disclose child's serostatus to people who can emotionally help me (1.78).
c. Disclose child's serostatus to people who can spiritually help me (1.91).
d. Disclose child's serostatus to people who can medically help me (3.70).

B. Expression of faith (0.80)

People who care for children with HIV/AIDS are at times tired of the caregiving demands and resort to other activities to boost themselves up. In what way(s) would you say you have done the following? Please answer each of the statements below by selecting the ones that best describes your case.

a. I go to church (mosque) when I'm tired with caregiving demands (2.72).
b. I pray more when caregiving demands get to me (3.37).
c. I sing Christian (religious) songs when caregiving demands become heavier (2.88).
d. I listen more to Christian (religious) songs when caregiving demands become difficult (2.91).
e. I ask people to pray for me when caregiving demands become heavier (2.15).

Response categories: (4) Very often; (3) Often; (2) Rarely; (1) Never.

C. Financial difficulties (0.88)

a. I have financial difficulty to feed the child (3.03).
b. I have financial difficulty to provide clothing for the child (3.31).
c. I have financial difficulty to provide leisure for the child (take the child out to the movies, beach, etc.) (3.32).
d. I have financial difficulty to provide sweet treats (candy, ice cream, cake, cookies, etc.) for the child (3.16).

Response categories: (4) Very often; (3) Often; (2) Rarely; (1) Never.

D. Family support (0.59)

Oftentimes, our family members provide different forms of support when we have difficulty, for instance when we are giving care to an ill person. However, we may be at times disappointed by the inaction of our family members. Please in what way(s) have you felt the following from family members?

a. Your brothers and sisters provide help and support in caregiving (1.86)
b. Other members of the family help with caregiving demands (1.26)
c. Your parents help you with caregiving (1.56)

Response categories: (4) Very often; (3) Often; (2) Rarely; (1) Never.

E. Impact of caregiving demands on other activities (0.47).

From your personal experiences, please give your view on the following statements regarding your activities (work or in market).

a. Since the beginning of caregiving of this child, I have stopped other income generating activities (1.78).
b. I have changed my income generating activities since caring for this child (1.30).
c. My income generating activities have declined since caring for this child (2.55).

Response categories: (4) Completely agree; (3) Agree; (2) Somewhat agree; (1) Disagree.

F. Personal and social norms (0.78)

We have our personal and social norms that usually guide our thoughts and actions. In caring for a child living with HIV/AIDS, how do the following propositions apply to you?

a. Due to my age, I shouldn't be caring for a child at this point in time (1.50).
b. Due to my health, I shouldn't be caring for a child (1.41).
c. Other members of my family should be caring for this child (1.81).
d. Members of the other family should be caring for this child (2.18).

Response categories (4) Completely agree; (3) Agree; (2) Somewhat agree; (1) Disagree.

G. Impact of antiretroviral drugs (alpha = 0.90).

Antiretroviral drugs (ARVs) have improved the lives of people living with HIV/AIDS. Please answer the following propositions regarding your sentiments toward ARVs.

a. I have less worry now knowing that the child is on ARVs (3.15).
b. I have hope for the future of the child because he/she in on ARVs (3.04).
c. I think my hope for the child to grow can be realized because the child is on ARVs (3.17).

Response categories (4) Completely agree; (3) Agree; (2) Somewhat agree; (1) Disagree.

H. Supplemental efforts made for the child (alpha = 0.91)

Oftentimes caregivers make supplemental effort because of the illness of the person they care for. Please answer the following questions by circling the answer the best suits you.

a. I give more love to the child because of her/his condition (3.55).
b. I am more empathetic toward the child because of her/his condition (3.58).
c. I am more worried about the child because of her/his condition (3.75).
d. The child I am caring for is more spoiled because of her/his condition (3.39)
e. The child I am caring for is more special because of her/his condition (3.33).

Response categories (4) Completely agree; (3) Agree; (2) Somewhat agree; (1) Disagree.

I. Coping with stress (0.80)

Caregivers adopt some behaviors due to stress of caregiving. How often to you as a caregiver do this?

a. I stay alone by myself (2.00).
b. I put all in God's (3.66).
c. I avoid people (1.81).
d. I keep to myself (2.10).
e. I cry (2.41).
f. I take painkillers (1.49).
g. I read the Bible (Koran) (2.48).
h. I listen to religious songs (2.91).
i. I pray (3.48).

Response categories: (4) Very often; (3) Often; (2) Rarely; (1) Never.

Table 2: Continued.

J. Positive comparison (alpha = 0.73)
Below are some thoughts that caregivers of children with HIV/AIDS have. How often do you think these thoughts?

a. You try to remember qualities that you have appreciated from the child's parents (2.95).
b. You try to remember good times that you had with the child (2.94).
c. You try to remember good qualities that you had appreciated in the child (2.70).
d. You try to remember good times that you had with the child's parents (2.64).

Response categories: (4) Very often; (3) Often; (2) Rarely; (1) Never.

K. Profound meanings of child's condition (alpha = 0.56)

a. You try to find a reason for the condition of the child (1.59)
b. You say to yourself that the child has HIV/AIDS because of destiny (1.31)
c. You believe there is a reason behind the condition of the child (1.23)

Response categories: (4) Very often; (3) Often; (2) Rarely; (1) Never.

Concepts and their measures are explained above. Reliability (alpha) is calculated for each scale: N=201.

The disclosure scale has two subscales: (1)--family member and (2)--provider of help. The family member scale is a three-item scale that assesses whether or not caregivers had disclosed child's serostatus to her/his own family members, the family members on the other side, and the siblings of the child living with HIV or AIDS. The provider of help scale taps the fact that caregivers disclosed to only people they knew would provide them some type of help. In fact, they reported disclosing to people who could help them financially, emotionally, spiritually, or medically.

The expression of faith scale measures ways and frequency caregivers boosted themselves up when they were tired of the caregiving burden. It consists of five items: go to church, pray more, sing religious songs, listen to religious songs, ask to be prayed for.

The financial difficulties scale reports ways and frequency that caregivers financially fall short regarding caring for the child. Participants mostly reported not being able to: (1)--feed the child, (2)—provide clothing for the child, (3)—provide leisure for the child, (4)—provide sweet treats for the child.

The family support scale is a three-item scale that assesses the source and frequency of help that caregivers receive. It is noteworthy to report that since most caregivers did not disclose the child's serostatus to others, even family; they did not receive support from them. Also, those who disclosed the child's serostatus reported not receiving much support either.

The impact of caregiving demands on other activities scale stresses the impact of caregiving on caregivers' income generating activities. While some caregivers had stopped their income generating activities, most had seen these activities decline due to caregiving demands.

The personal and social norms scale has four items that depict caregivers' personal and social values about whether or not she/he should be caring for the child. Old age and health impairment were mentioned as being reasons why caring for the child was seen as inappropriate by caregivers.

The impact of antiretroviral drugs scale assesses caregivers' grateful sentiments for having the drugs for the children. For example, participants reported that they had less worry now that the child was on ARVs. They also stated that they had hope for the future of the child because of the ARVs.

Another scale consists of the supplemental efforts caregivers made for the child because of her/his condition. They, for instance, reported showing more love to the child living with HIV or AIDS, being more empathetic toward the child or spoiling the child, in a special way because of the child's condition.

Coping with stress is a nine-item scale. Caregivers reported staying alone, avoiding people, keeping to oneself, crying, taking painkillers, reading Holy Scriptures, listening to religious songs, praying, and/or putting everything in God's hands.

The positive comparison scale consists of four items that assess ways caregivers remembered qualities they appreciated in the child and the child's parents, as well as the good times they had with both the child and the child's parents. Finally, caregivers searched for reasons and profound meanings of the child's condition.

Conclusion

Measures of informal caregiving to children with HIV or AIDS in Togo were developed in this study. Eleven dimensions that describe caregivers' experiences were: 1) disclosure, 2) expression of faith, 3) financial difficulties, 4) family support, 5) impact of caregiving demands on other activities, 6) personal and social norms, 7) impact of antiretroviral drugs, 8) supplemental efforts made for the child, 9) coping with stress of caregiving, 10) positive comparison, and 11) profound meaning of child's serostatus. Although cross-sectional data were used in the study and some of the findings may change in longitudinal data, this study is a beginning effort to examine this important issue of informal caregiving to children with HIV/AIDS, especially in Africa.

The findings in this study are based on both qualitative and quantitative research as well as the author's research studies with informal caregivers of children with HIV/AIDS in Togo. As with any new instrument, it should be considered as a heuristic tool that will need additional research for further validation.

Acknowledgements: Fulbright Program with the African Regional Research Program supported this study. The author would like to thank all the people that made this study possible, especially caregivers who participated in the study.

References

Aranda, M.P. & Knight. B.G. (1997). The Influence of Ethnicity and Culture on the Caregiver Stress and Coping process: A Sociocultural View and Analysis. *Gerontologist*, 37:342-354.

Atkins, R. & Amenta, M.A. (1991). Family adaptation to AIDS: A comparative study. *Hospice Journal*, 7:71-83.

Bettoli-Vaughan, E., Brown, R.T., Brown, J.V., et al. (1998). Psychological Adjustment and Adaptation of Siblings and Mothers of Children with HIV/AIDS. *Families, Systems & Health*, 16:249-266.

Carlisle, C. (2000). The search for meaning in HIV and AIDS: The carers' experience. *Qualitative Health Research*, 10:750-765.

Derogatis, L.R., Lipman, R.S., Rickles, K., et al. (1974). The Hopkins symptom checklist (HSCL): A self-report symptom inventory, *Behavioral Science*, 19:1-15.

Family Health International (FHI). (2001). Care for orphans, children affected by HIV/AIDS and other vulnerable children: A strategic framework. Retrieved May 24, 2007, from http://www.fhi.org/en/HIVAIDS/pub/fact/carorphans.htm.

Folkman, S., Chesney, M.A., Cooke, M., et al. (1994). Caregiver burden in HIV-positive and HIV-negative partners of men with AIDS. *Journal of Consulting and Clinical Psychology,* 62:746-56.

Foster, G. (2000). The capacity of the extended family safety net for orphans in Africa. *Psychology, Health, and Medicine,* 5(1):55-62.

Foster, G. & Williamson, J. (2000). A review of current literature on the impact of HIV/AIDS on children in Sub-Saharan Africa. *AIDS*:14 (suppl 3):S275-S284.

Graffi, S. & Minnes, P. (1989). Stress and Coping in Caregivers of Persons with Traumatic Head Injuries. *Journal of Applied Social Sciences*, 13:293-311.

Horowitz, A.V. & Reinhard, S.C. (1995). Ethnic Differences in Caregiving Duties and Burdens Among Parents and Siblings of Persons with Severe Mental Illness. *Journal of Health and Social Behavior*, 36:138-150.

Land, H. & Hudson, S. (2002). HIV serostatus and factors related to physical and mental well-being in Latina family caregives. *Social Science & Medicine*, 54:147-159.

LeBlanc, A.J., London, A. S. & Aneshensel, C.S. (1997). The Physical Costs of AIDS Caregiving. *Social Science and Medicine*, 45(6):915-923.

Lesar, S., Gerber, M.M. & Semmel, M.I. (1995). HIV Infection in Children: Family Stress, Social Support, and Adaptation. *Exceptional Children*, 62:224-236.

Lesar, S. & Maldonato, Y.A. (1997). The Impact of Children with HIV Infection on the Family System. Families in Society: *The Journal of Contemporary Human Services*, 78:272-279.

McCubbin, H. I. & Thompson, A.I. (1987). *Family assessment inventories for research and practice.* (Eds.) Madison: University of Wisconsin-Madison.

Merson, M. & Rosenfield, A. (2000). *The AIDS Epidemic: Lesson Learned.* Lancet, 356:1204.

Moore, A.R. & Henry, D. (2005). Experiences of older informal caregivers to people with HIV/AIDS in Lomé, Togo. *Ageing International*, 30:147-166.

Moore A. R. & Williamson, D. A. 2003. Problems with HIV/AIDS prevention, care, and treatment in Togo, West Africa: Professional caregivers' perspectives. *AIDS Care*, 15:615-627.

Pearlin, L.I, Aneshensel, C.S. & LeBlanc, A.J. (1997). The Forms and Mechanisms of Stress Proliferation: The Case of AIDS Caregivers. *Journal of Health and Social Behavior*, 38 :223-236.

Pearlin, L.I, Mullan, J.T., Semple, S.J., et al. (1990). Caregiving and the Stress Process: An Overview of Concepts and Their Measures. *The Gerontologist* 30 (5):583-594.

Radloff, L.S. (1977). The CES-D scale: A self report depression scale for research in the general population. *Applied Psychological Measurement*, 1:385-401.

Seeley, J., Kajura, E., Bachengama, C., et al. (1993). The extended family and support for people with AIDS in a rural population in southwest Uganda: A safety net with holes? *AIDS Care*, 5, 121- 126.

Turner, H.A. & Pearlin, L.I. (1989). Issues of Age, Stress, & Caregiving. *Generations* 13:56-59.

UNAIDS/WHO. 2000. Epidemiological fact sheet. Geneva: UNAIDS, The Joint United Nations' Program on HIV/AIDS and the World Health Organization.

UNDP. 2006. Human development indicators: Country facts sheets. Togo 2006. Retrieved 3 March, 2007, from http://hdr.undp.org/hdr2006/statistics/countries/ country_facts_sheets_cty_fs_TGO.html.

UNESCO. 2007. HIV impact on education clearinghouse. HIV/AIDS in Togo. (Retrieved 3 March 2007, from http://hivaidsclearinghouse.unesco.org/ ev.php?ID=2840_201&ID2=DO_TOPIC.

UNICEF. 2002. Orphans and other children affected by HIV/AIDS. Retrieved May 24, 2007, from http://www.unicef.org/publications/pub_factsheet_orphan_en_pdf.

Wikipedia. 2007. Economy of Togo, available at: Retrieved March 3, 2007, from, http://en.wikipedia.org/wiki/Economy_of_Togo.

In: Social Sciences in Health Care and Medicine ISBN: 978-1-60456-286-6
Editors: J. B. Garner, T. C. Christiansen, pp. 235-249

Chapter 11

REFERRALS TO SPECIALIST CARE AND FACTORS EXTRANEOUS TO CLIENT NEED: LESSONS FROM THE INTRODUCTION OF A PATIENT LIST SYSTEM IN NORWEGIAN GENERAL PRACTICE

Jon Erik Finnvold
Statistics Norway
E-mail: jef@ssb.no

ABSTRACT

Regardless of whether health care is funded by government or private insurance, general practitioners (GPs) often act as gatekeepers in restricting access to specialized medical resources in many countries. The current literature on referrals suggests that factors other than a patient's health care needs affect a doctor's decision to refer that individual to a medical specialist. This essay investigates a range of mechanisms that help explain the general practitioner's referral decisions in the Norwegian public health care system. In particular, the focus is on the consequences of a major health policy reform in Norwegian general practice, the introduction of a patient list system in 2001.

Data was obtained from the Statistics Norway's Level of Living Household Panel Study, which includes a representative sample of 3,500 individuals interviewed annually. After introduction of the patient list system, GP referrals appeared to be less influenced by the patient's health condition. In particular, after the reform and after accounting for health condition, patients with low educational qualifications were less likely to be referred to specialist treatment, and patients living in major city regions or using a female GP were more likely to receive a referral. The data also suggest that the incentive structure associated with a patient list system increases competition between practitioners. Consequently, a patient's request is more difficult to reject, and this diminishes the GP's commitment to the gatekeeper role.

This essay analyzed these changes further by exploring the physician's performance of the gatekeeping role within different institutional work settings and with different workloads.

1. INTRODUCTION

Physicians are expected to do everything within their power to help their patients. This fundamental ethic is manifest in the role of physician as patient advocate (Becker 1961, Schwartz 2002). The responsibility to guard a finite pool of scarce medical resources is also embedded in professional practice. The physician is therefore simultaneously an agent for the individual patient and for society at large (Willems 2001, Weinstein 2001, Rummery & Glendinning 2000). Each physician must negotiate these conflicting expectations. Decisions about referral to specialist care are made during encounters conducted in closed consulting rooms, which are protected by an official guarantee of professional confidentialty. Against this backdrop, the individual character of medical practice is reduced to the practitioner–client relationship. However, this impression may distract our attention from the fact that medical practice is organized within a framework that influences the behavior of both doctors and patients (Freidson 1970). Obviously, there is more to referral decisions than an individual physician's secluded weighting of the individual patient's benefit and public budgetary considerations.

The following discussion focuses on the influence of factors extraneous to the client's needs on referral rates, and in particular, on the consequences of a major health policy reform in Norwegian general practice. A patient list system (PLS) was introduced in Norway in 2001 following the examples of Britain, the Netherlands, and Denmark. During the implementation of the reform, citizens were invited to sign up for a physician of their preference. They could choose among all doctors who had entered into a contract with the local municipal authorities to participate in the PLS scheme. The regulations relating to the scheme state that there is a formal obligation on the side of the GP to provide general medical services to the persons on his or her list, and to accept a new patient if there is free capacity on the list. Although strengthening the rights to receive help from their GP, the contract does not imply that a citizen may walk into any waiting room of a GP and expect to be treated. Each individual is supposed to use the assigned GP. However, individuals may change doctor no more than once a year and have the right to a second opinion. It is easy to change doctor, and, in contrast to the situation before the reform, information about the capacity and list size of each physician is easily available to the public (i.a., through the internet). Under the new arrangement, a physician's income is partly dependent on a capitation component derived from the number of patients on the list (30%); the remainder derives from fee-for-service. The capitation component replaced a practice allowance from the municipality.

The major goal of the reform was to strengthen the personal continuity between patient and practitioner. Previously, citizens had no formal ties to any specific GP. A survey conducted less than a year after the reform found that 97 percent of citizens participated in the PLS scheme (Sandvik 2005), and at the end of 2003, 98 percent of physicians working in the municipal health services participated (Sandvik 2005).

Previous empirical evidence has suggested that improved continuity may increase the likelihood of referrals (Hjortdahl & Borchrevink 1991). Another study has argued that referrals are often not needed, and that as many as half of the referrals could be processed by a more competent general practice (Johansson & Westmann 1998). It follows that, insofar as the reform leads to a qualitatively more skilled general practice, fewer referrals may be generated.

The reform was also accompanied by a nine percent increase in physician person-years, a greater level of growth than in previous years (Finnvold, Svalund & Paulsen 2005). In countries with a well-developed primary health care system, the costs of specialist care are relatively low (Starfield 1994). It follows from this perspective that an overall strengthening of general practice may decrease the demand for specialist health care. On the other hand, it has been argued that the incentive structure associated with a patient list system increases competition between practitioners, making it more difficult to reject a patient's request, and thereby weakening the GP's commitment to the gatekeeper role (Carlsen & Norheim 2003, 2005).

To evaluate the reform, data from Statistics Norway's Level of Living Household Panel Study were used to monitor changes in referral rates. Using this empirical frame of reference, three related questions are asked:

- Was a change in the probability of being referred to specialist care observed after the reform?
- To what extent were people in different subgroups, institutional contexts, and geographical locations likely to experience different patterns of referrals in the aftermath of the reform?
- To what degree can the changes observed be interpreted as a reform or trend effect?

The essay begins with a discussion of previous studies to introduce the empirical investigation into variations in referral rates. Although the main goal of the analysis was to assess the significance of factors extraneous to client need, need has to be accounted for because it interacts with other factors, the prime examples being physician sex and patient social status (below). After all, physicians are trained to respond to medical needs. The most common way to analyze variations in referral rates is to compare general practices. The conclusion reached most often is that practices with high referral rates have less healthy patients (Reid, Cook & Majeed 1999). In any study of health care utilization, characteristics related to need must be taken into account. In studies using patients as the unit of study, the most common way to operationalize need is to use various measures of self-rated health condition or chronic disease. At more aggregate geographical levels, area characteristics have been used a proxy for health care needs. Medical practices in locations with varying degrees of "depressed" populations have also been compared to address the relation between referral rates and need (Hippisley-Cox et al 1997). The age and sex distributions of the physicians' patient populations have also been used as indicators of need.

2. Referrals and Factors Extraneous to Client Need

2.1 Patient Agency

A study from northern Norway showed that the patient's or the family's preferences regarding referrals are of medium to major importance in one-quarter of the investigated cases (Aaraas, Fylkesnes & Førde 1998). Another study reported that a significant minority of referrals was felt by the doctor to be slightly needed or not needed at all and that perceived patient pressure was a strong independent predictor of all doctor behaviors (Little et al 2004). It is likely that socioeconomic status is a proxy for patient agency. For example, low socioeconomic status is associated with a lower likelihood of referral (Gruen, Knox, Britt & Bailie 2002). A higher rate of referral of patients with higher educational achievements indicating a social status bias was found in a Norwegian study (Fylkesnes, Johnsen & Førde (1992).

2.2 Individual Decision-Maker Attributes

Physician's age and level of specialization: A Finnish study concluded that the level of referrals was negatively associated with the extent of the GP's professional experience and specialist training (Vehvilainen et al 1996). However, the opposite direction was found in a British study, reporting that individual doctors with a specialty referred more often (Reynolds, Chintis & Roland 1991).

Physician's gender: Several studies suggest that the practice of medicine may be gendered, in the sense that male and female doctors deliver a qualitatively different service (Arouni and Rich 2003, Boerma & Van den Brink-Muinen 2000, Cohen et al 1991, Meeuwesen, Bensing, & Van den Brink-Muinen 2002, Roter et al 1991). Female physicians are more likely to refer patients (Franks et al 2000, Vehvilainen et al 1996). Nevertheless, findings regarding gender differences in referral patterns are often difficult to interpret because female physicians serve a population of patients that are likely to have unique or additional needs compared with patients of male physicians. In Norway, about one-third of practicing GPs are female. Female patients have more frequent visits, present with a different pattern of disease, and often have preferences for using a female physician (Elstad, 1994). It follows that female physicians are more likely to experience a greater workload. During the implementation of the reform, when citizens were invited to sign up for a physician of their preference, it was feared that an explicit invitation to choose a regular GP would increase the pressure on female physicians (Skogsholm & Hasvold 1999).

2.3 Organizational Context of the Practicing Physician

Workload/list size: An important issue is whether the payment system has any implication for the tendency to refer patients to specialist care (Iversen and Lurås 2000). To increase income, the physician has an interest in having as long a list of patients as possible. To be able to handle the job strain associated with a long list, the physician may choose to refer patients instead. The economic incentive associated with a long list is, of course, present only in a situation with a capitation component. Data from a sample of GPs practicing with the new system before the reform provided evidence supporting the existence of such a mechanism. It is also possible that referrals are used as a strategy to deal with the job strain associated with long lists of patients. In this strategy, the mechanism is not economic motive, but a strategy to protect their work conditions. After all, referral is one of the least demanding ways of delivering services (Lipsky 1980).

Solo vs. group practice: A physician's everyday work setting tends to position him or her between two logically important extremes. At one end is true solo practice, which is a rare and unstable situation that often slips into informal cooperation with colleagues. Group practice entails formal cooperation. At the other extreme are the more complex organizational forms that include hospitals and elaborate medical bureaucracies. In a solo-practice, the professional works alone, funds the office facilities, and works with patients who freely choose the practice. To sustain a practice, a reasonable pool of patients must be recruited (Freidson 1970, p. 92). In this situation, the practitioner is wholly dependent on positive lay evaluation for economic continuance (client-dependent practice). To be chosen and to stay in practice, the practice must offer the patient something to make him or her feel the need to return. Freidson observed that '*emotional satisfaction on the part of the patient seems more likely to be gained from a physician who is in a position to be more immediately responsive to (and dependent on) the patient than are group physicians who have obligations to a work organization'* (Freidson 1970, p. 103). Freidson's assumption regarding referrals was that solo practitioners would be tempted to avoid making referrals. Patients using several sources of care might become attracted to any one of them and may not return to the initial source of care. The opposite was found in a Dutch study, which observed that referrals are lower for group practices (Wijkel 1985). The authors argued that professionals in larger practices have the opportunity to consult colleagues, as well as better prospects of purchasing diagnostic means.

2.4 Geographic Context

Rurality/centrality: GP-hospitals are considered a safe option to avoid long transport and substitute admission to a general hospital, referrals that would be unavoidable without this option, especially with elderly patients (Aaraas, Fylkesnes, and Førde 1998). Several studies suggest that rural and remote GPs are less likely to use specialists mainly because of the lack or scarcity of local specialists (Gruen, Knox, Britt, and Bailie 2002). A Canadian study found lower referral rates because of differences in local styles of practice, which resulted from differences in the rural practitioners' access to specialist care and lack of relationships with specialist consultants (Langley, Minkin, & Till 1997).

Trainees in local health service: In Norway, trainees are used to secure coverage by doctors in smaller and more remote municipalities. It follows that the population in these areas encounter a trainee more often when seeking help. A Finnish study found that these consultations are more likely to result in a referral (Vehvilainen et al 1997). However, Ingle and Levin (2004) found no differences in referral rates for trainees and trainers.

3. Materials and Methods

3.1 Study Population and Outcome Measure

The study was based on the Norwegian living condition panel data set established by Statistics Norway (Sundvoll 1999). Since 1997, a representative sample of 3,500 individuals has been interviewed annually about a range of aspects related to living conditions. The response rate is about 70 percent each year. To follow the same respondents over time, participation was required for each year of analysis. Because in each year a proportion of the panel does not participate for various reasons, the analysis presented in this study was based on a sample of 2,900 respondents. The data set included a number of items about the participants' use of and experience with health care in 2001 (before the reform) and in 2003 (after implementation). First, respondents who did not report a visit to a GP in the previous 12 months because of illness were excluded. About two-thirds of the study population reported to have visited a GP. This subsample was asked if they had been referred to specialist care by a GP during the previous 12 months.

3.2 Variation in Referrals: Relevant Measures

In addition to information collected in the survey itself, a number of public registers were used to obtain information about the participants. Following the reform in 2001, The National insurance (NAV) established a register that included all participating physicians. In the 2003 version of the panel, participants were asked to consent to having information about their regular doctor included in the panel. In this way, the reform made data about the characteristics of physicians and their work environment available for analysis. In addition to the physicians' age and specialist training, information about list size and preferred list size was included.

4. Results

4.1 Changes in Patterns of Referrals 2001–2003

A significant increase in the probability of being referred was observed during a relatively short time. Of the respondents asked about referrals, 41 percent (38.5–43.5, 95% confidence interval) answered that they were referred in 2001, and 46 percent (43.5–48.5, 95% confidence interval) were referred in 2003. Descriptive statistics are presented in Tables 1 and 2. The categorization of respondents belonging to physicians with different workloads (Table 2) was based on information about the physicians' actual and preferred list size. Most physicians represented in the sample (N = 1128) preferred to have more patients on their list. A "heavy" workload, meaning too many patients on the list, was not common.

Multivariate analysis was performed to identify significant correlations. Of the pattern of referrals in 2001, the only significant result was a marked trend related to self-evaluated health. Other characteristics that were not related to need did not influence the probability of being referred. The same analysis of an equivalent subsample of the panel in 2003 gave a different picture. The trend related to self-evaluated health was still significant but less distinct. Several factors not related to need influenced the probability of being referred. Female physicians referred patients more often under the new institutional arrangement. Patients with lower educational attainment were less likely to be referred in 2003, and respondents living in the most central city regions experienced a higher frequency of referrals after than before the reform. However, the referral rates did not differ from average rates for respondents living in the least central areas, patients using single practices, or patients living in municipalities with a high proportion of trainees.

Table 1. Characteristics of sub-sample reporting at least one visit to a GP in the previous 12 month because of illness. Frequency of respondents that was referred to specialist care during last 12 months. Percent. (N)

	2001		2003	
All	41	(1498)	46	(1477)
Age, patients				
16-24	31	(180)	41	(177)
25-44	39	(595)	44	(588)
45-66	43	(544)	48	(541)
67-79	46	(155)	51	(138)
80 +	52	(23)	41	(32)
Item nonresponse/missing	-	(1)	-	(1)
Gender, patients				
Women	43	(879)	46	(867)
Men	37	(618)	44	(609)
Item nonresponse/missing	-	(1)	-	(1)
Self evaluated health condition				
Very good	27	(298)	36	(278)
Good	37	(730)	43	(654)
Neither bad nor good	49	(313)	50	(359)
Bad/Very bad	64	(155)	61	(185)
Item nonresponse/missing	-	(2)	-	(1)
Duration of patients education[1]				
Primary school or less	45	(210)	40	(201)
Secondary school	38	(888)	46	(856)
University, lower level	43	(320)	49	(333)
University, higher level	42	(72)	46	(82)
Item nonresponse/missing	-	(8)	-	(5)
Centrality level of municipality[2]				
0. Least central municipalities	45	(189)	46	(166)
1. Less central municipalities	45	(143)	43	(134)
2 . Central municipalities	42	(299)	42	(344)
3. Most central municipalities	38	(866)	49	(832)
Item nonresponse/missing	-	(1)	-	(1)

Table 1. Continued.

	2001		2003	
Interns in General Practice				
> 20 % of municipal physician man-years interns	40	(150)	47	(115)
< 20 % of municipal physician man-years interns	46	(1347)	45	(1359)
Item nonresponse/missing	-	(1)	-	(4)
Gender of patients' physician				
Female	36	(312)	50	(358)
Male	41	(1153)	44	(1088)
Item nonresponse/missing	-	(33)		(1)
Organization of General Practice				
Patients using solo-practice	41	(290)	46	(219)
Patients using two-doctor practice	39	(154)	47	(152)
Patients using health-centre	40	(1015)	45	(1076)
Item nonresponse/missing	-	(39)	-	(30)

[1]University, higher level includes first stage of tertiary education and postgraduate education, code 7 and 8 in The Norwegian Standard Classification of Education (Statistics Norway 2003:7-8). University, lower level includes code 3, 4 & 5. Compulsory education include code 1 &2.

[2]For definitions of centrality, see Statistics Norway 1994).

Table 2. Characteristics of patients' general practitioners. Sub-sample reporting at least one visit to a GP in the previous 12 month because of illness. Frequency of respondents that was referred to specialist care during last 12 months. Percent. (N). 2003

All	46	(1477)
Age of physician		
> 37 years	45	(184)
37-60 years	44	(1135)
> 60 years	54	(157)
Item nonresponse/missing	-	(1)
Specialist competence		
Specialist in General practice/social medicine	46	(838)
No specialist training	45	(638)
Item nonresponse/missing	-	(1)
Work-load of patents physician[1]		
Low work load	46	(141)
Low/moderate work load	46	(987)
Moderat/high work load	46	(198)
High work load	45	(150)
Item nonresponse/missing		(1)
Number of patients on the physicians list		
> 1800 patients	41	(208)
< 1800 patients	46	(1267)
Item nonresponse/missing	-	(1)

[1]Low work load: At least 377 patients less than preferred on physicians list, Low/moderate work load: 0 - 377 patients less than preferred on physicians list. Moderate/high work load: 1 - 75 patients more than preferred on physicians list. High work load: 76 or more patients than preferred on physicians list.

4.2 Referrals, Institutional Context, and Physician Characteristics

The extended model of 2003 in Table 3 shows that patients using physicians over the age of 64 years were more likely to be referred. About half of the physicians were registered with a specialty in either social medicine or general practice. There was no indication that the referral performance was different for physicians with a specialist competence. A significant variation between individual physicians and between municipalities was observed regarding list size, workload, and capacity, but this variation did not have any significant effect on referral patterns.

Table 3. Probability of being referred to specialist care during last 12 months. Multivariate logistic regression. (N). 2001 and 2003. Odds-ratio

	2001	2003	2003 (extended model)
Age, patients			
16-24	0.8	1.0	1.0
25-44	Reference category	Reference category	Reference category
45-66	1.0	1.1	1.1
67-79	1.1	1.3	1.3
80 +	1.1	1.0	1.0
Gender, patients			
Women	1.2	1.0	1.0
Men	Reference category	Reference category	Reference category
Educational length[1]			
Primary education (< 10 years)	0.9	0.6**	0.6**
Intermediate education	Reference category	Reference category	Reference category
Tertiary education (> 17 years)	1.3	1.0	1.0
Self evaluated health condition			
Very Good	Reference category	Reference category	Reference category
Good	1,5**	1,3	1.3
Neither bad nor good	2.4**	1,9**	1.9**
Bad/Very bad	4.3**	2,8**	2.9**
Interns in General Practice			
> 20 % of municipal physician man-years interns	1.1	1.1	1.1
< 20 % of municipal physician man-years interns	Reference category	Reference category	Reference category

Table 3. Continued.

	2001	2003	2003 (extended model)
Centrality level of municipality[2]			
Least central municipalities	1.1	1.0	1.0
Residual municipalities	Reference category	Reference category	Reference category
Most central municipalities	0.9	1.3*	1.3*
Gender of patients' physician			
Female	0.8	1,3*	1.4*
Male	Reference category	Reference category	Reference category
Organization of General Practice			
Patients using solo-practice	0.9	1.0	1.0
Patients using two-doctor practice	0.9	1.2	1.2
Patients using health-centre	Reference category	Reference category	Reference category
Age of physician			
< 37 years	-	-	1.1
38-59	-	-	Reference category
> 60 years	-	-	1.6*
Specialist competence			
Specialist in General practice/social medicine	-	-	1.1
No specialist training	-	-	Reference category
Work-load of patents physician[3]			
Low work load	-	-	0.8
Low/moderate, moderate/high	-	-	Reference category
High work load			1.0
	(1423)	(N=1414)	(N=1413)

* significance level < .05 ** significance level < .01.

[1]Education, see Statistics Norway 2003:7-8.

[2]For definitions of centrality, see Statistics Norway 1994.

[3]Low work load: > 377 patients less than preferred on physicians list, Low/moderate work load: 0 - 377 patients less than preferred on physicians list. Moderate/high work load: 1 - 75 patients more than preferred on physicians list. High work load: 76 or more patients than preferred on physicians list.

5. Discussion

One conclusion often reached in previous studies is that a surprising number of referrals are unexplained (Haiko, Linden, & Kvist 1995); another is that need is the most successful predictor of variation in referral rates. This study confirmed these findings. Referral rates increased slightly after implementation of the reform, and the expected decrease in referral rates did not occur. However, interpreting the aggregate changes as a result of the reform is not straightforward because the capacity and rate of utilization within hospital care also expanded during the period of investigation (Statistics Norway 2004). The reform was introduced to physicians and patients with different individual attributes, geographic environments, and organization of the general practice. These changes occurred over a short time. The data indicated that self-assessed health condition is not as strong a predictor of referrals as it used to be, and several factors not related to need were significant after the reform. It does not seem plausible that changes occurring outside the institutional context of general practice altered the patterns of referrals in groups of patients with different educational background or self-assessed health condition, nor does it seem plausible that these changes affected the gendered nature of referrals. Nordheim & Carlsen (2003, 2005) found that physicians were less concerned with their gatekeeper role within the new patient list system and that they experienced a shift in the balance of power between physicians and patients in favor of the patient. Although the physicians' subjective understanding displayed in the interviews may not have consequences for their actual behavior, their statements are compatible with several of the observed changes.

Consider the finding that patients with lower educational attainment experience a lower than average referral rate under the new mode of organization. Several studies report that patient agency is important in referral decisions (Fylkesnes, Johnsen & Førde 1992, Little et al. 2004) and that pressure to refer explains some of the variation in referral rates between GPs. In general, welfare measures tend to benefit the middle classes rather than the least well off (Gal 1998). Any development in the direction of increasing patient autonomy will tend to favor those that have access to information and social networks that include physicians (Finnvold 2006).

After the reform, referral rates tended to have a gendered character not observed before the reform. This finding agrees with previous research (Arouni & Rich 2003). Some feared that the reform would increase pressure on female physicians (Malterud, Steinert & Mo 1995). However, information about the workload of female physicians before the reform was not available. In the analysis of the 2003 material, workload was not significant, suggesting another reason for the increased tendency of female physicians to refer patients. Gerrity et al. (1990) observed that male and female doctors respond differently to diagnostic uncertainty in the US, but findings from the American context do not necessarily apply to the Norwegian experience.

Implementation had no effect on the referral rates of patients by solo practitioners. Freidson (1979) argued that solo practitioners are dependent on a stable population of patients. It can be argued that this lack of incentive to refer might not be present within the context of a patient list system. Even if the physician decides to refer the patient to specialist care, the patient remains formally on the referring GP's list. It can also be argued that, by denying referrals, the physician risk losing the patient to another GP. Either way, the effect of solo practice on referral rates is not simple or clear, neither on empirical nor on theoretical grounds.

Why did workload fail to shed light on the variations in referral rates? A part of the answer can be found in a previous investigation that focused on the panels' experiences with the implementation of the reform in 2001 (Finnvold & Svalund 2005). Patients registered with physicians with a high workload in 2003 were more likely to continue a relationship with their previous doctor. These patients also reported the choice of doctor and the doctor's competence to be more important to them. These data suggest that physicians with a high workload are more popular. This would be unlikely if their referral behavior reflected an inability to deal with a relatively high workload.

Unlike the situation in many other countries, rurality was not associated with a lower chance of referral. At least on the level of rhetoric, equity in the geographic dimension has always been an important issue in Norwegian health policy. The geographic variables used in the analysis did not reveal any significant differences, except for the most central regions, which during the investigation experienced an 11 percent growth in physician person-years (Finnvold & Svalund 2004). Again this change is difficult to interpret and could have been influenced by several determinants including increased capacity within secondary care. It is noteworthy that inhabitants in the central city regions have a variety of doctors to choose from, which may have accentuated the competition between GPs, given that most physicians reported a shortage of patients.

6. Conclusion

The evidence put forward in this essay suggests that physicians are now less likely to compromise the wellbeing of their patients in favor of anonymous patients elsewhere. It seems that physicians have taken on the role of patient advocate rather than gatekeeper during the years of investigation. Faced with the difficult task of controlling health expenditure, it might seem problematic that the physicians' qualifications in terms of specialist competence in community and social medicine, added resources in terms of person-years in general practice, or the strengthening of continuity in physician–patient relations decrease or stabilize referral rates.

Expenditure on specialist health care increased from 56,500 million NOK in 2002 to 70,200 million NOK in 2005 (Statistics Norway 2007). Although Norway is fortunate in having a wealthy economy, referral rates might be of serious concern to the central authorities also for reasons other than financial. A recent white paper proposed a national strategy to reduce social inequalities in the distribution of health and health care (Ministry of Health & Social Affairs 2007). Such a strategy might include a conscious policy on referral practices by the front-line health care personnel.

ACKNOWLEDGEMENT

I would like to thank Kari H. Eika and Terje Wessel for valuable comments.

REFERENCES

Aaraas, I., Fylkesnes, K. & Førde, O.H. (1998). GPs' motives for referrals to general hospitals: does access to GP hospital beds make any difference? *Family Practice*, Vol. 15, 252-258.

Arouni, A.J. & Rich, E.C. (2003). Physician Gender and Patient Care. *Journal of Gender Specific Medicine,* 6, 24-30.

Becker, H.S. (1961). *Boys in white: Student culture in medical school.* Chicago: University of Chicago Press.

Boerma, W.G.W. & Van den Brink-Muinen, A. (2000). Gender-Related differences in the Organization and Provision of Services Among General Practitioners in Europe. A Signal to Health Care Planners. *Medical Care*; 10, 993-1002.

Carlsen, B. & Norheim, O.F. (2003). Introduction of the patient-list system in general practice: Changes in Norwegian physicians' perception of their gatekeeper role. *Scandinavian Journal of Primary Health Care,* 21(4): 209-13.

Carlsen, B. & Norheim, O.F. (2005). "Saying no is no easy matter" A qualitative study of competing concerns in rationing decisions in general practice *BMC Health Services Research*, 5:70.

Elstad, J.I. (1994). Women's Priorities Regarding Physician Behavior and their Preference for a Female Physician. *Womens Health*, vol 21 no. 4.

Finnvold, J.E. & Svalund, J. (2004). "Kontinuitet mellom lege og pasient: Blanda resultat av fastlegereforma". *Samfunnsspeilet*, 18, 1: 27-34.

Finnvold, J.E., Svalund, J. & Paulsen, B. (2005). *Etter innføring av fastlegeordning – brukervurderinger av allmennlegetjenesten*, Rapporter 1/2005, Statistisk sentralbyrå.

Finnvold, J.E. & Svalund, J. (2005). *Pasienterfaringer i allmennlegetjenesten før og etter fastlegeordningen. Del I Kronikeres erfaringer. Del II Kapasitetsforskjeller hos allmennlegene.* Rapporter 34/2005, Statistisk sentralbyrå.

Finnvold, J.E. (2006). Access to specialized health care for asthmatic children in Norway: the significance of parents' educational background and social network. *Social Science & Medicine*, 63, 1316-1327.

Freidson, E. (1970). *Profession of medicine: a study of the sociology of applied knowledge.* New York: Dodd, Mead & Co., 1970.

Franks, P. & Bertakis, K.D. (2003). Physician Gender, Patient Gender, and Primary Care. *Journal of Women's Health*; 12: 73-80.

Fylkesnes, K., Johnsen, R. & Førde, O.H. (1992). The Tromsø study: factors affecting patient-initiated and provider-initiated use of health care services. *Sociology of Health & Illness*, 14 (2), 275–292.

Gal, J. (1998). Formulating the Matthew Principle: on the role of the middle classes in the welfare state. *Scandinavian Journal of Social Welfare,* 7 (14) 42-55.

Gerrity, M.S., DeVallis, R.F. & Earp, J.L. (1990). Physicians' reactions to uncertainty in patient care: a new measure and new insights. *Med Care;* 28:724-36.

Goddard, M. & Smith, P. (2001). Equity of access to health care services: Theory and evidence from the UK. *Social Science & Medicine*, 53 (9) 1149-1162.

Gruen, R.L., Knox, S., Britt, H., & Bailie R.S. (2002). Where there is no surgeon: the effect of specialist proximity on general practitioners' referral rates. *Med J Aust,* 177: 111-115.

Grytten, J., Skau, I. & Sørensen, R. (2005). Kjennetegn ved solo- og gruppepraksiser i norsk allmennmedisin. *Tidsskrift for den norske Lægeforening* 10, 125: 1357-60.

Hart, J.T. (1971). The inverse care law. *The Lancet*, Saturday 27 February, 405-412.

Hippisley-Cox, et al. (1997). The effect of deprivation on variations in general practitioners' referral rates: a cross sectional study of computerised data on new medical and surgical outpatient referrals in Nottinghamshire. *British Medical Journal;* 314:1458.

Hjortdahl, P. & Borchrevink, C.F. (1991). General Practice. Continuity of care: influence of general practitioners knowledge about their patients on use of resources in consultations. *British Medical Journal,* vol. 303 1181-1184.

Iverson, G.D., Coleridge, S.T., Fulda, K.G., & Liccardone J.C. (2005). What factors influence a family physician's decision to refer a patient to a specialist? *Rural and remote health*, 5: 415.

Kerssens & Groenewegen (1990). Referrals to physioteraphy: the relation between number of referrals, the indication of referral and the inclination to refer. *Social Science and Medicine*, 30: 797-804.

Lipsky, M. (1980). *Street-level Bureaucracy: Dilemmas of the individual in public services.* Russel Sage Foundation, New York.

Little, et.al. (2004). Importance of patient pressure and perceived pressure and perceived medical need for investigations, referral, and prescribing in primary care: nested observational study. *British Medical Journal;* 328, 444.

Malterud, K., Steinert, S. & Mo, T.O. (1995). Kjønn, arbeidsbelastning og listeprofil i allmennpraksis. Tidsskr Nor Lægeforen 115: 2406-11.

Ministry of Health & Social Affairs (2007). *Nasjonal strategi for å utjevne sosiale helseforskjeller*. St.meld. nr. 20 (2006-2007)

O'Donnell, A. (2000). Variation in GP referral rates: What can be learnt from the literature? *Family Practice,* 17(6), 462-471.

Reid, Cook, & Majeed (1999). Explaining variation in hospital admission rates between general practices: cross sectional study. *British Medical Journal* 319:98-103.

Reynolds, G.A., Chitnis, J.G. & Roland, M.O. (1991). General practitioner outpatient referrals: do good doctors refer more patients to hospital? *British Medical Journal* 302: 1250–1252.

Roter, D., Lipkin, M. & Korsgaard, A. (1991). Sex differences in patients' and physicians' communication during primary care medical visits. *Medical Care,* 11: 1083-93.

Rummery, K. & Glendinning, C. (2000). Access to Services as a Civil and Social Rights Issue: The Role of Welfare Professionals in Regulating Access to and Commissioning Services for Disabled and Older People under New Labour. *Social Policy and Administration*, Volume 34, Number 5, 529-550.

Sandvik, H. (2005). *Evaluering av fastlegereformen 2001-2005. Sammenfatning og analyse av evalueringens delprosjekter.* Noregs forskningsråd.

Statistics Norway (1994). *Standard Classification of Municipalities.* Oslo/Kongsvinger

Statistics Norway (2003). *Norwegian Standard Classification of Education.* NOS C 751.

Statistics Norway (2004). Pasientstatistikk. Endelige tall, 2003. Sykehusene satser mer på dagbehandling. http://www.ssb.no/emner/03/02/pasient/ (12.05.04)

Statistics Norway (2007). Spesialisthelsetjenesten. Regnskap, 2006. http://www.ssb.no/speshelseregn/ (20.06.07)

Sturdy, Pereira, Hull, Carter, Naish, & Harvey. (1997). Effect of deprivation on general practitioners referral rates. Analyses should take age and sex into account. *British Medical Journal 315,* 883-884.

Starfield (1994). Primary care. Participants or gatekeepers? *Diabetes Care.* 17; Suppl 1:12-7

Sundvoll, A. (1999). *Samordnet levekårsundersøkelse 1999. Panelundersøkelsen.* (Coordinated Survey of Living Conditions 1999 - panel survey) Dokumentasjonsrapport. Notater 1999 / 66, Statistics Norway.

Vehvilainen, A.T., Voutilainen, S.O. & Takala, J.K. (1997). Does the doctors' professional experience reduce referral rates? Evidence from the Finnish referral study. *Scandinavian Journal of Primary Health Care,* 14 (1), 13-20.

Weinstein, M.C. (2001). Should physicians be gatekeepers of medical recources? *Journal of Medical Ethics;* 27, 268-274.

Willems, D.L. (2001). Balancing rationalities: gatekeeping in health care. *Journal of Medical Ethics;* 27: 25-29.

INDEX

A

B

C

D

E

H

I

J

K

L

M

N

O

P

Q

R

S

T